THE DOCTOR'S GUIDE TO
SURVIVING WHEN MODERN MEDICINE FAILS

THE ULTIMATE NATURAL MEDICINE GUIDE TO PREVENTING DISEASE AND LIVING LONGER

Dr. Scott A. Johnson

Skyhorse Publishing

Copyright © 2015 by Scott A. Johnson

All rights reserved. No part of this book may be reproduced in any manner without the express written consent of the publisher, except in the case of brief excerpts in critical reviews or articles. All inquiries should be addressed to Skyhorse Publishing, 307 West 36th Street, 11th Floor, New York, NY 10018.

Skyhorse Publishing books may be purchased in bulk at special discounts for sales promotion, corporate gifts, fund-raising, or educational purposes. Special editions can also be created to specifications. For details, contact the Special Sales Department, Skyhorse Publishing, 307 West 36th Street, 11th Floor, New York, NY 10018 or info@skyhorsepublishing.com.

Skyhorse® and Skyhorse Publishing® are registered trademarks of Skyhorse Publishing, Inc.®, a Delaware corporation.

Visit our website at www.skyhorsepublishing.com.

10 9 8 7 6 5 4 3 2 1

Library of Congress Cataloging-in-Publication Data is available on file.

Cover design by Georgia Morrissey

ISBN: 978-1-63450-052-4
Ebook ISBN: 978-1-63450-053-1

Printed in the United States of America

DISCLAIMERS OF WARRANTY AND LIMITATION OF LIABILITY

The author provides all information on an "as is" and "as available" basis and for informational purposes only. The author makes no representations or warranties of any kind, expressed or implied, as to the information, materials, or products mentioned. Every effort has been made to ensure accuracy and completeness of the information contained; however, it is not intended to replace any medical advice or to halt proper medical treatment, nor diagnose, treat, cure, or prevent any health condition or disease.

Always consult a qualified medical professional before using any dietary supplement, natural product, engaging in physical activity, or modifying your diet; and seek the advice of your physician with any questions you may have regarding any medical condition. Always consult your OB-GYN if you are pregnant or think you may become pregnant before using any dietary supplement, and to ensure you are healthy enough for exercise or any dietary modifications. The information contained in this book is for educational and informational purposes only, and it is not meant to replace medical advice, diagnosis, or treatment in any manner. Never delay or disregard professional medical advice. Use the information solely at your own risk; the author accepts no responsibility for the use thereof. This book is sold with the understanding that neither the author nor the publisher shall be liable for any loss, injury, or harm allegedly arising from any information or suggestion in this book.

The Food and Drug Administration (FDA) has not evaluated the statements contained in this book. The information and materials are not meant to diagnose, prescribe, or treat any disease, condition, illness, or injury.

Contents

Contents

Contents

CHAPTER 7

REDUCING THE RISK OF AMERICA'S TOP KILLERS   147

1

Introduction to the Best System of Wellness

Of all the wondrous and amazing inventions of man, none equal man himself. The human body is a magnificent interplay of systems, cells, tissues, and organs that all work to maintain homeostasis (the internal bodily process that maintains a relatively constant state). The body was designed to stay in this state. Homeostasis requires a delicate balance between the internal and external environments of the body. Everything that the body encounters both internally and externally can positively or negatively affect homeostasis. The body constantly monitors its internal environment and responds appropriately when conditions deviate from optimal circumstances. That the human body maintains all of these complex systems and processes simultaneously is quite remarkable. For example, the autonomic nervous system continues its duties and responsibilities without any voluntary control from us. It regulates heart rate, blood pressure, and breathing, to name just a few functions, without any thought or input from us required. Another extraordinary occurrence is conception—the creation of life by two human beings. When one considers all of the processes and conditions that must be met for life to form, it is a miracle that conception occurs so frequently. Despite all of our scientific research and experience with the human body, we have barely begun to understand all its complexities, capabilities, and power.

Unfortunately, this state of homeostasis is constantly under attack and must be maintained by our body while adapting to increasingly strenuous and difficult internal and external environments. The food we take into our body and the environment we subject it to can either facilitate or obstruct homeostasis, and today's world is heavily inclined toward a lack of homeostasis. When homeostasis is disturbed, illness and disease may take place.

Regrettably, to many the modern definition of health is the absence of disease or pain. But health is much more than the absence of adversity; it is a state of optimal spiritual, mental, emotional, and physical wellness. It is a state of oneness that comprises the whole person and all four dimensions of wellness. In fact, the Sanskrit word "svastha"—often used to indicate one's current state of health—literally means "standing in one's self" or "established in one's self," which means a balanced state between mental, spiritual, physical, and emotional health. The natural state of the body is wholeness and health, whereas disease is unnatural and unintended.

So how do we assist our body in its pursuit to remain whole and healthy? Many seek this assistance through modern health care or allopathic medicine. When a state of sickness and disease has set in, many seek treatment that relieves symptoms but ignores the cause. Modern approaches to disease and sickness largely ignore preventive measures. This is a very reactive and unproductive method to maintain homeostasis and optimal wellness. This reactive approach is akin to not performing any preventive maintenance for your vehicle, where you simply ignore the oil changes, tire rotations, and other necessary preventive services and wait for a failure to occur before you take your vehicle to a technician. If this approach were utilized, likely irreparable damage would occur, or at the very least a compounded problem. Vehicle manufacturers would call this neglect and potentially void any warranty that existed on the vehicle. The same applies to your body. You must take a more proactive approach and employ "preventive maintenance" to maintain optimal wellness. This doesn't mean that you will live your life disease-free, nor that you will avoid illness altogether. But, it does give your body the best chance to maintain homeostasis and achieve the best health you can as an individual. Just as failures can occur in well-maintained vehicles, failures do happen in a "well-maintained" body.

The saying "an ounce of prevention is worth a pound of cure" is an understatement. It may be more accurate to say "an ounce of prevention is worth one hundred pounds of cure." Let's look at it from a gardening perspective. A seed has the potential to become a thriving and healthy plant. It requires water, good soil, proper nutrients, and sunshine. Without these things it simply remains a seed, never realizing its full potential. Your body is like the seed. It has the potential to flourish with vitality and optimal health if cared for appropriately. If nutrition, physical activity, protection from harmful chemicals, and management of negative emotions and stress are observed, the body will flourish and reduce the occurrence of disease. Conversely, disease is like a weed, which seems to grow with very little support, and takes nutrients from life that surrounds it. Nevertheless, if you focus on providing healthy food and fuel for your body, reduce and mitigate exposure to harmful chemicals, and participate in regular physical activity, you will be in a state of well-being. Indeed, you can create an internal environment that is hostile and inhospitable to disease, rather than being open and inviting to it.

The goal and purpose of this book is to provide information and knowledge that will help you create an ideal environment for optimum health to thrive and to encourage you to develop the healthiest you possible. Its primary focus is that of preventive care, or maintenance of the wondrous body each of us possesses. It is much better to avoid getting a dreadful or deadly disease than to treat it after it has taken hold of your body.

Thomas Edison is quoted as saying, "The doctor of the future will give no medicine, but will instruct his patient in the care of the human frame, in diet and in the cause and prevention of disease. There were never so many able, active minds at work on the problems of diseases as now, and all their discoveries are tending to the simple truth—that you can't improve on nature." Unfortunately his prediction has not quite come true. Modern allopathic doctors spend more time prescribing drugs and surgery and little, if any time, sharing information with patients about eating better and disease prevention. On the contrary, the goal of naturopathy is to educate and empower people with the knowledge necessary to achieve and maintain optimum health, with prevention at the forefront.

Naturopathy is a system of health that builds, supports, and sustains optimal health and wellness through natural means: water, nutrition, exercise, massage, and herbs to name a few. The focus of naturopathy is to educate and empower people with the knowledge necessary to maintain good health naturally and in collaboration with the innate healing power within us all. One of the major focuses of naturopathy is to support the various systems and processes of the body that prevent or handle disease. The ideas and suggestions contained in this book incorporate many of the different forms of healing encompassed under the naturopathy umbrella. This does not mean that naturopathy has the answer to all health concerns. There is no perfect single health care system, nor one that has the answer to all health conditions that man experiences. The best health care system combines the strengths of the most effective health care approaches available with a preference for the least invasive options. For example, it is not reasonable to take a person hit by a bus to the local health food store for herbal remedies. Nor, is it reasonable to immediately perform surgery on a person with back pain. In many cases physical therapy, anti-inflammatory supplements, and essential oils could relieve the back pain without the surgery. In order to appreciate the medicinal recommendations in this book it is important for you to understand the many available forms of health care that exist.

ALLOPATHIC OR WESTERN MEDICINE: STRENGTH IN TECHNOLOGY

The first form of health care is **allopathic medicine**, also known as Western medicine, conventional medicine, or traditional health care. This is the form of health care that most citizens of the United States are familiar with. It trusts heavily in science and technology; almost entirely relying on surgery and pharmaceutical drugs as treatment methods. These means are intended to redirect the body rather than assist the body in its restoration process.

The primary focus of allopathic medicine is to treat the disease, not the person, by alleviating symptoms. Methods are employed that counteract a symptom, meaning that if spasms are the problem an antispasmodic method will be used. Most conventional drugs work by preventing cells of the body from performing a function that appears to be hyperactive. Allopathy holds to the theory that disease is a result of one single cause—an attack from a foreign invader such as a virus, germ, or bacteria, or body systems gone awry. Allopathy views the mind and body as separate entities and treats them as such. It pays little attention to the inseparable union between the two. Regrettably, most allopathic medical schools teach very little about preventing disease or more natural approaches to healing.

Allopathy excels in its diagnostics abilities and in the treatment of acute trauma. It is a "heroic" or a lifesaving medical system and definitely has its place and merits. It is indispensable during life-threatening situations (think heart attack) and after traumatic injury (think car accident). In these situations, allopathy is critically important because if you employ a natural method that takes time to produce an effect you could put the life of the injured or ill person at risk. Modern technology has supplied a plethora of tools for the allopathic physician to diagnose disorders and identify disease. These tools are often beneficial in choosing the appropriate treatment approach and are better at identifying underlying causes of ill-health. For example, lower back pain can have numerous causes. The ability to conduct X-rays, computed axiom tomography scan (CT scan), magnetic resonance imagery (MRI), and perform blood tests makes finding the cause of back pain significantly easier. Many surgeries and advanced medical techniques have been developed to help provide people with normal lives (think organ transplants). Allopathy is a superb emergency medicine and many lives have been saved because of the advances in this system of medicine and the doctors who dedicate their lives to it.

A complete and integrative approach to health care would certainly include allopathy. Unfortunately, its heavy reliance on technology often compels it to shun any "simple" means of disease treatment or prevention. Allopathic medicine is the antithesis of naturopathy in theory, but savvy practitioners from both naturopathy and allopathy realize the two methods of thought can coexist peacefully and appreciate that both methods can offer benefits when it comes to human health. Allopathy is certainly a valuable member of an integrative health approach with significant virtues to offer.

NATUROPATHY: A RETURN TO NATURE

Naturopathy is a system used to prevent and treat disease without drugs or surgery through diverse natural modalities—from herbs to homeopathic remedies and nutrition to tissue manipulation. The methods used in this system have been employed for thousands of years, in every area of the world. The methodology of naturopathy believes in the healing power of nature and the body. A perfect example of the healing power within each of us is a laceration or cut. If there is no foreign particle or infection located in the wound, the body will heal and repair the area. The process of wound healing involves a complex set of biological responses controlled by the body. Blood is released from the wound to cleanse it of bacteria, debris, or possible causes of infection; new blood vessels are formed, and collagen and fibronectin are released to form new tissue; the smooth muscle cells work with epithelial cells to contract, close, and cover the wound; and new skin layers are grown to cover the once open part of the body. This is just one example of the many systems and inherit protocols the body has in place for virtually everything that ails us.

Naturopathy is founded on utilizing the power of nature to bring about this internal healing response. The body has a set limit wherein it will make repairs and restore homeostasis. However, naturopathy works to create the most favorable environment for healing to take place, as well as stimulates the body to work at its optimal level. The body has amazing innate healing powers, but sometimes requires the assistance of another natural method to synergistically enhance the healing process.

Naturopathy believes in a holistic approach, which means the spiritual, mental, emotional, and physical sides of poor health are all factors. Complete wellness and health will not be established if one of these systems is not nourished properly. While substituting a natural product for a pharmaceutical drug can be effective, it is not the intent of naturopathy or a reasonable approach to genuine health.

A practical health and wellness plan will do more than prescribe a cure. It will establish new lifestyle habits, modify eating behaviors, teach ways to combat stress and emotional upset, and help the person grow spiritually by connecting with our inner self. This is often a challenge for those accustomed to Western-ized medicine to overcome because of ingrained perceptions and a long history of doing things a certain way—often called a paradigm. Modern medicine has given us the expectation that we go to a doctor who is all-knowing and receive a prescription for a medicine that will "cure" us. For the most part, little or no time is spent in educating the clients about their disease, what factors may have contributed to it, dietary and lifestyle changes that may be beneficial, valuable information to avoid the condition in the future, and supplementary measures that may be useful. In fact, insurance companies and the way many physicians are paid encourages just the opposite—a quick diagnosis and appointment leading to a quick recommendation so the next patient may be attended to. Many of us thrive on this approach of modern medicine, and in fact, demand it. It does not force us to make corrections in our life, nor require as much effort to be effective. It simply is easier than taking accountability for our lifestyle.

Naturopathy is an individualized approach, not a one size fits all approach. Each of us is biologically different with unique requirements. One person may respond better to homeopathic remedies, while another will have better success using herbs, and another will see greater success with essential oils. In addition, a person with a chronic illness requires a different health plan than one who is mostly well.

Naturopathy strives to use the least invasive and least harmful method that results in the fewest side effects but will still produce the desired results. Just because a method is simple doesn't mean it isn't effective. In fact, herbs used in their whole form are far more complex than the synthetic drugs that are meant to imitate them; as are essential oils that contain dozens to hundreds of con-stituents in oils. Chicken noodle soup is often eaten when a person has a cold because that is what mom or grandma did. We do this because it is tradition, not necessarily because we understand the reason why. In reality, the reason why this simple food is effective is because the hot broth promotes expectoration of mucous. Thus we feel better because we have assisted the body's built-in process to eliminate mucous. Simple, but a time-honored and effective tradition for the minor cold that countless numbers of people have benefited from.

Naturopathy does not view symptoms as part of a disease, but rather regards them as warning signs or attempts by the body to heal itself. Someone may have diarrhea and vomit as the body attempts to eliminate a harmful substance in the gastrointestinal system. A runny nose is likely the body's efforts to eliminate built-up mucous or prevent a perceived threat from entering through the nasal cavity. A fever makes the body less hospitable to certain harmful organisms that can only operate within a narrow temperature range. A cough is the body's way to expel mucous or other foreign substances from the throat and lungs. Pain provides a warning to prevent further harm to the body. Instead of trying to suppress these corrective events, naturopaths help the body more effectively complete these processes. Naturopathy believes that suppression of symptoms leads to deeper problems later in life, called iatrogenic illness.

Prevention is the key to naturopathy. Frankly, the prevention of chronic disease is much easier than its treatment. By establishing proper eating and lifestyle habits, the body builds an environment that is less hospitable to disease. This is why when one person in your family catches a cold, not everyone in the family catches it. Some people have stronger immune systems or have established an internal environment that doesn't allow the disease to take hold. The goal of naturopathy is to help individuals establish a personal optimal level of health and maintain it.

Naturopathy encompasses a broad range of modalities some of which are discussed in greater detail below.

HOMEOPATHY: LIKE CURES LIKE

Homeopathy is its own health care system, but it is also a modality often used by naturopaths. It is a health practice based on the opposite of allopathic medicine, "like cures like." Homeopathy was founded in the eighteenth century by Samuel Hahnemann who believed that symptoms caused by a harmful or poisonous substance in healthy people would cure those same symptoms in those who are not well. In other words, if poison oak causes hives in a healthy subject, the highly diluted form may cure hives in another person. In fact, Hahnemann determined many of the indications for remedies based on "provings." Provings were conducted when healthy individuals took a diluted dose of a poison and then the symptoms they experienced were observed. This information was compiled and turned into a remedy profile.

One of the primary advantages of homeopathy is that there are virtually no contraindications and very rarely any adverse reactions. Remedies can be given to infants, the elderly, and to pregnant and nursing mothers. This is in contrast to most prescription and over-the-counter medications and even some herbal products, which are used as remedies to prevent the occurrence of a specific symptom or set of symptoms (think anti-inflammatory).

Homeopathy is very individualized in administration and nature. The totality of all symptoms are used to determine a specific remedy, thus a person with

7

the common cold could have numerous remedies that would result in a cure. This makes each case uniquely different despite the fact that the healer could be treating the exact same disease, even among family members. Homeopathic remedies can be so specific to a person that they often result in an aggravation, or a temporary worsening of symptoms, before a cure takes place. This is sometimes termed a healing crisis, and though the symptoms that present during this period of time may be unpleasant, it is a positive sign that the correct remedy was selected and it will effectively reverse the disease. The remedy is given not to counteract a symptom but to assist the body in its own healing process. Much like a vaccine is given for the body to build up immunity to a specific disease, homeopathic remedies are given to strengthen the body's ability to heal.

Homeopathic remedies are diluted by mixing the substance with greater parts of another substance, generally lactose or alcohol, then assigned a potency rating based on the number of times the remedy is diluted. For example, you will find remedies labeled 6X, 30C, 10M, or LM. The number indicates the number of times the remedy is diluted. The letter indicates the dilution ratio or proportion of active to inactive substance. X=1/10, C=1/100, M=1/1,000, and LM=1/50,000. After the substance is mixed with the inactive substance, it is shaken. The shaking potentiates the substance into a therapeutically active medicine. Some remedies are diluted to the infinitesimal amount (parts per million and beyond) where virtually none of the original substance is present. However, because homeopathy works on the theory of vital force, the dynamic or vital portion of the medicine remains curative in nature. Hahnemann believed the vital force regulated and maintained everything within the living organism and without it the organism was incapable of any sensation or function.

Homeopathy works on basic laws, the first being the "Law of Similars" or "like cures like." Another law is the "Law of Cure." This law states that the cure will happen in a predictable manner and order; from above downward, from within outward, from a more important to a less important organ, and in the reverse order the symptoms occurred. If this pattern or order occurs, the homeopath can be confident that a cure is taking place and not simply palliation or suppression of symptoms. Another law is the "Law of the Minimum Dose." A remedy should be given in the smallest dose and for the shortest duration possible to elicit a cure. In addition, in classical homeopathy, only one single remedy should be used at a time. If the remedy does not work, the wrong remedy has been administered and the homeopath must rework the case to find the correct remedy.

Traditional homeopaths follow these laws, but many modern homeopaths use "combination remedies," which have a few of the most common and effective remedies combined into one remedy for a specific condition or symptom. Many homeopathic remedies found at your local health food store are combination remedies. The advantage of these remedies is that they remove much of the analyzing involved in finding the exact or specific remedy. The disadvantage is the healing process may not be as deep as is necessary to avoid subsequent reoccurrence.

Many practitioners and users of homeopathic remedies can testify that you can achieve remarkable results with both single and combination remedies. The *Materia Medica*, the book containing the remedy profiles and provings, is intimidating to say the least. If you look up a particular symptom, you are likely to have more than a dozen remedies to choose from. Some remedies are considered "specifics," such as *arnica montana* for sore or bruised muscles, and *chamomilla* for teething. But most of the remedies have a plethora of different symptoms or conditions that they treat. Therefore, traditional homeopathy is best practiced by the experienced homeopath with expertise in case taking.

HERBALISM: THE WORLD'S MOST COMMON FORM OF HEALTH CARE

Like homeopathy, **herbalism** can be its own form of health care, but the naturopath frequently relies on herbs to restore homeostasis. It has been practiced since the origin of humankind and in virtually every culture on earth. The use of herbs is predominant among non-industrialized societies. In fact, the World Health Organization estimates that 80 percent of the world's population currently uses herbs for some facet of primary health care.[1] This statistic makes one wonder why herbalism is considered an "alternative" medicine if the vast majority of the world population uses it as a means to maintain or restore health. Tablets of clay found in Mesopotamia indicate that the Sumerians used herbs for healing over five thousand years ago. Ayurvedic medicine, founded in India, was set forth in writings called the Vedas, which originate from the second century B.C. Hippocrates (c.460-377 B.C.), the man credited as the "Father of Modern Medicine," was indeed an herbalist. He is credited with the statement "Let your foods be your medicines, and your medicines your food." An "ice man" dating back 5,300 years found frozen in the Swiss Alps was discovered to be carrying medicinal herbs evidently used for the parasites found in his intestines. The *Pen-ts'ao*, credited as the first written record of herbal medicine, was written by the Chinese emperor Shen Nung approximately in 2,800 B.C. You can see that herbalism has a long history of use.

Like homeopathy, herbalism works to stimulate the body's innate healing ability, strengthening the body as a whole. Many of today's pharmaceutical drugs are derived from plants and herbs. However, pharmaceutical drugs use

9

just one active constituent among the hundreds of constituents that the plant contains to palliate symptoms. The primary problem with this approach is that the drug is then isolated from the dozens of other compounds naturally found in the plant, many of which may act as a buffer for or reduce any side effects caused by the primary or active constituent. Man's arrogant attempt to produce a more effective treatment than one created by nature creates dangerous side effects in drugs. In contrast, herbalism leaves all the constituents intact, believing that nature provides the best forms of healing. The one exception to this rule is when an herbal or natural product is standardized for one or more active constituent in order to increase the remedy's effectiveness. For example, milk thistle is often standardized for silymarin flavonoids content because these flavonoids are considered the active constituent that produces pharmacological effects. While standardizing herbs is a hotly debated topic among traditional herbalists and those who advocate standardization, anecdotal evidence suggests that standardization does increase effectiveness.

Many herbalists have learned the proper use of medicinal herbs through observation and research. They noted the plants animals consumed when they were sick. Moreover, they used plants based on the doctrine of signatures. The concept behind this principle is that the shape, color, smell, taste, and appearance of a plant will indicate how the plant can be used medicinally. For instance, red plants are medicines for blood and plants in the shape of a particular organ were effective in treating that organ, and so on.

Herbalism was pioneered in America by men like Samuel Thomson, a self-taught herbalist. He was exposed to herbalism after his wife nearly died as a result of the conventional medical treatment of the time. During his lifetime, conventional medicine included the use of poisonous mercury, bloodletting, and purgation all of which caused serious side effects and even death. He consulted two herbalists who taught him some of their methods and began using these methods on his sick family members and neighbors. Soon his reputation grew and he introduced a system of medicine called Thomsonian Medicine, based on the fact that the origin of disease came from a lack of heat within the body. In order to restore the body's natural heat, he used steam baths and laxatives and was particularly fond of the herb lobelia.

TRADITIONAL CHINESE MEDICINE AND ACUPUNCTURE: QI RESTORATION

The focus of **Traditional Chinese Medicine (TCM) and Acupuncture** is to restore or improve the flow of energy (Qi or chi) within the body. TCM theory believes that when energy does not flow properly or is stagnated within the body disease occurs. Originating in Asia, both modalities have been practiced and fine-tuned for thousands of years. TCM is based on the philosophical foundation that human beings are intimately connected with their environment. The human body is considered a small "universe" in and of itself, with many interconnected systems and organs that must remain in balance to maintain health. The balance of yin and yang is crucial. If the body is too yin or too yang, disease occurs. Yin and yang are considered both complimentary and opposite forces, with everything having a part of each. Yang is associated with male, light, hot, dominance, and so on; whereas yin is associated with female, darkness, cold, submission, and so on. They represent a complete circle without beginning or end, in complete balance, complementary and interdependent.

The basic concept of TCM is that energy flows within the body on meridians (channels that connect all parts of the body and allow energy, yin, yang, blood, and biological information to flow throughout the body) which maintain bodily functions and activities. When this flow is interrupted, blocked, or insufficient, the body becomes more susceptible to disease. There are twelve primary meridians in the human body that run vertically. Each meridian is paired with a meridian on the other side of the body. TCM uses a variety of natural healing methods to restore balance and the flow of qi. Acupuncture inserts tiny needles at key meridian points to enhance or restore the flow of qi. The strength, speed, rhythm, quality, and depth of the pulse at both wrists helps the practitioner determine the course of action to take to help restore qi.

Another foundation of TCM which fundamentally contrasts from Western medicine is the organ system. In TCM, the organs don't necessarily represent a specific tissue within the body; instead they represent a functional system of the body. This complex system divides organs into yin (or zang) organs with corresponding yang (or fu) organs, of which the yin organs are considered most important. The zang organs are as follows: the heart circulates blood and transports fluids; the spleen regulates the transportation of and extracts energy from nutrients; the kidney organ is the foundation for all other organs and governs birth, growth, reproduction, and development; the lung governs respiration and the extraction of qi from the air; the liver stores blood and ensures proper flow of qi; and the pericardium protects the heart and houses the mind. The fu organs are as follows: the stomach is responsible for digestion of food and drink; the gallbladder stores and excretes bile; the large intestine is responsible for excretion of feces; the bladder governs urinary excretion; the small intestine receives processed food from the stomach further processing and separating it; the San Jiao organ, or three compartments that comprise the mid-section of the body from the chest to the abdomen, assists in the process of water metabolism.

In addition, TCM identifies six extraordinary organs including: the uterus, which regulates conception, pregnancy, and menstruation; the brain, which governs intelligence, memory, and the senses (sight, smell, hearing, touch); the marrow, which fills the bones, brain, and spinal cord; the blood vessels, which circulate the blood; the bones, which store bone marrow and provide structure to the body; and finally the gallbladder, which doubles as both a fu organ and an extraordinary organ because it stores bile.

The five elements of TCM are earth, wood, fire, water, and metal, and represent the cycles of nature. A variety of characteristics relate to each element and therefore with the organ they are associated with. These characteristics are used to help identify disease and understand the cause of symptoms. They help the practitioner determine what organ to treat. As with other concepts in TCM, the elements are interrelated. Wood feeds fire. Fire creates ashes that become earth. Metal within the earth is heated and liquefies creating water vapor. The water that is produced nourishes the trees (wood). Wood comprises the liver/gallbladder meridian. Fire includes the heart, pericardium, triple warmer, and small intestines meridians. Earth corresponds with the spleen and stomach meridians. Metal includes the lins and large intestines meridians. Water comprises the kidneys and bladder meridians. In addition, each element is associated with an emotion. TCM believes balancing the organ associated with the emotion will balance the emotion. When an organ is out of balance, emotional changes or disturbance occurs. According to TCM theory, wood is associated with anger, fire with joy, water with fear, metal with grief, and earth with pensiveness.

Acupressure is a manual therapy that follows TCM theory of restoring proper energy flow through the manual stimulation of specific points along the body. Instead of inserting needles as in acupuncture, acupressure applies pressure to points along meridians to restore the flow of qi and restore health.

MANUAL THERAPIES AND BODYWORK: RESTORE ALIGNMENT AND BALANCE

Manual therapies or bodywork are general terms used for hands-on body manipulation therapies to promote relaxation, encourage proper posture, relieve pain, and diminish stress. The philosophy is that people learn unnatural postures and ways of moving their body because of stress or injury. This causes misalignment of bones and muscle soreness, contributing to health problems. The goal of manual therapies and bodywork is to realign the body, promote natural movement, increase the range of motion of the joints, relieve muscle tension, and reduce musculoskeletal pain.

There are many forms of manual therapy and body work, each with its own unique techniques and methods. Osteopathy uses low velocity movements to restore proper function of the autonomic nervous system and musculoskeletal system. The theory is that defects in the musculoskeletal system such as subluxations (very slight offsets or misalignments of joints) or weakness of the ligaments that support the joint influence the natural function of the internal organs, resulting in pain and poor health. Adjustments are made and proper body movement and posture is taught to restore correct alignment, increase range of motion, provide joint support, and eliminate pain. Modern doctors of osteopathy often practice alongside MDs and can prescribe drugs and other medical treatments.

Chiropractic views are similar to that of osteopathy in that chiropractors believe we are more susceptible to disease when balance is disturbed by subluxations or misalignments of bones and joints or tissue damage to muscles. These disturbances cause malfunction and interruption of proper nervous system function. Manipulations are employed to improve mobility, support the joints, improve nervous system function, and reduce pain. Two primary manipulations are utilized, low velocity and high velocity. Low velocity adjustments are slow movements that stretch, compress, push, or pull. While high velocity adjustments move joints to their full range of motion and end with a quick precise thrust. As with osteopaths, chiropractors advise clients in proper use of the body in relation to the environment, such as posture and body movement. Of critical importance when receiving chiropractic treatment is to retrain muscles. When joints or the spine are misaligned, muscles and other soft tissues "learn" to be in that position, like a memory. You need to retrain these muscles and tissues to help maintain adjustments and correct anatomical positioning.

Massage is a manual therapy applied to the muscles and soft tissue of the body through many different forms and techniques. There are hundreds of techniques ranging from Swedish massage to shiatsu and from deep tissue massage to Rolfing. Massage is very relaxing but has beneficial physiological effects as well, such as increased blood flow, activation of pain suppression mechanisms, relief of tension, removal of toxins, and improved lymph drainage. Massage is an excellent way to relieve stress and anxiety.

Spinal or joint manipulation involves the passive movement of a joint within or slightly beyond the normal range of motion. The aim is to achieve a therapeutic effect such as pain relief, reduced recovery time after injury, increased range of motion, and improved central nervous system function. Most manipulation therapies are performed by a trained physical therapist.

CLINICAL NUTRITION AND ORTHOMOLECULAR MEDICINE: THE USE OF NUTRIENTS TO PROMOTE HEALTH

Clinical nutrition and orthomolecular medicine utilizes nutrition and nutrients to promote optimal health within the body. There is a definite relationship between proper nutrition and well-being. The way the body digests, absorbs, metabolizes, stores, and eliminates nutrients directly correlates with good health. Indeed, if you are not absorbing nutrients from your food your digestive tract becomes little more than a tube for food to enter through the mouth and pass out through the anus. Nutrients are used in the creation of every molecule within the body. If the body is deficient in a nutrient, disease may occur. Orthomolecular medicine uses vitamins, minerals, and amino acids to treat and prevent illness. It attempts to create a proper balance of these nutrients to reach optimal physical, mental, and emotional health. Both methods recognize the biochemical individuality of human beings and the unique requirements for nutrients we all have.

ESSENTIAL OILS

Essential oils, aromatic plant essences, and resins have been used for thousands of years by a number of cultures for medicinal, ritual, beauty, and food purposes. These natural aromatic compounds and volatile liquids extracted from the seeds, roots, barks, stems, leaves, flowers, and other parts of plants merge potency with naturally effective. Often consumers feel they have to choose between a drug that is fast acting but will carry greater risk of side effects, or a natural product that will work slower but not produce as many side effects. This is not the case with essential oils as they are both rapidly effective and very safe. They are most commonly obtained from plants through distillation—often by using steam, but may also be expressed mechanically or cold-pressed—or extracted by solvents.

A great deal of evidence has emerged that demonstrates essential oils possess myriad properties beneficial to human health, including anti-inflammatory, antimicrobial, antispasmodic, immunomodulatory and immune stimulating properties, and more.

Few remedies can match the potency and rapid effectiveness of essential oils. Aromatherapy works simultaneously on the emotional, physical, mental and spiritual aspects of well-being, which makes them ideal natural remedies. They have great versatility, with each essential oil possessing a variety of uses. Another advantage to essential oils is their ease of use. Unlike homeopathy with a daunting *materia medica*, essential oils can be used with a basic understanding and common sense.

Only a few of the naturopathic therapies have been discussed, but you should have a good idea now of what naturopathy is and how it endeavors to promote health. The best form of health care truly is an integrative and all-encompassing approach that includes all forms of health care that are effective and safe. If there is hope that a treatment or prevention method will be successful, it should be utilized, particularly if it is noninvasive and nontoxic.

The goal of this book is not to convert you to a particular form of health care, but to empower you to make better choices in your life to allow you to realize your optimal well-being. The focus is disease risk reduction and prevention. As noted earlier, it is easier to avoid disease than to treat it once it has occurred. For some, these protective methods will require a whole new way of thinking and drastic changes. Others will require only minor changes. Change will not occur overnight and may take months or even years to accomplish, but if you follow the guidelines in this book, your body will establish a suitable environment to encourage optimal health and you will be more likely to realize improvements in the quality of your life. Change is constant and those who are willing to adapt to change will often grow stronger and ultimately be more successful.

2

You Are What You Eat

Proper nutrition is the foundation of good health. It is the fuel for your body. Nutrients from food are essential building blocks for our bodies, providing for energy maintenance and repair requirements. When you make a conscious effort to eat better, you provide the body the nutrients it needs to carry out necessary functions. When you drink or eat something, your body breaks down the food or beverage, which enters the bloodstream and then becomes literally part of you. The old adage "you are what you eat" is very literal—more literal than some of us would like to believe. For some, this does not conjure a pretty picture and these individuals may wonder just how bad their insides look because of the food choices they have made.

What you eat affects your health as well as your risk for certain diseases and illnesses. If your body is taxed and overloaded because of poor eating habits, it has less time to function optimally and your immune system may weaken. When you overindulge in one food category, while ignoring another, it can lead to nutrient deficiencies and disease. Eating a wide variety of nutritious foods will give your body a wide variety of beneficial nutrients, but making poor food choices deprives your body of important nutrients. Too much refined sugar, high calorie foods, or the wrong kinds of fats increase the possibility of weight issues or obesity. Too much weight on the body places a significant burden on your system and increases your risk of many chronic diseases, including heart disease, diabetes, arthritis, cancer, and stroke.

Despite a plethora of studies that correlate poor nutritional habits with disease, nutrition is rarely taken seriously as a means to reduce or correct disease in Western doctors' offices. Instead Western doctors prescribe, and patients expect, a drug to "fix" their problem. It is easier for the patient to continue their health-disintegrating eating behaviors and lifestyle than to take the necessary steps to prevent disease reoccurrence. Our expectation is that we must do nothing more than take a drug or undergo surgery to "cure" us. If you go to a surgeon expecting a recommendation other than surgery, you may leave disappointed. One example of this unconscionable practice is promoting surgical procedures to combat obesity. Instead of educating patients about proper diet and lifestyle measures that could potentially change their weight for the better, dangerous surgeries that modify the natural shape and function of the stomach are encouraged. These bariatric surgeries can be successful and may even be necessary in the severely obese, but they carry with them significant risks and, worse, they teach no new behaviors to avoid regaining all the pounds that were lost and more.

If you provide junk for your body through unhealthy food and beverages, you may promote an array of diseases. Conversely, if you fill your body with highly nutritious food, you can effectively reduce the risk of disease and even reverse disease (think back to the chicken soup discussion). Many foods can have an immediate beneficial effect on the body. To support health and prevent disease follow these six fundamental philosophies:

1. Fruits and vegetables are the cornerstone of eating well.
2. Drink clean, filtered water and drink it often.
3. Eat meat and animal foods sparingly.
4. Eat whole grains sparingly and avoid refined or hybridized grains.
5. Consume the right types of fat for the body.
6. Avoid harmful substances and foods.

FRUITS AND VEGETABLES: THE CORNERSTONE OF EATING BETTER

Fruits and vegetables are the most potent disease-fighting and nutrient-dense foods available. The phytochemicals (chemicals produced by plants that have protective or health benefits when consumed by humans), vitamins, and minerals found in fruits and vegetables are essential to good health. More and more evidence is mounting that the greater your consumption of fruits and vegetables the lower your risk for chronic degenerative diseases.[2] Vegetables, in particular, provide the most extensive collection of nutrients and phytochemicals.

Research suggests that the more vegetables you eat, the lower your risk for chronic and degenerative disease.[3] Numerous studies have indicated that when more vegetables are consumed you can realize a reduced risk of heart disease,[4,5] stroke,[6] diabetes,[7] and even cancer.[8-11] Vegetables can help you look and feel better and promote an overall feeling of well-being.

The more fruits and vegetables consumed, the more disease resistant your internal environment and the less friendly it will be to harmful microorganisms. Eating better should include at least five to seven servings of fruits and vegetables every day, with a heavy focus on vegetables, to promote optimum health and reduce mortality risk.[12] An understanding of serving sizes is important so that you can account for how many servings you get each day. Some general guidelines to follow for serving sizes are:

- One half cup of fruit, one half cup of raw or cooked vegetables.
- One cup of leafy green vegetables.
- Three quarters cup of one hundred percent fruit or vegetable juice.
- One quarter cup of dried fruit.
- One medium piece of fruit.

An even better way to customize servings to your specific body size is to base a serving size on the size of your hands. For example:

- A serving of protein should fit in the palm of your hand.
- A serving of fruits or vegetables would cover your entire hand.
- A serving of wholesome carbohydrates (grains, for example) should fill your cupped hand.
- A small serving of added fat equals roughly the size of your thumb.

It doesn't seem so hard to reach the ideal number of fruits and vegetables after all, does it?

Besides consuming enough vegetables, it is important for you to eat a wide assortment of them. Each of the colors you see in fruits and vegetables represents a specific nutrient, with the darker colors generally containing the most beneficial nutrients. Each fruit or vegetable has its own nutrient composition, providing different essential vitamins, minerals, and building blocks for the body. Eating a broad array of fruits and vegetables stimulates the senses with a diversity of colors, smells, and tastes. No one fruit or vegetable contains all the nutrients a person needs—though some superfoods come very close—so we need to consume many different kinds each day. People may become accustomed to or find a favorite, but this denies the body the nutrients that other fruits and vegetables will provide. Besides, eating the same fruits and vegetables every day would get boring.

What makes a superfood super? These foods, such as dark chocolate, berries, kale, and chlorella are nutrient powerhouses that provide the lion's share of vitamins, minerals, amino acids, antioxidants, and phytonutrients. Because they are so nutrient-rich they may help reduce the risk of a number of diseases, promote graceful aging, and even foster longevity.

Fruits and vegetables provide noteworthy amounts of beneficial fiber. Fiber is not just for the elderly or those who are not "regular," it is useful and necessary for all ages. Optimum fiber intake supports the gastrointestinal system, may slow the breakdown of carbohydrates and the absorption of sugar (soluble fiber), is useful as part of a weight loss or management program, supports cardiovascular health,[13-15] and promotes regular function of the bowel. Soluble fiber—found in beans, seeds, nuts, oat bran, barley, and some fruits and vegetables—soaks up water and becomes gel-like during digestion. Insoluble fiber—found in vegetables, wheat bran, and whole grains—is resistant to digestion, moving through the digestive system virtually unchanged. It adds bulk to stool, which helps food pass through the stomach and intestines more rapidly. If waste stagnates in the intestinal tract too long, it places more pressure on the intestines, which increases the risk of constipation, diverticulosis (a bulging pouch forms by herniation of the mucous lining of the digestive tract), and diverticulitis (the painful inflammation or infection of these pouches).[16] If wastes are allowed to accumulate in the intestines or get stuck in diverticula, it provides an excellent breeding ground for bacteria and infection to thrive. Over time, this process can lead to malnutrition and to chronic disorders like reactive arthritis,[17] irritable bowel syndrome,[18] and Crohn's disease.[19]

Soluble fiber also helps remove cholesterol—particularly LDL (bad) cholesterol—from the body and may reduce the risk of high cholesterol.[20,21] Soluble fiber does this by binding to cholesterol as it travels through the intestines, preventing it from entering the bloodstream and instead sending it to the colon for excretion in the feces. In order to enjoy this benefit you should aim for about ten grams of soluble fiber daily. Some foods that contain soluble fiber and that are known to lower cholesterol levels include oatmeal, walnuts, almonds, beans, apples, grapes, and strawberries.

High fiber foods encourage satiety, while helping one consume fewer calories. Indeed, some fibers like glucomannan can absorb significantly more times their weight in water;[22] in effect, your stomach sends signals to the brain that it is satiated because of this effect. If you feel full, you are less likely to consume more than your daily calorie requirements, and are more likely to maintain a healthy weight. Vegetables and fruits (especially fruits) naturally contain water, which increases the flow of urine and aids the elimination of toxins. The water content of produce also helps remove excess fluids from the body, speeds metabolism, and may accelerate your weight loss efforts.

Many vegetables, particularly dark green leafy vegetables, contain abundant amounts of carotenoids. Carotenoids are substances that give plants their vibrant yellow and orange pigments and supply a vast array of human health benefits. Some carotenoids, such as beta-carotene, alpha-carotene, and cryptoxanthin, are converted to vitamin A within the body.[23,24] The unique property of these provitamin A carotenoids is that they terminate the conversion process when enough vitamin A (retinol) is present in the body, which reduces toxicity risk. When your mother told you to eat your carrots because it would promote healthy vision she was right. With vitamin A supporting night vision, and the carotenoids lutein and zeaxanthin protecting the sensitive tissues of the eyes, preserving or improving eye health is possible. Vitamin A and carotenoids also support immune system function, promote healthy skin, repair and restore tissues, and act as antioxidants.

Eating potassium-rich fruits and vegetables—sweet potatoes, peas, bananas, greens, oranges, etc.—decreases the effects of sodium and may help maintain normal blood pressure.[25] Some experts suggest that the potassium counterbalances the effect of sodium intake and may lower blood pressure more effectively than salt reduction alone. Potassium is an electrolyte (meaning it carries an electrical charge), which helps regulate water balance within the body as well as the acid-alkali balance in the blood and tissues. This mineral performs several very important functions including blood pressure regulation, helping to generate muscle contractions, being essential for proper nerve function, and assisting in the regulation of cardiac function. The best way to maintain optimal and beneficial levels of this mineral is to eat potassium-rich foods. Most fruits and vegetables have a potassium to sodium ratio of at least 50 to 1 and some contain ratios as high as 696 to 1.

Besides eating enough fruits and vegetables it is important to eat them in season. This allows us to acquire nutrients from them when they are at their peak nutritional value. Eating fruits and vegetables in season ensures the freshest produce, may help support farmers in your local community, and provides key nutrients intended to be consumed during that season. For example, leafy greens, onions, and garlic harvested in the spring help detoxify the body after the winter. Juicy melons like watermelon, honeydew, and cantaloupe supply good quantities of water during the hotter summer months. Fall harvest provides hearty squash that not only keep well and can be stored for use during winter, but provide loads of antioxidants and disease-fighting nutrients like vitamin C and beta-carotene. This doesn't mean that we can't consume fruits and vegetables out of their normal season, but it does suggest that when eaten in their season fruits and vegetables have superior nutrient density. Even better is to eat locally grown fruits and vegetables, because most produce from outside your local area is picked before it is fully ripened (thus not fully developed nutritionally), and then shipped to your location, sometimes from hundreds of miles away. Some of this produce is irradiated (exposing food to radiation to kill microorganisms) during the journey to the grocery store to prevent spoilage and eliminate harmful germs, further depleting nutrients.

The best way to eat fruits is raw and vegetables raw or steamed. This protects many of the delicate nutrients and natural enzymes that are often damaged with cooking or boiling. Steamed vegetables are softened making them easier to digest with minimal destruction of nutrients. Uncooked, raw, plant-based foods are often called live foods, while cooking them reduces their nutrient value and some go as far as to say diminishes the plant's "life force." A reduction in enzymes from food may increase the burden on the body to create additional enzymes for proper digestion and to make use of vital nutrients. On the other hand, too many raw vegetables in the diet may cause indigestion and gas, particularly if your body is not used to this type of eating.

The availability of organic produce is growing rapidly as the demand for healthier choices increases. Organic produce is grown using soil mixed with natural fertilizers (organic matter, such as decaying plant and animal waste) and responsible weed and pest control. Moreover, organic farming is environmentally friendly by encouraging water and soil conservation. The debate about the benefits of non-organic versus organic produce is intense, with farmers on both sides vehemently defending their position. The primary advantage of organic produce is the fact that it helps one avoid exposure to harmful chemicals—toxic pesticides, harmful weed killers, synthetic fertilizers, waxes, or irradiation—commonly used in conventionally grown produce. Even if you wash your produce, pesticides leach into the skins of the produce causing consumption of small quantities of these poisons each time you eat non-organic produce. Organic farming practices often produce a more nutrient dense produce as opposed to non-organic produce with higher water content. If you compare an organic apple to a non-organic apple, the non-organic apple will be more aesthetically appealing because it is often sprayed with wax or even dyed to make it more visually attractive. You can't judge a book by its cover because the organic apple will often have a better flavor. We convince ourselves that a better looking fruit will be more delicious and healthy, when in reality this is not always the case.

Human anatomy provides some evidence for a diet heavy in plant consumption. There is no question that the human body is designed to consume both animals and plants, but some telltale signs point toward an affinity to plants. When you examine the teeth of a carnivore, you will find an impressive set of long, sharp teeth made for tearing, ripping, grabbing, and shredding meat. In contrast, the human mouth has four relatively pathetic canine teeth coupled with twelve molars for grinding and crushing plant foods. In addition, our eight front incisors are excellent for biting into crisp fruits and vegetables. A carnivore's jaws can only move up and down, which is superior when you want to rip and tear raw meat. Conversely, human jaws will move slightly side to side and up and down, which is ideal for the efficient consumption of both meat and plant foods.

The human intestinal tract and stomach also differ from that of carnivorous animals. Because days can pass between the meals of carnivores, they have large stomachs to store significant quantities of meat. A carnivore's stomach makes up about two-thirds of the digestive tract, whereas the human stomach makes up approximately one-quarter of the digestive tract. Carnivores have short intestinal tracts and smooth bowels with fewer twists and turns in order for meat to pass through quickly before it putrefies—the process whereby organic matter decays—and can cause illness. Humans have long intestinal tracts with many twists and turns—similar to herbivores. This causes plant foods to pass through the intestinal tract more slowly and maximizes nutrient absorption. The human intestinal tract is not as suitable for meat consumption, given that the pockets created by multiple twists and turns provide excellent breeding grounds for the putrefaction of meat and a breeding ground for harmful microorganisms. Moreover, a carnivore's stomach contains acid about ten times as strong as human stomach acid (hydrochloric acid) with a pH near one when food is in the stomach. The harsh acidic stomach environment of carnivores proficiently breaks down flesh and kills dangerous bacteria that would otherwise cause disease. Human stomach acid has a pH of about four to five with food in it, the same as herbivores.

Although the nutrient and disease-fighting power of fruits and vegetables, combined with an anatomy that favors plant consumption, strongly suggests humans would benefit from a mostly plant based diet, it doesn't mean you need to become a vegan or vegetarian. Indeed, some people subjectively report that they feel and function better when they include meat in their diet. For example, vegetarian women have poorer mental health and increased menstrual problems when compared to women who are omnivores.[26] Similarly, teenage vegetarians tend to report more alcohol use, poorer self-rated health, and poorer social adjustment in relation to their omnivore peers.[27]

Furthermore, there is a greater risk of nutrient deficiency—vitamin D, DHA, vitamin B12, iodine, and riboflavin associated with an exclusively plant-based diet.[28-30] A vegetarian or vegan diet can be very healthful and has advantages but it may require supplementation to maintain adequate to optimum levels of particular nutrients.[31] You should transition slowly to a more plant-based diet to avoid significant digestive upset. Some digestive upset and overall adverse feeling is to be expected as your body adjusts to a different way of eating and different nutrient intake. Continue to enjoy meat, just in smaller quantities and certainly not every day. This switch can help make a significant difference in your overall well-being.

DRINK CLEAN, AND HYDRATE OFTEN

Next to the air we breathe, water is the most important life sustaining element. It is essential for survival and myriad body processes. A person can die after only three days without water and is unlikely to survive more than ten days. Approximately 55 to 60 percent of the adult human body is made up of water.[33] In fact many of the major tissues and organs of the body are near or above 75 percent water, including the lungs, kidneys, brain, heart, liver, and the muscles.[32] The body simply can't function without adequate amounts of water. Every cell and organ in the human body depends on proper hydration to function. Water transports nutrients and oxygen in the body and is the primary component of blood. It participates in the breakdown of what is eaten so nutrients can be absorbed. Water serves as a lubricant during digestion and helps cushion and lubricate your joints. It helps form saliva and keeps the mucous membranes of the mouth moist. Water helps regulate and boost metabolism. Water works synergistically with the skin to help maintain body temperature. It facilitates waste elimination and is vital for cellular growth, reproduction, and survival.

Even mild dehydration may cause impaired body function. Dehydration occurs when the amount of water lost from the body is greater than the amount consumed. We lose water through many normal body functions including respiration, perspiration, urination and fecal excretion. A constant stream of clean water is required to replenish what is lost daily through normal body processes. Those who live in hot climates or are more physically active will require more water.

Mild to moderate dehydration can cause symptoms such as muscle weakness, headache, dry mouth, light-headedness, or tiredness. Severe dehydration can result in shriveled and dry skin, irregular heartbeat, delirium, low blood pressure, and even unconsciousness. Persistent dehydration can contribute to chronic health problems such as arthritis, asthma, diabetes, back pain, high cholesterol, and colitis. It is obvious that proper hydration is a key to optimal health and disease prevention.

If you haven't been convinced of the importance of sufficient water consumption yet, how about adding anti-aging and weight loss support to water's benefits? Water is an excellent weight loss tool. If you drink water approximately half an hour before meals it may provide a feeling of satiety and prevent overeating. Water participates in the metabolism process and studies indicate that the consumption of water increases metabolism. One study observed a significant increase in metabolism when seventeen ounces of water were consumed at one time, increasing metabolism 30 percent only ten minutes post-consumption.[33] Interestingly, the study also observed that the increased metabolism was different among males and females. Men increased their fat burning rate, whereas women burned more carbohydrates after the water consumption.

Sufficient quantities of water are essential to avoid unsightly early wrinkling of the skin. If insufficient water is consumed, toxins are allowed to accumulate in the skin contributing to fine lines and dry skin. Additionally, water is necessary to transport essential vitamins and minerals to keep skin healthy. Collagen also relies upon water to maintain skin elasticity. So if you want youthful and healthy skin or want to lose weight, water should be part of your daily regimen.

It is important to drink water throughout the day and before you feel thirsty. If you feel thirsty your thirst mechanism is signaling that your body is becoming dry. A good general rule to follow when it comes to water intake is to consume half your body weight in ounces daily, and adjust for outside temperature and physical activity level. Following this simple guideline means that a 150-pound person who lives in a relatively mild climate and participates in average physical activity would consume seventy-five ounces of water per day. A practical way to ensure adequate water intake is to keep a water bottle with you and take frequent drinks throughout the day. What's important is that you drink plenty of water, not how you go about it.

It is also important to keep in mind some beverages increase your need for water. Coffee, for example, is a diuretic and can actually cause greater water loss than it contains.[34] Some teas (originating from the *Camellia sinensis* plant, including black and green teas) and alcoholic drinks deplete water supply rather than replenish it. When tea or alcoholic beverages are frequently consumed, your water loss can rapidly increase.

Soda is another abused beverage all too frequently used as the primary fluid and even as a water substitute for many adults. Soda, particularly caffeinated soda, upsets your water balance in two ways. Not only is caffeine a diuretic (a substance that promotes urine excretion), but the high levels of sugar in soda causes your body to rob water from other parts of the body to dilute the sugar for elimination. The same applies for most commercial juices that are full of added sugar. A savvy label reader can identify just how much sugar is in typical beverages. Every four grams of sugar listed on the label is about equivalent to one teaspoon of sugar. Some drinks will both amaze and disgust you with the amount of sugar they contain.

Proper water is important for efficient elimination of wastes and toxins. Sufficient water stimulates the kidneys and liver, both organs of detoxification. The kidneys depend upon adequate amounts of water to perform their vital function of filtering and removing waste and toxins through the urine. Without sufficient water, toxins and wastes are allowed to accumulate within the body rather than being flushed out in urine and feces. If your urine is dark yellow and/or has a foul odor, this may be a sign you are drinking insufficient amounts of water.

The type of water you drink is also important. There are many types of water to choose from. Unfortunately tap water, the most readily available and inexpensive source, is not the best choice. Tap water is often exposed accidentally to harmful substances such as chemicals, fertilizers, pesticides, radon, nitrates, mercury, arsenic, and environmental pollutants. Moreover, tap water may be contaminated with lead, primarily from corrosion of pipes and lead solder in plumbing. This is particularly a concern for people living in homes built before 1980. Of great concern is the fact that pharmaceuticals enter drinking water supplies through excretion and bathing.[35] This leads to a vast assortment of drugs—antibiotics, synthetic hormones, antidepressants, and pain relievers—that are consumed by those who drink unfiltered tap water with unknown long-term consequences to human health. This fact is quite revolting and alarming when you think about it. If you want to avoid consuming post-consumed pharmaceuticals it is best to drink water that has been processed by reverse osmosis or nanofiltration, which removes more than 85 percent of pharmaceuticals commonly found in tap water.[36]

Tap water is processed with minerals and chemicals such as chlorine, but this may not sufficiently clean the water of contaminants, poses its own health risks (asthma and dermatitis),[37,38] and certainly alters its taste. Most experts believe that tap water does not pose immediate health risks unless it is contaminated with harmful organisms. However, some research is beginning to link tap water with adverse health effects[39-42] such as gastrointestinal illnesses and bladder cancer, and the long-term ramifications can't be ignored.

Filtered water is a good choice for clean drinking water. There are many different filtering methods to sort through. The best type of water filter is dependent on the type of contaminant you need to remove. Carbon (commonly used in refrigerator water dispensers) and reverse osmosis filters are the most popular filters. Carbon filters absorb impurities and trap chemicals and some microorganisms, but they ineffectively remove fluoride and lead. The main advantage of carbon is that it leaves the trace minerals found naturally in water intact. Reverse osmosis filters use membranes that allow water molecules to pass through but prevent harmful materials from successful penetration. Reverse osmosis systems will remove much smaller particles than carbon filters. The downside is they also remove the beneficial trace minerals, increase costs per gallon, and generally decrease water pressure.

Distilled water is popularly used in detoxification programs and to elicit the medicinal properties in herbal formulas because it is the purest form of water. The distillation process removes most minerals, chemicals, and organisms, which leaves only oxygen and hydrogen. There is some debate about the regular consumption of distilled water. Some believe drinking distilled water for long periods may leach minerals from the body, while others believe it only flushes excess minerals from the body. It is likely wise to limit your consumption of distilled water if a mineral deficiency already exists.

MEAT: IT'S AT DINNER TOO OFTEN

A great deal of scientific evidence suggests that the more animal products you consume, the greater your risk for ill health and chronic diseases.[43-47] On the contrary, those who eat a more plant-based diet generally experience better health and a decreased risk of disease. And this benefit is not exclusive to vegetarians or vegans, individuals who consume fish and lean poultry in place of red and processed meats have lower risks of disease and death.[48-52] Meat seems to be the main course in most meals among Westernized cultures, when a healthy diet would actually make it a smaller portion of most meals and a less frequently found food on the plate

The average American consumes about half a pound of meat every single day, adding up to an astounding 180 plus pounds of meat per year.[53] That is equivalent to a person eating a 250-pound hog each year, because that 250-pound hog yields about 180 pounds of meat. In reality, many people may be consuming more than their own body weight in meat per year. Half a pound, or eight ounces, of meat daily is about three to five times the amount—eleven to eighteen ounces per week—recommended by the World Cancer Research Fund.[54] It takes planning to reduce the amount of meat you consume, but if you organize your meal menu to include a few meatless meals each week and possibly a day or two without any meat at all, it can be accomplished. Americans who consume large quantities of meat are simply eating themselves to death. Short-term the consequences of this dietary habit are hard to detect, but long-term adverse health effects are highly likely. More and more scientific evidence is linking excess meat consumption—especially processed and red meat—to an increased risk of cancer, diabetes, asthma, arthritis, and heart disease, as well as the likelihood of mortality from these diseases. A study of the patterns, causes, and effects of diseases in a well-defined population concluded that the consumption of an average of 3.7 ounces of meat per day among pre-meno-pausal women caused a 12 percent increased risk of breast cancer. Conversely pre-menopausal women who consumed less than 3.7 ounces daily benefited from a 32 percent decrease in breast cancer risk. Findings of the same study suggest that post-menopausal women should be even more cautious with how much meat they consume. Even small quantities of meat consumption resulted in a 52 percent increase in breast cancer, while higher levels of meat consumption increased risk 63 percent among post-menopausal women.[55] The choice of meat is also very important according to the available scientific research. One study linked the consumption of red and processed meats to a 35 and 49 percent increased risk of colorectal cancer accordingly.[56] Eating red meat regularly is associated with a significantly elevated risk of esophageal, liver, and lung cancers.[56] There is a correlation between arthritis, particularly flare-ups, and meat consumption.[57,58] Including so much meat in our diet is very likely a contributing factor to the increase in chronic diseases in the United States. Next time you are in a restaurant you may want to reconsider that 16-ounce steak and order a healthy vegetable salad instead. As discussed earlier, the human gastrointestinal system is an ideal place for meat to putrefy, decompose, and rot, which provides a perfect environment for bacteria and pathogens to develop. Do your gut and overall health a favor and opt for the salad or another meatless option.

Pork and red meat—processed or cured—pose the greatest health risks.[59-64] If you want to include meat in your diet, choose healthier meat options like fish, seafood, turkey, and chicken. Keep in mind that even these choices can be made unhealthy depending on how they are cooked (think fried chicken). Fried and smoked meat may increase the risk of adverse health conditions associated with this practice, including premature aging and cognitive disorders.[65-67] One of the primary dangers of smoked and cured meats are the nitrates or nitrites they often contain. These preservative chemicals add flavor to the meat and help prevent botulism, but they are extremely dangerous to humans. Nitrates and amines—the chemical precursors to the formation of nitrosamines—commonly occur in cured meats. When these meats are consumed, a reaction occurs that joins the two compounds and forms carcinogenic nitrosamines. Bacon may taste good, but it is one of the least healthy meats to eat, because the cooking process promotes the formation of nitrosamine. If you choose to include red meats in your diet, purchase lean cuts (95 percent lean or greater), preferably grass fed, and limit consumption to two to three ounces or less of meat per day. A healthier alternative would be to substitute other protein sources such as beans or nuts at least occasionally.

Protein is made of hundreds of smaller units called amino acids and is necessary for multiple bodily functions, including formation of enzymes and hormones, manufacture and repair of body tissues, and is also is an effective energy source for the body. Protein is necessary not only for proper bodily functions, but for survival. When most people hear protein they automatically think of animal products like meat and dairy, which are significant sources of protein. But, the question is: are these the right sources of protein for the body to function optimally? Researchers set out to answer this question through an animal study. The researchers administered carcinogenic aflatoxin to rodents and then fed them a diet consisting of either a 5 or 20 percent animal protein diet. Rodents that received the 20 percent protein diet experienced considerably greater levels of cancer. Conversely, many of the rodents who consumed a smaller percentage of protein in their diet remained cancer-free.[68] The researchers concluded that diet, particularly the percentage of animal protein in the diet, was a significant predictor of cancer risk. In other words nutrition was the "trigger" that caused the rodents to develop cancer, not the exposure to a carcinogenic agent. This rodent study correlates with some human studies and clinical observations that also suggest what we eat impacts our risk of cancer.[69,70]

Another interesting conclusion of this study was the observation that plant-based protein did not cause the same increased incidence of cancer. Even when rats were fed plant-based proteins at very high levels, they did not experience the same incidence of cancer as those fed animal protein in similar percentages. Interestingly, the researchers noted that plant-based foods decreased tumor development, which suggests plant-based proteins provide a protective effect against cancer. Based on these findings, it can be concluded that the type and quality of protein is vastly more important than quantity. In addition, the evidence suggests that protein from animal sources foster an optimal environment for cancer initiation and growth, while proteins from plants have the opposite effect.

Despite the fact that smoking is the most preventable cause of cancer and it is well known that cigarettes contain thousands of harmful chemicals, not all people who smoke get cancer. This also suggests that other factors such as diet, lifestyle, environment, and to some extent, genetics play a significant role in triggering cancer.

Milk is often glorified as an essential health food that strengthens bones and nourishes the body. This may be true for calves, but it is not completely accurate when it comes to human health. While milk is beneficial for young children—especially breast milk, cow's milk can be harmful and disease promoting for adolescents, teens, and adults. For most babies, mother's milk is the primary baby food and necessary for survival, growth, and development. Mother's milk is the healthiest food for newborn babies and provides complete and necessary nutrients. Human milk and cow's milk both contain the sugar lactose. However, human milk also provides the lactase enzyme necessary to digest lactose, whereas cow's milk does not. Approximately 80 percent of proteins in cow's milk are caseins, with the other 20 percent being whey protein. Caseins supply an appropriate level of nutrition for the nursing and developing young. Whey is a better and healthier protein because it contains all of the essential amino acids required by the body in a highly absorbable and fast digesting form. Whey is often used by bodybuilders to increase muscle mass, and for good reason.

Going back to the rodent study, the animal protein administered to the rodents was the milk protein casein. It is remarkable that human beings are the only mammals that continue drinking milk even after it is no longer necessary for growth and development. When consumed by humans, cow's milk appears to promote congestion in the body, depresses the immune system, and is associated with greater disease risk,[71] including diabetes,[72] heart disease,[73,74] acne,[75] neurological disorders,[76] cancer,[77,78] and increased mortality and fractures.[79] A Harvard review observed a positive association between increased consumption of dairy products and prostate cancer in men. Those who consumed the most milk increased their risk for prostate cancer 50 percent compared to those who consumed fewer dairy products.[80]

Because cow's milk promotes clogging and mucous formation, it is associated with constipation, especially in children. Some health care professionals have found that if dairy products are simply eliminated from a child's diet, constipation is reduced or eliminated. If this is a concern among your children, it may be worth a try to eliminate dairy foods for several days. If it alleviates the constipation consider a cow's milk substitute such as coconut, almond, or rice milk.

A significant number of the world population (estimated to be 65 percent of the human population after infancy) is lactose intolerant.[81] This means they are unable to digest the milk sugar lactose. It is normally a result of the small intestine producing insufficient amounts of the digestive enzyme lactase. Production of this enzyme decreases with age because before humans became dairy farmers, milk was not readily consumed during adulthood. Consequently the body was not required to produce significant quantities of lactase throughout adulthood. For those who are lactose intolerant, consuming dairy products causes uncomfortable gastrointestinal symptoms such as bloating, stomach cramps or pain, gas, and diarrhea.

The Dairy Council boldly claims and promotes drinking cow's milk as the best way to strengthen bones because of milk's high calcium content. We all grew up hearing this from our parents, school teachers, and the various athletes and celebrities hired to promote this ideal. We have all seen a celebrity or athlete on a billboard proudly display a milk mustache!

The idea that if you drink milk you will experience stronger bones and teeth is somewhat misleading. A number of organizations and government bodies suggest consuming 800 to 1,500 mg of calcium daily—much of it from dairy sources—to encourage strong bones and teeth. Nevertheless, the evidence for this recommendation is lacking and contradicted in studies, even among young children and adolescents.[82] While an eight-ounce serving of milk provides significant amounts of calcium, approximately 300 mg, only about one-quarter of it is actually absorbed by the body.[83] Furthermore, pasteurizing dairy products—a process required by the US Food and Drug Administration to remove harmful organisms from dairy products—has been shown to reduce calcium absorption rates even further.[84] Pasteurization heats dairy products, or other liquids, to a temperature that destroys nearly 90 percent of bacteria, which leaves up to 10 percent of the pathogenic bacteria present when consumed. Moreover, pasteurization is not selective in its destruction and destroys both beneficial and harmful bacteria. There simply are better ways to get your daily requirement for calcium from food. Plant sources with good quantities of absorbable calcium are green leafy vegetables, sesame seeds, beans, almonds, and broccoli.

Many find that if dairy products are eliminated and meat consumption limited they feel better. Give it a try for two to four weeks—especially dairy—and see how you feel. The evidence suggests this practice may provide substantial benefits in the long term. However, if trying this diet, be aware that animal products are a significant source of vitamin B12. Dietary deficiencies in this vitamin are generally the result of a vegan diet that is continued for many years without supplemental B12.

Animal products can be part of a health-promoting and disease-preventing diet if eaten in moderation and if healthier meat options are chosen. Eating less animal products can significantly reduce your risk of heart disease and certain cancers. This will require much effort and adaptation for many who have incorporated meat as a primary food in their diet. However, the health benefits are worth the effort of redesigning meals and menus, retraining the body to eat better, and changing our dietary habits.

GRAINS: TO EAT OR NOT TO EAT

Grains are the dietary staple of many cultures and have been historically import-ant for man's survival throughout the ages. Grains can be stored for many years and still retain their beneficial nutrients for later consumption, which makes them ideal food storage items. There are numerous grains to choose from but the primary grains consumed worldwide are wheat, rice, corn, and oats.

Today most grains are consumed in refined, hybridized, and unnatural states. We consume empty calories from commercially prepared and refined white bread and pasta. We experience increased inflammation, weight gain, autoimmune disorders, and sensitivities to hybridized grains. Unfortunately, this single dietary habit is taking an enormous toll on our health.

Whole grains are grains that have not been processed; the bran, germ, and endosperm are intact. Whole grains are significant sources of fiber, potassium, iron, the B vitamins, selenium, magnesium, and other essential nutrients. The grain refining process removes the bran and germ of grains and takes with it most of the fiber and many vitamins and minerals. White flour is produced by refining and usually bleaching whole wheat. This process destroys more than half of the nutrients whole wheat contains in its original form. This includes vitamins B1, B2, B3, E, folic acid, calcium, zinc, iron, phosphorus, copper, and fiber. That is a long list of healthful nutrients being destroyed and removed from wheat all in the name of improved appearance, texture, volume, and a longer shelf life. Wheat is thus placed in an unnatural, damaged, and less nourishing state. It is interesting that weevils (a very small beetle known to infest grain stores) are far more likely to infest whole wheat flour than refined flour—the same is true of white versus brown rice. Even this insignificant and seemingly unintelligent creature knows whole wheat will provide better nourishment and life-giving nutrients compared to refined flour.

Manufacturers have tried to overcome the loss of nutrients that occurs when grains are refined by "enriching" them. Enriching means to improve upon or enhance, neither of which occur during the "enriching" process of refined grains. Using the word "enriched" for this process is erroneous, since the enrichment process only adds vitamins B1, B2, B3, and iron back to the processed grain. Other essential nutrients, which were stripped from the whole grain such as fiber, calcium, phosphorus, zinc, and folic acid are ignored.

Whole grains are complex carbohydrates, which means that they are broken down in a controlled, regulated manner during the digestive process. This is in contrast to refined carbohydrates, which are broken down so quickly that they provide a rush of energy followed by a decline. "Complex" might not be the best word for determining what carbohydrates or grains you should choose. The preferred word is "wholesome" because technically, depending on the way you bake a chocolate cake, it could be considered a complex carbohydrate. The bulk of carbohydrates in your diet should be wholesome. Simple carbohydrates, such as refined sugar and flour, are empty calories (high calorie, low nutrition) and result in increased caloric intake, weight gain, and create nutrient deficiencies. Wholesome carbohydrates like quinoa, brown rice, oats, and barley are also more satisfying when compared to simple carbohydrates like white sugar, flour, and rice. They provide a feeling of fullness that helps reduce one's appetite and cravings.

When whole grains are consumed instead of refined grains, common diseases of our day are reduced including coronary heart disease, atherosclerosis, stroke, obesity, and diabetes.[85-87] When consumed in moderation, whole grains can be a tool for weight management. Increased consumption of whole grains is inversely associated with weight gain, largely due to the high fiber content in whole grains, which supports regular elimination and helps maintain normal fluid balance.[88,89] The caveat here is that they shouldn't be a major portion of your eating plan because it is also clear that excess consumption of grains—particularly today's wheat—promotes visceral, or belly fat, storage. Those who choose refined grains fare even worse, as refined grains are strongly associated with weight gain.[90,91] Whole grains may even be beneficial for babies during the fetal development stage. Whole grains are a good source of folate and folate is indispensable during pregnancy to prevent neural tube defects in the developing fetus. Without proper levels of folate the developing fetus can experience significant neural tube defects.

The B vitamins in whole grains are essential for metabolism and help release energy from the foods we consume. Magnesium, found in whole grains, helps the body better absorb calcium, which builds strong bones and teeth. It is also a cofactor for enzymes involved in the body's use of glucose and insulin secretion, is essential for the transmission of nerve impulses, and supports the immune system. The trace mineral, selenium, found in whole grains, is a powerful antioxidant that protects cells from oxidative damage, supports normal thyroid function, and helps promote healthy immune system function.

You can clearly see that when you eat more whole grains you can experience many health benefits. Whole grains contain polyphenols that are converted to enterolignans, enterodiol, and enterolactone by bacteria normally found in the gut. These substances are known to produce biological effects because they weakly mimic or block the action of estrogen. When they occupy estrogen receptors in the body, lignans may encourage the maintenance of bone density[92] and help protect against breast cancer in women.[93] Lignans may also benefit men, though this connection is still poorly understood. Some research suggests that lignans may bind to testosterone, helping to remove it from the body, which may offer protection from the growth of prostate tumors.[94] Scientists have linked the consumption of lignans to a reduction in the risk of myriad diseases, such as cancer, diabetes, cardiovascular disease, and kidney disease.[95-98] The fiber from whole grains provides a protective factor against breast cancer as well. In fact, for every 10 grams of fiber consumed per day, women may reduce their risk of breast cancer by 5 percent.[99]

A conglomeration of nutrients found in whole grains may help support normal cholesterol levels.[100] Examples of these nutrients in whole grains are polyunsaturated fats, plant sterols, saponins, fiber, and oligosaccharides. A lack of whole grains in the typical Western diet may be a casual factor in the number of Americans that suffer from high cholesterol. All too often, cholesterol drugs with significant side-effects are prescribed rather than educating the person about dietary and lifestyle factors that can contribute to or prevent high cholesterol. High cholesterol is not the result of a statin deficiency; it is the result of years of nutrient deficiency and an overload of antinutrients. When it comes to high cholesterol levels, the single most important preventive factor may be what you eat. Eating more whole grains to reduce cholesterol levels, may result in a significant protective effect against the number one killer among both men and women—heart disease. Beyond their interaction with estrogen receptors and influence on hormone levels, phytoestrogens are also known to benefit the cardiovascular system and possibly reduce the risk of cardiovascular disease because they support normal cholesterol levels, protect LDL cholesterol from oxidation, and enhance blood vessel elasticity.[101-103]

Clinical trials have indicated that whole grains are associated with increased insulin sensitivity, one of the factors associated with type 2 diabetes.[104,105] If you improve your body's sensitivity to insulin, cells uptake sugar for energy more efficiently and blood sugar levels are balanced. Refined grains produce quite the opposite effect and decrease the body's response to insulin.

Corn, wheat, and rice make up the majority of grain production globally, which totals 1,972 million tons of harvested grain. Three countries—China, the United States, and India—account for almost half of the global grain production. Rice is the grain of choice in Asian and Indian cultures, while wheat seems to dominate Westernized cultures.

Wheat is a vital cereal crop that provides nourishment for millions of people worldwide. Whole wheat bread contains more than fifteen times the amount of vitamin E and three times as much fiber as refined white bread. Most grains provide inadequate amounts of protein, but wheat has a respectable amount of protein at 8 to 15 percent. The consumption of whole grain products—like whole wheat—is associated with a lower incidence of coronary heart disease[106] and colon cancer,[107] promotes regular bowel function, and reduces the risk of diverticular disease.

Unrefined wheat contains a plethora of beneficial nutrients including fiber, manganese, vitamins B1, B2, B3, B5, B6, E, folic acid, calcium, phosphorus, zinc, copper, protein, iron, and magnesium. Gluten is a protein found in many grains but there are greater quantities in wheat. It provides elasticity and structure to bread. Many prefer the taste and texture of white bread over wheat bread, but over time this taste will change as you become accustomed to wheat bread. A properly baked loaf of wheat bread can be vastly more flavorful and desirable than white bread.

One of the disease-preventing nutrients found in whole wheat is its metabolite betaine. Betaine helps reduce inflammatory markers, improves vascular function, decreases homocysteine levels, and protects internal organs. This helps reduce the risk of several chronic diseases including heart disease, diabetes, osteoporosis, and reduced cognitive function.[108-110] Wheat bran is a dietary fiber and considered an anti-cancer food and has been linked to a reduction in colon, stomach, and breast cancer.[111-114] Wheat germ contains appreciable amounts of oil along with the antioxidant, vitamin E, which protects the oil from oxidizing too quickly.

The primary disadvantage of today's wheat is its hybridization and modification. Today's wheat hardly resembles the wholesome and beneficial wheat of our ancestors. In an effort to improve yield and make wheat more pesticide resistant, man has modified wheat resulting in changes in the way wheat affects humans biologically. Modern hybridized wheat promotes excess inflammation, causes skin problems, promotes obesity, increases the body's acidity, disrupts the digestive system, spikes insulin levels, rapidly increases blood sugar levels, and is a factor in autoimmune disorders. With the exception of ancient grains, like einkorn wheat—an ancient wheat that has avoided tampering by man—most wheat products should be limited or avoided, particularly if you have diabetes, an autoimmune disorder, or a chronic inflammatory condition. Besides einkorn, sprouted breads, quinoa, and amaranth are good substitutes.

A recent trend is to eliminate gluten from the diet because of its association with gastrointestinal symptoms, disruption of immune system function, excess inflammation, and autoimmune disorders.[115,116] Gluten causes intestinal cells to release too much zonulin—a protein that regulates intestinal permeability.[117] It allows or prevents nutrients and other substances into the bloodstream from the intestines. If too much zonulin is present, permeability increases, which allows larger molecules like toxins, microbes, bacteria, and peptides to exit the intestine and enter the bloodstream. Once there, these substances disrupt immune function and may increase the risk of autoimmune and autoinflammatory disorders in susceptible people.[118] Based on the available evidence, it is wise to limit gluten in the diet.

Rice is the staple food for more than half of the world's population. Some cultures are dependent on rice as a source of food, make it an integral part of everyday life, and consume it frequently during meals. Three of the most population dense areas of the world—China, India, and Indonesia—are rice-based societies. Indeed, the word used for rice is the same word used for food in China. Like wheat, most of the rice consumed worldwide is refined and adulterated, and has been stripped of vital nutrients. Interestingly, studies suggest that we prefer white and polished rice over brown rice based on its color, appearance, texture, taste, and overall quality.[119,120] Unfortunately this preference for white rice has been associated with an increased risk of diabetes,[121] metabolic syndrome,[122] and heart disease.[123]

White rice is milled to remove the husk, germ, and bran that naturally occurs in brown rice and then polished to improve appearance. The complete process of milling and polishing destroys significant quantities of vitamins B3, B1, and B6, the minerals manganese, phosphorus, iron, and all of the dietary fiber and essential fatty acids. In contrast, brown rice retains all these vital nutrients and is considered a good source of protein—5 g per cup. In fact, one cup of cooked brown rice contains about 90 percent of the recommended daily allowance of manganese—a critical nutrient for nervous system function—and more than one-third of the recommended selenium. Interestingly, brown rice has an amino acid profile similar to whey protein, but with greater quantities of arginine and glutamine. More arginine in the diet may positively influence cardiac function. This is because arginine converts to nitric oxide in the body, which helps blood vessels relax, improves blood flow, and aids circulation.[124] It may also decrease blood pressure, though evidence to prove this is weak.[125]

Brown rice is a good source of soluble fiber, which may keep cholesterol levels in the normal range. It also helps prevent rapid increases in blood sugar post-consumption, encourages the normal function of the bowel, may help prevent breast cancer due to its lignin content, and is a good source of antioxidants. Brown rice is firmer, less sticky, and has a nuttier flavor when compared to white rice.

Say the word corn and people are likely to immediately think of popcorn or corn on the cob. Corn is a versatile grain widely cultivated in America, featuring an assortment of kernel colors, such as yellow, white, red, pink, black, purple, and blue. Today, most corn doesn't make it onto our dinner plates though. Instead, it is fed to livestock or used to produce ethanol fuel, sweeteners (like the nasty high-fructose corn syrup), and oils. Millions of people consume popcorn while enjoying a movie every year, and just as many slather an ear of corn in butter, salt, and pepper each summer. In fact, one study found that moviegoers who normally buy popcorn while watching a movie will eat stale popcorn because it has become a deeply entrenched habit.[126] Popcorn is considered a low calorie snack when it isn't drowned in butter and topped with copious amounts of salt, and can even be a healthy snack when flavored with garlic or other herbal spices. Experiment with spices until you find a flavor that you enjoy rather than coating it with butter and salt.

The nutrient composition of corn varies according to the color of the kernels. This goes back to our earlier discussion about choosing a variety of colors in your fruits and vegetables because each color represents a different nutrient. For example, yellow corn is high in the carotenoids lutein and zeaxanthin, whereas blue kernels have measurable levels of anthocyanins. Lutein has been linked with protection against heart disease and macular degeneration.[127,128] The most common corn, yellow corn, contains good levels of vitamins B5, B3, and B6, and the minerals phosphorus and manganese, as well as fiber and essential fatty acids. When the major grains were compared for antioxidant activity, corn came in just slightly below wheat for antioxidant activity.[129] Corn is not generally the staple food consumed by societies any longer because of its association with an increased risk of pellagra—a disease caused by a deficiency of niacin—in the 1920s. The niacin content in corn is not very absorbable thus it creates a greater risk of the deficiency disease. Common manifestations of pellagra include dermatitis caused by sun exposure, diarrhea, cognitive decline, and in rare cases, death. Interestingly, the Native Americans reportedly avoided pellagra by mixing corn with mineral ash from their fires, which increased the bioavailability of niacin. Early pilgrims observed this practice but did not follow it and later fell victim to pellagra.

Starting the day with a warm bowl of oatmeal is becoming a customary practice for those striving to maintain normal cholesterol levels. A hearty cereal grain that grows well even in poor conditions, oats are growing in popularity due to their published health benefits. As with corn, a significant portion of oats are fed to livestock rather than to humans. It is predominantly used as a breakfast cereal, like oatmeal, and this is what is most frequently thought of when oats are mentioned—at least among those who have never had a no-bake cookie with oats. Naturally gluten-free, oat bran is a good substitute for wheat for those who are sensitive to gluten.

Despite the fact that oats are hulled for consumption, the nutrients of oats remain intact because the bran and germ are not removed. Oats supply almost 100 percent of the daily value of manganese, more than 60 percent of molybdenum, and good quantities of phosphorus, copper, biotin, vitamin B1, magnesium, chromium, magnesium, and zinc. Oats also contain about 13 percent protein, good amounts of fiber, balanced amounts of essential fatty acids, and a high percentage of complex carbohydrates, which may help reduce the risk of certain cancers, diabetes, and bowel irregularity. Oats are an excellent source of amino acids, except lysine and threonine.

Oats help balance blood sugar levels and increase insulin sensitivity, which is essential to prevent diabetes complications and control blood sugar spikes after a meal.[130,131] Oats contain the polysaccharide, beta-glucan, which may enhance immune system activity against harmful microorganisms,[132,133] encourage satiety,[134] and lower cholesterol levels.[135,136] Many studies have demonstrated that frequent consumption of oats can significantly reduce high cholesterol levels.[137-140] finnish researchers reported that the early introduction of oats in a child's diet reduced the child's risk of asthma at age five.[141]

Although often cooked and treated like a grain, quinoa is not technically a grain; it's actually a seed botanically similar to spinach, beets, and chard. Notwithstanding quinoa is unflamiliar to many people and not a primary ingredient found in many recipes, it is a nutrient-dense food with significant health benefits. It contains all nine essential amino acids so it is considered a complete protein source. It is high in manganese and phosphorus and contains good amounts of copper, magnesium, folate, and zinc, as well as excellent quantities of fiber—about 20 percent of the daily value. Quinoa is also rich in the flavonoid quercetin, which is beneficial for allergies (by inhibiting histamine release),[142] asthma (opens the bronchiole tubes and airways),[143] heart disease,[144] high cholesterol,[145] rheumatoid arthritis,[146] and cancer.[147] Quinoa is a good choice for those with celiac disease (CD), and doesn't appear to exacerbate symptoms like digestive problems.[148]

Amaranth is commonly used by those who prefer a gluten-free diet or are gluten intolerant. Often referred to as a pseudo-cereal because it doesn't belong to the true cereal botanical family Poaceae, there are more than 60 known varieties of amaranth. Amaranth is native to Peru and served as a staple food among the Aztecs. It contains good levels of calcium, iron, magnesium, phosphorus, and potassium. Amaranth is the only grain to have documented levels of vitamin C. It contains more protein than most other grains—about 13 to 14 percent— and the protein is high quality which is considered similar in nutritive value to animal proteins. Several animal studies suggest that amaranth helps lower cholesterol,[149,150,151] which makes it a heart-healthy grain.

Barley has a nut-like flavor and a chewy, pasta-like consistency. It is naturally high in maltose—an uncommon sugar found in plants. Fermented barley is used to make beer and other alcoholic beverages. Barley contains more fiber than any other grain, up to 30 percent in some varieties. It is also a good source of molybdenum, manganese, selenium, copper, vitamin B1, chromium, phosphorus, magnesium, and vitamin B3. Like other grains, it has cholesterol-lowering effects[152] and research suggests that it enhances glucose and insulin responses.[153] The benefits of barley are largely attributed to its beta-glucan content, which also has been investigated for its ability to enhance immune system activity and prevent cancer.[154,155]

FATS: THE GOOD, THE BAD, AND THE UGLY

Fat has become a villain and now has a terrible reputation as the leading contributor to obesity and a host of chronic diseases. But in reality, fat is a crucial nutrient that performs many essential functions within the body and is a valuable part of a balanced eating plan. Fat does more than add flavor to your food. It is a more efficient source of energy than protein—energy is generally measured in calories and fat provides more calories per ounce than any other food constituent. Fat helps the intestines absorb and the body to utilize fat-soluble vitamins A, D, E, and K. Fat is a fundamental part of the membrane that surrounds each cell in the body. It also makes up the covering that protects nerve cells and is a structural component of cell membranes in the brain. Fatty acids promote healthy skin and regulate body temperature because they nourish the insulating layer of fat just below the skin. Vital organs, such as the kidneys and heart are surrounded and protected by fat. Fat obviously plays a very important role within the human body and is necessary in small quantities in one's diet.

Over the last few decades dieticians, government agencies, and health care professionals have attempted to limit fat in the diet to decrease the obesity, cardiovascular, and disease burden affecting most industrialized nations. However, these attempts have been unfruitful and have not produced the desired outcomes. Indeed, studies have found low-fat diets (those that attempt to limit all forms of fat in the diet) do little to decrease overweight symptoms and obesity.[156-160] Ironically, the obesity epidemic accelerated dramatically at the peak of the low-fat dietary guidelines' reign during the 1990s. While this hardly means that you can go load up on butter, bacon, and cheese, it does suggest that the type of fats you provide for your body is of great importance. The growing body of evidence suggests that the most beneficial fats for the body are omega-3 fatty acids, particularly DHA (docosahexaenoic acid) and EPA (eicosapentaenoic acid).

Excessive intake of the wrong kinds of fats is a contributing factor in multiple diseases.[161-167] According to the available research and clinical observations, saturated and trans fats are the "bad" and the "ugly" of dietary fats and major contributors to these diseases. These fats should be restricted to a very small portion of or eliminated from the diet. Predominantly made and manufactured by man, trans fat, hydrogenated, or partially hydrogenated fat, is also naturally found in small amounts in beef, pork, lamb, and butter. Artificial, or manmade trans fat, is created by adding hydrogen to liquid vegetable oils to make them more solid. This process is called hydrogenation. Companies manufacture and use trans fats in foods because they are easy to make, inexpensive, and have a long shelf life. Some experts suggest that trans fats make foods more addictive in nature because they may enhance the flavor and texture of foods they are added to. Trans fats raise blood cholesterol—perhaps at a greater rate than saturated fats, increase LDL cholesterol, and decrease HDL cholesterol levels.[168] The consumption of trans fat is strongly associated with an increased risk of cardiovascular disease and stroke and all causes of mortality, which caused many experts to call for an absolute ban.[169-173] This action may benefit the hearts and health of millions of Americans according to observations from Denmark. Twenty years after banning trans fats, Denmark experienced a 50 percent reduction in the number of deaths due to coronary heart disease.[174] A large variety of processed foods contain trans fats, including potato chips, fried foods, shortening, margarine, frosting, pancake and waffle mixes, microwave popcorn, ice cream, cookies, pies, and cakes. Carefully read food labels and watch for the words "hydrogenated," "partially hydrogenated," and "shortening" in the ingredients. Even doing this you may still consume trans fats though, because food manufacturers are not required to list it on the label if one serving contains less than 0.5 grams of trans fat.

Saturated fat is predominantly acquired from animal sources and its excess consumption is associated with increased LDL cholesterol levels.[175] However, this does not necessarily directly correlate saturated fat to heart disease risk, especially if starches and refined carbohydrates are substituted for saturated fats.[176] Saturated fats are found in animal products like beef, lamb, pork, poultry with skin, cheese, butter, and many dairy products (unless they are labeled fatfree). Adhering to a low-saturated fat diet may produce weight loss in the short term, but so does following a high-protein, low carbohydrate diet. The truth is, just about any diet that restricts calories will result in temporary weight loss.

The *Dietary Guidelines for Americans, 2010,* suggest consuming less than 10 percent of total calories from saturated fat,[177] and trans fatty acid intake should be as low as possible.[178] Based on these guidelines, a person with a calorie requirement of 2,000 calories daily should only consume 200 calories from saturated fat, or roughly 22 grams. To put that in perspective, dishes at several major American restaurant chains would put you way over that total after just one meal.

- The Cheesecake Factory's French Toast Napoleon—51 g saturated fat.[179]
- Red Robin's A.1. Peppercorn Burger (no fries, drink, or anything else with it)—83 g fat and 1,381 calories.[180]
- Outback Steakhouse's Blooming Onion—48 g saturated fat, almost 2,000 calories.[181]
- IHOP's Hearty Ham and Cheese Omelets—32 g saturated fat.[182]
- Applebee's Quesadilla Burger—45 g saturated fat and 3.5 grams trans fat.[183]

Most fast food is virtually devoid of beneficial nutrients but packed with harmful or excessive fat and disproportionate salt, sugar, and calories. Don't give up on eating out, but do limit the number of times you do. When you do eat out, make a conscious effort to choose healthier alternatives by adhering to the following guidelines:

- Ask to see calorie and nutritional information—most reputable restaurants will provide this information for you or have it available online.
- Share a meal—most portions provided at restaurants are twice what is considered a reasonable portion; choose tomato based sauces rather than cream based.
- Ask for sauces on the side so you can choose how much you want to eat.
- Ask if the restaurant has a low-calorie or healthier menu.
- Order steamed vegetables as a side dish instead of French fries or a baked potato.
- Avoid the soft drinks and choose water instead—add some lemon if you need flavor.
- Skip the appetizer.

As consumers increase their desire for and demand healthier options, restaurants will have no choice but to increase the availability of healthy options. Make "going out" a special occasion and choose to cook at home instead—this way you'll know what ingredients are included in your meal.

Essential fatty acids—meaning they must be obtained from food—are vital to human health, particularly omega-3 fatty acids. Americans currently consume far too many omega-6 essential fatty acids from vegetable oils. This disproportionate consumption of omega-3s and omega-6s is detrimental to human health, increases inflammation, and may increase the risk of multiple adverse health conditions. Conversely, maintaining a balanced ratio between these two fatty acids, thought to be anywhere from 2:1 and 5:1, is vital to optimum health and reduces the risk and symptoms of many diseases. Most Western diets are thought to be closer to a ratio of 15:1 and 17:1. To eat better requires a focused effort to bring this ratio into better balance, increase omega-3s, and simultaneously decrease omega-6s, trans fats, and saturated fats. Research suggests you can't just decrease total fat, or even just bad fats. To achieve the greatest health benefits, you need to replace them with healthy fats. Good sources of omega-3 fatty acids include seafood (salmon, trout, herring, sardines, and tuna), flaxseed, chia, red algae, and walnuts.

The major omega-3 fatty acids include alpha-linolenic acid (ALA), eicosapentaenoic acid (EPA), and docosahexaenoic acid (DHA). In healthy individuals, ALA is converted to DHA and EPA after ingestion. However, unhealthy individuals may not convert ALA as readily. Interestingly, research suggests that women more readily convert ALA to EPA and DHA than men. They convert approximately 21 percent of dietary ALA to EPA and 9 percent to DHA; whereas men convert only 8 percent of ALA to EPA and less than 4 percent is converted to DHA.[184,185] To skip the conversion process it is best to consume DHA and EPA instead of ALA, because research suggests plant-based sources may not be as beneficial as consuming the superior DHA and EPA sources predominantly found in animals. One benefit to plant-based omega-3 fatty acids is that they usually supply vitamin E, which helps to protect the fatty acids from rancidity, whereas an antioxidant generally needs to be added to animal-based sources to prevent lipid peroxidation. One example of the superiority of animal-based omega-3s is the findings from a study that compared the reduction in breast cancer risk of plant-based omega-3s (ALA) and marine omega-3s (DHA/EPA). This study concluded that for every 0.1 g per day increment increase in marine omega-3s, women experience a 5 percent reduction in breast cancer risk.[186] Sadly, the same results were not observed for ALA during the study.

Omega-3 fatty acids play a vital role in normal growth and development as well as brain function. They are highly concentrated within the brain and appear to be very important for cognitive and behavioral function, memory, and learning ability. Remarkably, scientists discovered that when DHA is taken with vitamin D3, the immune system's ability to clear amyloid plaques from the brain is optimized.[187] This is a significant finding for dementia and Alzheimer's disease.

Scientific studies have concluded that omega-3 fatty acids are valuable for human health in the following ways:

- DHA and EPA are precursors to the production of anti-inflammatory compounds resolvins and protectins. Omega-3s may help reduce inflammation in the body—particularly in the cause of autoimmune inflammation—and reduce the need for anti-inflammatory medications.[188-190]

- Omega-3s help normalize blood pressure, decrease plasma triglycerides, improve vascular function, decrease inflammation, and enhance endothelial function, which may help reduce the risk of cardiovascular disease.[191,192]

- Given their ability to affect autoimmune disorders and inflammation, omega-3s are a good option for rheumatoid arthritis.[193]

- When combined with regular physical activity, marine omega-3s may aid blood flow and fat utilization, which aids weight loss.[194]

In fact, a deficiency in DHA is a contributing factor in many illnesses both physical and mental.[195,196] The best way to get these healthy fats is through cold water fish consumption, but if you don't like the taste of fish, don't fret, studies indicate you can achieve the same benefit by using fish oil supplements.[197]

Clinical evidence suggests consuming DHA and EPA in the range of 250–500 mg each per day may reduce risk factors for heart disease.[198] Some scientists now recommend this intake be established as the Dietary Reference Intake (DRI) for these important EFAs.[199] Clinical research suggests a marked reduction in cardiovascular disease risk is achieved through omega-3 consumption.[200,201] Some emerging research suggests that triglyceride (TG) forms of fish oil may be the most beneficial, although most clinical studies have utilized the ethyl ester (EE) type.[202] Unrefined fish oil in its natural state contains triglycerides with DHA and EPA that are attached to glycerol. When fish oil is processed to remove harmful substances, the glycerol molecule is also removed, which converts the fish oil to the EE type. Some manufacturers add the glycerol molecule back into the fish oil after processing, which returns it to a TG form.

The bulk of omega-6 fatty acids obtained from Western diets come from vegetables oils—such as linoleic acid—and some from animal sources (eggs and meat). The two most common omega-6 fatty acids are linoleic acid (found in corn, sunflower, safflower and soybean oils) and arachidonic acid (from eggs and meat). Linoleic acid converts to arachidonic acid in the body, and if there are insufficient quantities of omega-3s to balance it, inflammation increases.

Omega-6s are also essential for good health but should be consumed sparingly. Omega-6s are required for cell growth, brain and muscle development, support nervous system function, and help produce chemical messengers. However, it is rare for Westerners to have a deficiency in omega-6s and too much of them may promote inflammation[203] and increase the risks of many chronic diseases.

Omega-9 fatty acids are a third but not often mentioned category of essential fatty acids. The body can produce them in small amounts as long as sufficient quantities of omega-3 and omega-6 fatty acids are present. They may support heart health and improve the balance of LDL to HDL cholesterol and are important for blood sugar control. They are commonly found in olive oil, peanut oil, canola oil, sunflower oil, safflower oil, avocados, almonds, hazelnuts, peanuts, eggs, cashews, and poultry.

Fat is essential to human health and the right kinds of fats (omega-3s) should be included in the diet and in proper proportion with omega-6 (about 2–4 omega-6 to 1 omega-3).[204] Rather than trying to avoid fat, strive to eliminate trans fat, reduce saturated fat, increase the consumption of omega-3 fatty acids, and better balance omega-6/omega-3. The right types of fat promote health and prevent disease, while the wrong kinds do exactly the opposite.

THE HARMFUL SUBSTANCES LURKING IN YOUR FOOD

There is an abundance of substances that are harmful to our health. Some of these substances are found commonly in foods and/or beverages consumed on a daily basis. It wouldn't be sensible or easy to list every unhealthy substance that should be avoided, and it would be equally difficult for the average consumer to abide by all these restrictions. Instead common sense and careful thought will generally lead you to the answer as to whether you should consume a food that contains a particular ingredient or not. Keeping this in mind, this book will list some of the most commonly consumed harmful substances that according to available knowledge should either be eliminated or severely restricted when striving to eat better.

Refined sugar, or sucrose, is devoid of all nutrients and is nothing more than a pleasing sweet taste of empty calories. Aside from the quick burst of energy it provides, it has only detrimental effects on health. It promotes tooth decay, leaches calcium from the body, destroys the balance between calcium and phosphorus, is addictive, depletes the body of vitamins and minerals, causes mood swings and uncontrollable personality changes, and contributes to degenerative conditions.

Despite the recommendation by the Unites States Department of Agriculture (USDA) that we consume no more than ten teaspoons of sugar per day, it is estimated that the average American consumes roughly forty teaspoons of sugar daily.[205] In fact, some juices, soft drinks, and even yogurts contain more than the recommended ten teaspoons of sugar in one serving. Drinking one twelve ounce can of regular Mountain Dew provides over eleven teaspoons of sugar alone.[206] Sonic Drive-in's Route 44 Cherry Limeade supplies over thirty teaspoons of sugar—almost two-thirds of a cup.[207] If you want to find out how much sugar you are consuming, read the nutrition facts panel on the product and look for the number of grams of sugar it contains; divide this number by four and you have the number of teaspoons of sugar contained in the product. Be prepared, you will likely be astounded by the sugar content in some foods.

When refined sugar is consumed, it quickly enters the bloodstream triggering the pancreas to release insulin in an effort to encourage the cellular uptake of sugar for energy and to reduce the amount of sugar in the blood. Unfortunately, if too much sugar is consumed, over time the body is no longer able to control blood sugar levels through insulin release because the cells of the body fail to respond to insulin efficiently. This is termed "insulin resistance," meaning the body is resistant to the effects of insulin. Thus the body's blood sugar control system has been damaged and the risk of diabetes increases. This process also depresses the immune system making the body more susceptible to disease. Sugar depresses immune system cells such as macrophages and natural killer (NK) cells.[208] NK cells are innately ready to recognize and neutralize infected cells and cancer cells within the body. Macrophages recruit other cells to areas of infection and ingest bacteria, foreign cells, and damaged or dead cells. Dysfunctions or inefficiencies of either of these cells reduce the body's chances of finding and eliminating harmful organisms.

According to John Ely's Glucose-Ascorbate-Antagonism theory, glucose (blood sugar) and vitamin C share similar chemical structures. Therefore, he suggests that significant levels of glucose in the blood stream compete with vitamin C to enter cells. Quite simply, the more glucose in the blood stream, the less vitamin C that will be absorbed.

Sugar may be a significant factor in many of the diseases we suffer with. Tooth decay is definitely associated with sugar intake,[209] particularly when we eat hard candies that stay in the mouth for long periods and constantly coat our teeth with sugar (think suckers). Long-lasting over-consumption of sugar may damage the millions of filtering units within the kidneys, and excess consumption of sugar (fructose) has been linked to kidney diseases.[210] Consumption of sugar by the mother immediately preceding and after birth has been associated with an increased risk of severe asthma among her children.[211]

The empty calories of sugar combined with its sweet taste contribute to obesity as we consume more and more sweet tasting goodies and increase caloric intake. The over-consumption of sugar even affects our mood and may promote mood swings and irritability and contributes to depression.[212] Interestingly, researchers have observed that drinking a sugary soda rapidly increases blood sugar levels, followed by a steep decline about four hours later. The body responds to this decline in blood sugar by significantly increasing the release of adrenaline (up to ten times normal levels), which could trigger anxious feelings and hyperactivity.[213] Many nutritionists believe the increase in attention deficit and attention deficit hyperactivity disorders are directly correlated with sugar intake. Even cancer has a sugar connection. Too much sugar contributes to insulin resistance and weight gain, both of which are associated with an increased risk of cancer and cancer progression (tumor growth).[214] All cells feed off of sugars and use it to maintain vital bodily functions—even cancer cells. What is important to remember in this situation is that it's *added* sugars that need to be avoided, not naturally occurring sugar found in fruits and vegetables. Discontinuing the consumption of all foods, even fruits and vegetables that contain sugar, would deprive the body of phytonutrients, fiber, and antioxidants that may be beneficial in reducing the risk of cancer and cancer progression.

High-fructose corn syrup (HFCS) is sweeter and cheaper than table sugar and therefore added to countless foods and beverages. It is commonly found in: soda/soft drinks, baked goods, candy, sauces, salad dressings, yogurt, and cereals. High-fructose corn syrup (HFCS) is in so many food products it is virtually unavoidable if you eat processed foods or beverages that have been sweetened. This sweetener and preservative is associated with a surplus of health problems including obesity, diabetes,[215] metabolic syndrome[216,217] (a group of risk factors that increase the risk of heart disease and diabetes), atherosclerosis,[218] elevated triglyceride levels,[219] increased LDL cholesterol levels,[220] may depress your immune system, and even accelerates the aging process. Many brands of high-fructose corn syrup have been found to contain the toxic heavy metal mercury, which has been linked to heart disease in adults and learning disabilities in children.[221] High-fructose corn syrup is metabolized by the body differently than normal sugar and blocks the ability of the body to regulate appetite. It does this largely because it inhibits the hormone used by the body to tell you that you are full—leptin. In other words when you consume HFCS your brain doesn't receive the same signal it receives when consuming regular sugar and therefore doesn't process that the body has acquired calories. In addition, fructose encourages the storage of fat in the abdominal region. Consequently, we may consume excess calories that get stored in everyone's least favorite place for fat—the belly—and increase our weight. When metabolized by the liver, fructose is converted to triglycerides or stored as body fat, not converted to blood glucose like other sugars.

Agave is portrayed as a wholesome alternative to sugar, but in reality it is a glorified HFCS. The process by which it is produced is similar to that of HFCS and agave is a highly concentrated source of fructose—70 percent or more, compared to about 55 percent for HFCS. Concentrated sources of fructose should be high on the list of food additives to avoid. You can accomplish this by carefully reading labels—watch for hidden HFCS names like glucose-fructose syrup and isoglucose on labels, avoiding foods that contain them, and by substituting natural sweeteners like stevia.

Like alcohol or cocaine, caffeine is a drug of abuse. In fact, it is the most popular behavior modifying drug used and abused in the world. It is found in soft drinks, coffee, tea, energy drinks, chocolate, and some plants. The tell-tale signs of excessive caffeine consumption include a rapid heartbeat, insomnia, increased urination, heartburn or acid reflux, headache, anxiety, indigestion, muscle tremors, malnutrition, and hypertension—due to an increase in the production of adrenaline. Too much caffeine can lead to reduced liver function, infertility in women, and excretion of B vitamins, adrenal exhaustion, osteoporosis, elevated cholesterol levels, and depletion of essential minerals (especially calcium). After initial ingestion, caffeine rapidly enters the bloodstream and causes an increase in energy levels and mental alertness. This juiced-up state subsides as caffeine clears the system, often leading to fatigue and mental depression—termed a "caffeine crash." A person has to continually pump their body full of caffeine in order to maintain energy levels and peak mental fitness. Some become so addicted to this false state of alertness and increased energy that they only "feel well" when they are under the influence of caffeine. Their body is now dependent on caffeine, requiring it to feel normal.

Ask anyone who has quit or tried to quit drinking caffeinated beverages cold turkey and most will say they experienced symptoms such as headache, difficulty concentrating, muscle stiffness, and irritability. A much better option is to slowly reduce the amount of caffeinated beverages you consume by 25 percent each week or two until you reach your desired level of caffeine consumption. A slow reduction of caffeine may help to avoid some of the undesirable effects of withdrawal. The FDA's current recommended safe level of caffeine consumption is 400 mg per day for adults. That is roughly the equivalent of four to five cups of coffee or two energy drinks. Other experts consider 300 mg of caffeine moderate consumption. But, keep in mind that these levels are based on statistical averages among populations and your tolerance to caffeine may be lower.

Energy drinks appear to be the beverage of choice among teens and college students who want to increase energy levels or use it as an alcohol substitute or to help keep them awake after insufficient sleep. Consuming these beverages frequently has been associated with the participation in more unhealthy behaviors like smoking, unwholesome beverage choices, and excess media usage (TV, video games).[222] Teens aren't the only ones who enjoy these drinks though.

Adults partake freely to maintain alertness as well. These drinks provide energy through a surge of caffeine—as much as 300 mg per 8.4 ounce serving. They also include other ingredients from natural and artificial sources that stimulate the nervous system like guarana, taurine, and ginseng that may enhance the stimulating effects of caffeine. If the caffeine occurs naturally from ingredients such as green tea or guarana, manufacturers are not required to list the caffeine content on the nutrition facts label. Without knowing it, consumers, including teenagers and young children, may be consuming a dangerous amount of caffeine through oversized and caffeine-laced energy drinks. In sensitive people an overdose of caffeine can occur with as little as 250 mg. Soda and other foods are limited to a maximum of 71 mg of caffeine per twelve ounce serving by the FDA, but energy drinks are exempt from this limitation because they are labeled as dietary supplements. Manufacturers know that caffeine is an addictive substance so the more they can load into their product—up to five times the amount found in a cup of coffee[223]—the greater the chance they will create an addicted customer who requires their product daily.

Every person has their own level of caffeine tolerance. For some, 500 to 600 mg of caffeine can cause anxiety, muscle tremors, and abnormal heart rhythms. Other individuals, who are more sensitive, experience adverse reactions with as little as 50 to 100 mg of caffeine. As consumption of these harmful beverages rise, so do the trips to emergency rooms, hospitalizations, and even deaths related to them. Emergency room visits related to energy drinks more than doubled from 2007 to 2011,[224] and a number of deaths have now been reported that allegedly involved energy drink consumption. Even athletes in superb shape are not immune to an overdose of caffeine. Disappointingly, some athletes rely on these drinks to give them an extra edge in competitions. The fact is energy drinks have even been implicated as a contributing factor in a few deaths even among seemingly very healthy athletes. Studies suggest large doses of caffeine cause decreased cardiovascular function in predisposed individuals, which may contribute to the serious adverse events often associated with energy drink consumption.[225,226]

Black, white, and green teas are often recommended as healthy substitutes for coffee and caffeinated beverages. These teas all originate from the same plant, the *Camellia sinensis* plant, and differ only in the way they are processed. White tea is the least processed—the leaves are steamed and then dried, which leaves the antioxidant polyphenols intact. Green tea leaves undergo minimal processing, whereas black tea is oxidized through fermentation—the oxidation of the plant polyphenols in the tea leaf. Green tea has received a great deal of publicity and has been flaunted as a cure for everything from memory loss to cancer because of the significant antioxidant properties it possesses. Because it can boost metabolism, enhance thermogenesis, and remove excess fluids from the body, it is frequently advertised as a weight loss miracle. Green tea has great value as a medicinal plant but it should be used prudently because of the thexanthine alkaloids it contains—caffeine, theobromine, and theophylline —and its fluoride, tannin, and some oxalate content. The three xanthine alkaloids create a trio of compounds that cross the blood-brain barrier and stimulate the central nervous system and heart, as well as act as diuretics. Excess blood levels of xanthines may cause diarrhea, dizziness, trembling, frequent urination, and insomnia. Theobromine is suspected of being toxic to the reproductive system[227,228] and may increase the risk of prostate cancer.[229] Theophylline is a bronchodilator and sometimes used medicinally in the treatment of respiratory disorders. It is associated with diarrhea, nausea, vomiting, muscle tremors, and irregular heartbeat. The chlorogenic acid content in black tea increases plasma homocysteine levels, a predictor of cardiovascular disease.[230] Premenstrual syndrome may be aggravated by excess tea consumption.[231] The *Camellia sinensis* plant naturally concentrates fluoride it obtains from soil and the air. It takes as few as four cups of tea per day to provide1 to 1.9 mg of fluoride. This level of fluoride approaches the Environmental Protection Agency's secondary safety standard, which limits fluoride to 2 mg per liter or less daily to avoid the risk of dental fluorosis.[232] If the water that the person uses to make the tea in is also fluoridated the levels could increase above the secondary standard safe levels.

A recent trend by dietary supplement manufacturers is to concentrate green tea for its antioxidant polyphenol EGCG (epigallocatechin gallate) content because of its chemopreventive properties.[233] Manufacturers don't always inform the public when they do this, which makes it more difficult to identify a concentrated product. Both animal and human studies have demonstrated that this practice can cause harm to the liver, particularly if green tea is consumed for prolonged periods and on an empty stomach.[234-237] It appears that EGCG accumulates in the liver, leading to hepatotoxicity—chemically caused liver damage. In one rare case an individual required an emergency liver transplant after taking a weight loss supplement that contained green tea, guggul, and usnic acid.[238] The liver damage is usually reversed after discontinuance of the green tea product. If your product says it is the equivalent to several or more cups of green tea, then it is a concentrated extract. Based on the current available research, it is wise to use green tea for medicinal purposes only or in great moderation. In addition, it should only be used for short periods of time and should be taken with food.

It is customary for millions of people worldwide to start their day with a cup of coffee and some can't imagine starting a day without it. Scientific research has been mixed regarding whether this practice is harmful or beneficial. Like tea, coffee contains varying amounts of caffeine depending on the type of bean used and how it is brewed, though it usually has significantly higher levels of caffeine than green tea and up to fourteen times more caffeine than black tea.[239] Coffee contains the same three xanthine alkaloids (theobromine, theophylline, and caffeine) that tea does, but it seems to provide more of a kick or jolt than tea.

Your body produces large amounts of hydrochloric acid (HCl) when you drink a cup of coffee, particularly if consumed on an empty stomach. It is thought that the extra production may decrease future production of HCl when it is actually needed for a meal, which may significantly impair the digestion of proteins. Compounds found in coffee may irritate gastrointestinal tissues and cause digestive upset and even ulcers. Coffee may relax the lower esophageal sphincter that prevents food and beverages from regurgitating up the esophagus. If this sphincter remains in a relaxed position acid reflux may occur. Coffee has also been linked to increased cardiovascular disease and all causes of mortality (when four or more cups are consumed per day),[240] increased risk of heart attack (more than three cups per day),[241] and increased cholesterol levels (boiled not filtered).[242] It also may cause rheumatoid arthritis (decaffeinated only)[243] and inhibit iron absorption (especially plant-based iron).[244] But, as was stated, the research is mixed with other reports that suggest coffee consumption reduces the risk of cardiovascular disease and all-cause mortality,[245] reduces type 2 diabetes risk,[246] reduces inflammatory markers,[247] and modestly reduces stroke risk.[248] Coffee is a complex beverage with hundreds of constituents, making it important to consider both the positive and negative effects of its consumption.

Decaffeinated coffee is often the beverage of choice for those who enjoy its flavor but don't want the caffeine found in regular coffee. However, decaffeinated coffee is not without risks, especially when you consider the chemicals used to extract the caffeine. The majority of decaffeinated coffees are processed with solvents to remove the caffeine, which leaves solvent residue on the coffee beans. Robusta beans are generally the beans of choice when making decaffeinated coffee because they retain more of the coffee flavor than other beans. Sadly, robusta beans are highly acidic producing a more acidic internal environment and throwing off the body's optimal pH balance. To consider coffee a safe or even healthful beverage purely because the caffeine is eliminated discounts the many other harmful chemical compounds it contains. If you would like a hot drink, consider a more wholesome beverage such as Pero made from barley, chicory, and rye.

Alcohol seems like an innocent drug when consumed responsibly, but sadly this is not completely so. The National Institute on Drug Abuse considers it a drug because it is a depressant. Besides the consequences to the individual, families are frequently torn apart and lives are lost from the abuse of alcohol. Alcohol is a central nervous system depressant, poison, and harmful to the organs of the body.[249] Abuse of alcohol is also associated with cognitive impairment and short-term mortality among the elderly.[250] It suppresses your inhibitions, moral sense, increases reckless behavior, provides a false sense of well-being, slurs speech, causes drowsiness, decreases motor skills, diminishes muscle control, reduces coordination, impairs judgment, may cause respiratory distress, and hinders cognitive abilities

Alcohol consumption is the fourth leading preventable cause of death in the United States[251] and results in the deaths of more than 241 people every day.[251] Many people consume alcohol to cope with life's problems or to numb the pain of feeling bad, which unwittingly creates a dependence. Once addiction sets in it can be very difficult to give up the psycho-physiological need for this harmful drug.

The physical, social, and economic impact of alcohol abuse is huge. Astonishingly, up to 40 percent of all patients in general hospital beds (not maternity or intensive care units) were there for alcohol related complications according to a report published in 1994.[252] Heavy drinkers experience higher health care costs—approximately 42 percent more annually[253]—and are more likely to require emergency room care when compared to light to moderate drinkers.[254] The economic costs of alcoholism are estimated at almost $185 billion yearly.[255]

Alcohol is a diuretic and causes the body to excrete more water than it takes in and increases the risk of dehydration. Alcohol inhibits absorption of nutrients in the small intestine, which may cause deficiencies in vitamins and minerals.[256] Excessive alcohol consumption can lead to liver cirrhosis,[257] various cancers,[258] and unintentional injuries that occur without the intent to harm. After consumption, alcohol travels down the esophagus and into the stomach, where up to 20 percent of it is absorbed and enters the bloodstream. The rest continues through the gastrointestinal (GI) tract and is absorbed with other nutrients. Once inside the GI tract alcohol can cause dysfunction, such as a weakened esophageal sphincter, which promotes heartburn. It also damages the lining of the esophagus and increases the risk of esophageal cancer. Alcohol irritates the intestines and may cause diarrhea.[259] The liver is the primary organ of detoxification and prioritizes the metabolism of alcohol above all other substances. Contrary to other nutrients the body does not have a specific place to store alcohol, so it must metabolize alcohol first. If too much alcohol is consumed, or if the liver is already compromised from prolonged alcohol consumption, it can quickly overwhelm the liver, and lead to damaged or destroyed liver cells, fatty deposits in the liver, liver inflammation, or permanent scarring (cirrhosis). If the liver is damaged, body toxicity can result as the liver is unable to rid the body of the toxins it is exposed to regularly.

An abundance of pesticides and herbicides are applied to produce in the United States at a rate equivalent to about four pounds of pesticides and herbicides for every man, woman, and child each year. This adds up to an astounding 1.2 billion pounds of pest-controlling chemicals used every year.[260] Sadly much of this remains on fruits, vegetables, and other food crops when consumed. In fact, virtually all non-organic produce has a detectable amount of pesticide or herbicide when sent to market for consumption. This obviously leads to human consumption of substances made to kill unwanted pests. Beyond the consumption of these chemicals in our food we are also exposed to them via the air we breathe and the environment we live in. In the short-term this will generally have no discernable effect on a person. The jury is still out on the long-term effects of pesticide exposure; however, evidence is mounting that continued exposure to pesticides is directly related to various cancers[261] and neurological disorders.[262] Moreover, the constant onslaught of chemicals may inhibit the proper functioning of the body's detoxification systems.

Some foods such as animal products, peaches, strawberries, grapes, juices, bananas, and potatoes have a higher concentration of pesticides than others. These food products should be purchased organic whenever possible. Another way to avoid pesticide-laced produce is to buy organic produce that is locally grown and in season. Produce purchased out of season often travels great distances, which requires heavy amounts of pesticides to avoid infestation by insects as it is transported to your area. Most pesticides are stored in the outer layer or skin of produce, so removal of the skins may not eliminate all of the pesticides. However, this practice also removes vital nutrients found in the skins of produce. You can also remove much of the surface pesticides if you wash the produce in a mild additive-free soap or a cleanser available at most health food stores.

The bottom line is don't avoid healthy fruits and vegetables because you are afraid of pesticide exposure. Do what you can to limit your exposure and encourage organic farming by purchasing organic products. It is better to limit your exposure and still get the benefits of the produce.

Food additives and preservatives are added to foods to generate a longer shelf life, make them more convenient, improve taste or flavor, or enhance the appearance of food. Unfortunately many of these additives and preservatives have negative health consequences and contribute to attention deficit disorders and allergies, cause hyperactivity, encourage mood disorders and depression, promote headaches, and increase cancer risk. The less packaged and canned foods you eat, the more you will avoid these risks. Of particular concerns are the following:

- Monosodium glutamate (MSG) is a flavor enhancer commonly found in Chinese food, canned soups, processed and packaged foods, snack foods, and chips. It is known to cause short-term reactions such as headache, chest pain, nausea, shortness of breath, and numbness around the mouth. Experts believe it is toxic to the nervous system and it has been associated with neurological disorders.[263] A rodent study suggested that high consumption of MSG results in obesity.[264] MSG gets such bad press lately that food manufacturers have attempted to hide this ingredient by using other names such as autolyzed yeast, textured protein, natrium glutamate, and glutamic acid.

- Artificial sweeteners like aspartame and sucralose were created to provide a substitute for sugar that does not so readily raise blood sugar levels, but the question is are we providing a healthy alternative to sugar? The current amount of scientific research suggest the answer is no. In 1995, aspartame was responsible for 75 percent of adverse reactions reported to the FDA Adverse Reaction Monitoring System.[265] Because aspartame contains phenylalanine, people with phenylketonuria should particularly avoid aspartame as they will have increased sensitivity to this artificial sweetener. Although these sweeteners can be used by diabetics to sweeten foods without an increase in blood sugar levels, they may pose other health risks. Some doctors believe there is a correlation between aspartame and declined cognitive function, especially memory. There is also a question about whether artificial sweeteners form toxic compounds in the stomach. If you must satisfy your sweet tooth, try a natural sweetener like stevia, which is currently recognized as a safer alternative to artificial sweeteners, provides zero calories, and is significantly sweeter than sugar when compared ounce for ounce.

- High-fructose corn syrup has already been mentioned, but it is worth reminding you here that it is definitely an ingredient to avoid.

- Sodium, or salt, is required for proper body function and helps maintain normal fluid balance and nerve impulses. It is the primary electrolyte (an electrically charge ion) found in body fluids and utilized by your cells to carry electrical impulses that regulate nerve and muscle function. Electrolytes are lost on a daily basis and must be replenished through diet. However, far too many Americans consume considerably more sodium than they are losing each day, thus creating an imbalance. A recent report suggests that favorable health outcomes can be achieved if most individuals stayed within a sodium range of 2,645 mg to 4,945 mg per day.[266] Intakes of sodium above or below this range resulted in an increased risk of all causes of mortality.

AVOID EXCESS SALT INTAKE:

- Don't put the salt shaker on the table. Sometimes it is a psychological thing and we grab the salt to "flavor" our food before we even taste it. If you eliminate added salt at the dinner table you will not only reduce salt intake, you will be able to taste and learn to enjoy the true flavor of foods.
- Reduce salt when you prepare meals. This may need to be a gradual process in many traditional family recipes, but a worthy endeavor.
- Flavor foods with herbs and spices instead.
- Limit or avoid canned foods and prepared condiments.
- Limit consumption of processed cheese and smoked meats.
- Read food labels carefully and try not to fall over in shock when you find out just how much sodium is in that can of beef stew.

- Found commonly in processed meats, hot dogs, sausage, bacon, beef jerky, deli meats, and canned soups, sodium nitrite (sodium nitrate) has been linked to certain cancers[267] and may decrease blood vessel function, which increases the risk of heart disease. Research suggests that those who eat the most processed meat (known to contain sodium nitrite) have a greater risk of cancer and heart disease than people who eat red meat. During digestion, this ingredient combines with amino acids to form nitrosamines, which are very harmful to the liver and pancreas and are highly carcinogenic.

There are a few additional recommendations to be mindful of as you strive to eat better.

- Chew your food thoroughly. When you chew, it begins the digestive process and breaks down food into smaller pieces that mix with saliva. Saliva lubricates food and makes it easier to pass through the digestive process. Saliva also releases enzymes that help to break down food and inhibit bacterial growth in the mouth.

■ Eating several small meals a day rather than three large ones helps the body digest food more effectively. It also facilitates the optimal absorption and use of nutrients. Frequent small meals helps keep metabolism operating efficiently and helps avoid binge eating that may occur when you eat three large meals a day. This practice also helps prevent extreme blood sugar swings that can occur when large meals are consumed. You can incorporate these principals if you eat a mid-morning snack like fruit and a protein or fat, and a mid-afternoon vegetable snack with a healthy dip. This will help you reduce what you eat for the "normal" three large meals of breakfast, lunch, and dinner. To learn more about this way of eating refer to my book *TransformWise: Your Complete Guide to a Wise Body Transformation.*

■ Portion sizes are completely out of control in the United States. It seems most restaurants are supersizing our plates as well as our midsections as a standard practice. Often what is provided as a single portion is actually a suitable and more sensible portion for two people. At home, use medium-sized dinner plates rather than the large ones. Furthermore, fill one-third to half of your plate with vegetables to avoid the excess intake of less healthy foods, which also helps you to meet your daily vegetable requirements. Avoid buffets. You have to eat way too much food to get your money's worth and this often encourages you to eat more than you should. If you must have seconds, have a second helping of vegetables.

■ As the most important meal of the day, breakfast should never be skipped. If you skip breakfast after prolonged abstinence from foods overnight your body triggers the appetite control center's feeling of hunger. In fact, this appetite control center may send the brain a signal that the body is starving. Breakfast provides a break from the fast that occurred while you slept and provides essential fuel for your body and mind to function properly. Some people skip breakfast as a weight loss measure, but evidence suggests that those who eat breakfast are more likely to maintain a healthy weight than those who don't.[268]

■ The time of day you eat is also important when it comes to healthy eating. Digestion is considered at its peak during midday because the digestive enzymes are at their maximum during this time. This is a great time to eat harder to digest foods like raw vegetables. The largest meal is best consumed at midday when digestion is functioning optimally. It is preferable to avoid eating two to three hours before going to bed to allow your body a rest period to rejuvenate the body, rather than focus on digestion of your late night meal or snack. If you eat too close to bedtime, your body will still be working hard to digest food. If efforts are diverted to digestion, your body may not properly mobilize immune system cells that track, identify, and eliminate harmful substances. Your immune cells are most active at night and require this sleep period to perform their duties more effectively.

ENHANCE DIGESTION AND MAKE THE MOST OF WHAT YOU EAT

Optimum health starts in the gut and requires proper digestion, efficient metabolism, and the productive absorption and utilization of the nutrients you eat. If your digestive system is sluggish you may not assimilate all the beneficial nutrients that you eat. In fact, inefficient digestion could mean that the food you eat is simply going for a ride through the digestive tract before exiting out the other end. This deprives your cells, tissues, organs, and body systems of vital nutrients they rely on to function well. It is estimated that up to 70 million Americans are affected by digestive diseases and that this results in almost $142 billion spent in medical care for these diseases.[269,270] The primary symptoms of indigestion include abdominal pain, nausea, bloating, expansion of the abdominal region, and belching after you eat a meal.

The inability to digest foods properly may be caused by a deficiency in enzymes. Digestive enzymes break down food into nutrients that can be absorbed and utilized by the body. Inadequate production of enzymes may lead to malnutrition. The pancreas and small intestines produce the majority of digestive enzymes but if either is not working optimally insufficient enzymes may be produced. Chronic stress, decreased stomach acid production, inflammation of the intestinal tract, and pancreatic disorders can all reduce production of enzymes.

The bottom line is that enzymes help you make use of the nutrients you ingest from food and supplements. There are a variety of digestive enzymes, each with a specific purpose.

- **Proteases** aid the digestion of protein and support healthy digestion, circulation, and immune function.
- **Amylase** promotes the digestion of starchy foods (i.e., potatoes, rice, bread, and pasta). Starchy foods are used abundantly in the typical American diet.
- **Cellulase** helps to break down part of the cellulose—an insoluble plant carbohydrate—obtained from eating plant foods and converts it to beta-glucose. Beta-glucose affects blood sugar to a lesser degree than glucose because it is absorbed more slowly.

- **Lipase** helps digest fats or lipids, and improves the absorption of essential fatty acids.
- **Peptidase** helps break down chains of amino acids called peptides.
- The body uses **phytase** to release phosphate and other essential minerals from grains and seeds.
- **Lactase** is the enzyme that helps you digest the milk sugar lactose.
- **Invertase** aids the break down of sugar (table sugar).

It takes representation from each of these digestive enzymes to make the most of the food you eat.

Some foods also contain measurable amounts of enzymes. Two of the most well-known are papain and bromelain, which are found in papayas and pineapples. Both aid the digestion of proteins but bromelain is often used to help reduce inflammation as well.[271] Bromelain appears to exert widespread inflammation control in the airways, digestive tract, and throughout the body.[272,273] In fact, its pain-relieving and anti-inflammatory effects rival that of prescription drugs.[274,275,276]

Digestive enzymes can be particularly beneficial when you overeat (think Thanksgiving) or eat too many sweats. To maximize your digestion, take a full-spectrum enzyme supplement with each meal. A full-spectrum enzyme provides a blend of multiple enzymes that will help break down and absorb the nutrients from various foods such as fats, carbohydrates, protein, and fiber.

Essential oils are also known to aid digestion. Ginger is prized for its ability to support digestion. It protects the gut and encourages the rhythmic contraction of the gastrointestinal system. It is often used to calm nausea, relieve motion sickness, soothe an upset stomach, and alleviate diarrhea. Peppermint stimulates the gallbladder to release its store of bile, which helps digest fats. It soothes the muscles of the stomach, relieves abdominal cramps, and helps relieve gas. Fennel has been used for centuries to support healthy digestion. It contains the compound anethole, which helps digest rich foods and may help settle the stomach. It also is used to help relieve constipation. Rosemary helps balance digestion, encourages the expulsion of excess gas, and is believed to enhance the production of digestive juices and bile. Because essential oils are concentrated plant extracts, very little is needed to relieve indigestion. Just a few drops of any of the mentioned essential oils, alone or in combination and diluted in a carrier oil, can be rubbed over the stomach to relieve indigestion.

One of the most common digestive disturbances is gastroesophageal reflux disease (GERD), or simply acid reflux, which is a condition where stomach contents and acid come back up the esophagus. This condition affects about 20 percent of Americans and causes a burning sensation in the lower chest behind the breastbone. Millions of Americans rely on antacids or prescription medications to avoid this uncomfortable condition. These over-the-counter and prescription drugs modify the production of acid within the stomach. This is less than ideal because not only does it reduce the digestive capabilities of your stomach, prolonged use encourages bacterial overgrowth, impairs nutrient absorption, and may increase your risk of fractures.[277]

For those who suffer from heartburn or GERD frequently, natural remedies can provide great relief. Deglycyrrhizinated licorice (DGL) very effectively relieves heartburn and GERD because it soothes the digestive tract and encourages the formation and repair of the protective lining of the stomach.[278-280] For the greatest relief, DGL should be taken on an empty stomach approximately twenty minutes before meals. The typical dosage ranges from 380 to 750 mg in chewable tablet form. Alternately, you may find relief if you drink several drops of lemon essential oil in water.

Don't expect to drastically change your eating habits overnight. It is not practical nor healthy to do so. Instead make small, gradual changes to produce the best environment for your body to achieve optimal health and wellness. If you make changes, you need to do them gradually to allow your body the necessary time to adjust. Symptoms such as diarrhea and upset stomach are common, but temporary, as your body acclimates to a new diet. Remain faithful to eating better and you may realize noticeable benefits to your health and well-being.

3

Nutritional Supplements: Infuse the Body with Optimum Nutrients

In the perfect world, we would get all the vitamins, minerals, and nutrients we need to maintain optimum health from our food. However, several factors make this virtually impossible including modern farming and agriculture practices, environmental pollution and toxin levels, elevated stress levels, and known nutrient deficiencies (it is estimated that 250 million preschool children are vitamin A deficient,[281] and 40 percent of preschool children are anemic, many due to iron deficiency).[282] The evidence is undeniable that dietary supplements are essential for those who want to realize optimum health and reduce disease risk. Supplements are not just for those who have deficiencies or chronic illnesses, they can benefit virtually anyone who seeks greater wellness.[283] Think of your daily multivitamin and mineral as insurance or extra protection against disease and illness and a daily infusion of valuable nutrients.

The optimum infusion of micronutrients is the amount that maximizes a healthy life span and will vary based on age and constitution. Without a daily infusion of micronutrients (above the Recommended Dietary Allowance), DNA damage, cognitive dysfunction, and accelerated aging may occur. Your body uses the nutrients it receives from food and supplementation to improve cellular efficiency, organ function, and overall well-being. If you provide your body insufficient nutrients, inefficiencies in body functions and systems will lead to ill health. In contrast, a daily infusion of essential nutrients helps create an environment for optimum health to thrive. Natural health practitioners have long advocated for the inclusion of essential dietary supplements, and scientific evidence supports this claim.

Even Western physicians have started to realize the importance of dietary supplements. In 2002 research published in the *Journal of the American Medical Association* recommended that all adults take a daily multivitamin to reduce disease risk.[284] Seventy-nine percent of physicians and 82 percent of nurses recommend dietary supplements to their patients, while 72 percent of physicians and 89 percent of nurses personally take dietary supplements.[285] This is remarkable considering Western physicians generally disregard supplements as useless. If the majority of physicians choose to take a multivitamin, despite indifference or indignation toward them, shouldn't we all be taking a daily multinutrient?

DIETARY SUPPLEMENTS: A NECESSITY FOR A HEALTHY LIFE SPAN

The evidence is growing stronger that dietary supplements are essential to optimum health and wellness and may even prolong life. Research demonstrates that reasonable doses of vitamins and minerals play a crucial role in preventing oxidation—reducing the risk of oxidative disease such as cancer and cardiovascular disease.

While dietary supplements are necessary components for anyone who desires to realize optimal health and wellness, they are not meant to replace proper dietary habits and lifestyle choices. If you have skipped to this chapter hoping you can just take supplements and forget about everything else, you will be disappointed. No amount of supplementation will make up for poor nutrition or lifestyle choices. Dietary supplements are meant to be just that, supplements not replacements, meaning they are supportive, not substitutive. Frankly, eating better is necessary for dietary supplements to be effective. Without a proper nutritional foundation your body will not have the ability to absorb and utilize dietary supplements properly.

Many contend that we get enough nutrients from our food and supplementation is unnecessary. However, this outdated philosophy is contrary to what many leading natural health experts recommend. They strongly encourage a quality, optimum-potency, multivitamin and mineral be taken daily to encourage optimum health. Quite simply, eating better does not guarantee sufficient quantities of nutrients to prevent chronic illness and disease, or a healthy life span. Even if you eat healthily you may have less than optimum key nutrients in your body. Unfortunately, minor deficiencies may not exhibit any noticeable adverse effects, while your cells are slowly being deprived of the nutrients they require to function efficiently and correctly.

A common statement from those who oppose dietary supplements is that they only create "expensive urine." While much of dietary supplements is eliminated through the urine because your body can only absorb a certain quantity of nutrients at any given time, this is a normal body process. Your body is designed to efficiently assimilate and utilize nutrients and just as efficiently eliminate unused nutrients. In reality, the same is true for any meal you consume—your body uses some of the food for fuel and sends the rest for waste. Blood tests indicate that when you take a vitamin supplement it measurably increases blood levels of the nutrient the particular supplement contains, even though the nutrient is also detected in the urine. For example, if you take a vitamin C supplement, blood tests confirm that your blood levels of vitamin C will have indeed increased as a result. In other words, if you take a supplement, it can enter the bloodstream, and your body efficiently eliminates any excess it doesn't need.

Many articles and scientific studies have trivialized and even scared the general public away from dietary supplements. Much of this anti-supplement literature is flawed, faulty, irresponsible, and borders on pseudoscience rather than legitimate science. Specifically, these studies often use insignificant amounts of vitamins that are not likely to produce a noticeable therapeutic benefit. They also use doses no higher than RDA levels that are incapable of demonstrating a benefit for diseases, administer unusual, synthetic, less effective, or poorly absorbed forms, or include health-compromised or overweight people, which precludes the study from ascertaining results that could have occurred had they used healthy individuals. Unhealthy individuals require more vitamins and minerals because they often have deficiencies in specific nutrients.

Another problem often associated with these studies is they allow subjects to self-report whether they actually took the supplement and don't track the exact nutrients, or forms included in the supplements taken. All of this leads to inaccurate and erroneous data and conclusions.

Much of this irresponsible research focuses on the benefits of antioxidants. The truth is the secret to optimal antioxidant support lies in balance and specificity. Proper antioxidant support is a major key to optimum well-being, and supports cardiovascular, cellular, joint, eye, respiratory, and brain health to name a few.

To better appreciate the importance of antioxidants we have to understand how they interact with free radicals. Normally molecules have paired electrons to improve stability. Free radicals are very unstable molecules with unpaired electrons, which form during normal metabolism, cellular processes, and from external factors. When a molecule is missing a paired electron—as is the case with free radicals—it attacks the nearest stable molecule to steal an electron. The attacked molecule then becomes a free radical itself, which can quickly cascade and result in the disruption of cellular function.

THE SECRETS TO CREATING AN OPTIMUM ANTIOXIDANT DEFENSE SYSTEM

The body's defense system against this cascade of events is antioxidants. Antioxidants neutralize free radicals through the donation of one of their own electrons to prevent the free radical from stealing an electron. These defenders basically sacrifice themselves to protect your body from damage without becoming an electron-scavenging free radical as well.

Now, more isn't always better, and this is the case with antioxidants, especially if it is too much of any single antioxidant. When it comes to research of antioxidants, it is important to know the form (synthetic or natural), whether antioxidants were taken alone or in combination with other antioxidants, and whether a therapeutic or preventive dose was administered. This may be why many researchers call two studies that concluded vitamin E increased prostate cancer risk by 17 to 63 percent flawed and inappropriate.[286,287] What we can learn from these studies, and other studies like them, is that the growing body of evidence suggests that you shouldn't supplement with too much of any single isolated antioxidant. If you focus on one single antioxidant it may be more risky than getting too few antioxidants.

One of the major keys to optimal antioxidant support is balance. Antioxidant balance requires the consumption of a wide variety of the major groups of antioxidants. You wouldn't eat just one macronutrient (fat, protein, or carbohydrate) because it isn't reasonable and would leave your body with significant nutrient deficiencies, so why take just one antioxidant. In 2012, a news report of a seventeen-year-old female who consumed virtually nothing but McDonald's chicken nuggets went viral. Reportedly her dangerous diet required her to be hospitalized for nutrient deficiencies, anemia, and inflammation of the veins in her tongue that caused her to collapse and struggle to breathe.[288] Her deficiency in key nutrients was so substantial doctors had to administer them intravenously. As impractical as a diet with only one type of food or macronutrient is, the same is true with antioxidants—they work better together and each group should be consumed. The major antioxidant groups will be defined as follows for the purpose of this text:

- **Vitamin C**
- **Vitamin E complex** (tocopherols/tocotrienols)
- **Carotenoids** (astaxanthin, beta-carotene, alpha-carotene, lutein, lycopene, beta-cryptoxanthin)

- **Thiols** (sulfur-containing compounds like alpha lipoic acid, methylsulfonylmethane, glutathione, and cysteine)
- **Enzymatic antioxidants** (superoxide dismutase, catalase, glutathione peroxidase, glutathione reductase)
- **Antioxidant coenzymes** (PQQ and CoQ10)
- **Antioxidant minerals** (selenium, zinc)
- **Bioflavonoids** (polyphenols, xanthones, catechins, anthocyanins, flavones, isoflavones, flavanones)
- **Antioxidant hormones** (melatonin, Vitamin D)

Forget the idea of taking large doses of a single antioxidant, no matter how powerful it is. Your cells need representatives from each of these antioxidant groups to mount the strongest defense against free radicals. Antioxidants work together and can greatly enhance the power of one another. For example, CoQ10 enhances the action of vitamin E and alpha lipoic acid recycles both vitamin C and glutathione back into their active antioxidant form. When antioxidants support one another, your antioxidant defenses are bolstered to help prevent illness and disease, and encourage a healthy life span.

Just as a healthy diet includes a variety of fruits and vegetables, when you choose to supplement your diet with antioxidant supplements you should aim for a balanced mix of antioxidants from multiple sources. Think of it like a football team. Even if you have a star quarterback, he will not be effective without a supportive offensive line, receivers, and running backs. He may be able to make some big plays occasionally, but long-term he is highly unlikely to win the game alone or, in this case, the battle against free radicals.

The second significant key to optimal antioxidant support is antioxidant specificity. This is related to antioxidant balance because certain antioxidants are better to support specific cells, organs, and systems of the body. To achieve optimum health you need antioxidants that support multiple cells, organs and systems. For example, CoQ10 and resveratrol are excellent for the heart, ergothioneine and turmeric are beneficial for the joints, and PQQ and anthocyanins support brain health. So, you can see that obtaining a variety of antioxidants from both food and supplementation is necessary for optimum health and a healthy life span. This list provides a few of the antioxidants and their specificity to organs or body systems:

- **Cells:** Limonene, turmeric, vitamin A, vitamin C, vitamin D, vitamin E.
- **Heart:** CoQ10, resveratrol, vitamin E, beta-carotene, vitamin D.
- **Brain:** Pyrroloquinoline quinone (PQQ), astaxanthin, anthocyanins, resveratrol, L-carnitine.

- **Joints:** Astaxanthin, anthocyanins, ergothioneine, turmeric, methylsulfonylmethane.
- **Skin:** Astaxanthin, beta-carotene, vitamin A, vitamin C, vitamin E, selenium.
- **Kidneys:** Resveratrol, L-carnosine, silymarin, CoQ10, glutathione (GSH), superoxide dismutase (SOD).
- **Immune:** Methylsulfonylmethane, vitamin C, vitamin D.
- **Eyes:** Beta-carotene, astaxanthin, vitamin A, vitamin C, lutein, zeaxanthin, bilberry.
- **Liver:** Lycopene, milk thistle, N-acetyl-cysteine, alpha lipoic acid, vitamin A, vitamin C, vitamin E.

In review, optimum levels of antioxidants are essential for optimum health and a healthy life. But, they need to be the right quantities—not extreme, but not inconsequential. Last, a variety of antioxidants that supports a diversity of cells, organs, and systems ensures you are targeting all aspects of your well-being. When it comes to the secrets of antioxidant support, balance and specificity are a crucial part of your strategic plan to achieve peak vitality and longevity.

One of the key reasons a multivitamin and mineral (multinutrient) is necessary is the diminishing nutrients in the modern diet. Americans eat greater quantities of food today than in past years and thus more calories. More calories does not mean we receive the same amount of nutrition people did thirty or more years ago. According to one report, adult women fail to meet the Recommended Dietary Allowance (RDA) for calcium, vitamin E, vitamin B6, magnesium, and zinc from diet alone; while adult men get insufficient vitamin E, magnesium, and zinc.[289] The International Micronutrient Malnutrition Prevention and Control Program estimates that at least half of the children worldwide ages six months to five years suffer from at least one micronutrient deficiency, affecting more than 2 billion people.[290] Deficiencies in key nutrients can result in birth defects, mental retardation, blindness, and delayed growth and development.

Not only are our foods processed to the point of diminished nutrient values, modern agriculture practices also reduce the nutrient content of fruits and vegetables. High-nitrogen chemical fertilizers are the modern choice in agriculture for plant growth. While nitrogen will indeed produce rapid plant growth and increased crop yield, this is mostly due to increased water intake by the fruits and vegetables. This "dilution effect" means you get larger fruits and vegetables with more water, not more nutrients.

In contrast, organic foods are generally smaller in size and yield lower quantities of crops. But pound for pound, organic produce have more nutrients, because they contain less water. More importantly, you are not getting pesticide laced foods. USDA testing has found numerous pesticide compounds on fruits destined for store shelves, some of which exceed exposure limits set by governments.[291] In addition, pesticide compounds that are banned or not approved for use because of their negative health consequences have been found in produce in the United States. Next time you go to the grocery store, look for smaller produce, rather than larger, which may have less of a "dilution effect."

A careful review of fifty years (1950–1999) of USDA food composition data suggested the following decreases in food nutrients have occurred in some foods: a 16 percent loss of calcium, a 20 percent decline in vitamin C, and a 15 percent loss of iron.[292] This study only names three of the nutrients that have decreased over time. Another study indicated similar nutrient losses in fruits from 1975 to 2000.[293] It is clear that our most nutritious foods, fruits and vegetables, have declined in nutrients, which makes it that much harder to get the necessary amounts without supplementation.

Travel time from farm, orchard, or field to your plate or the grocery store is also of great concern. Produce is often picked before it is fully ripe in order to withstand long travel miles without spoiling. When the produce is picked earlier than nature intended, it is not fully mature, nor does it contain all the nutrients it normally would if it had been left to ripen on the vine. Not only is the taste and freshness compromised, quality is reduced. According to one study, the average American meal travels approximately 1,500 miles from farm to plate.[294] More and more of the foods Americans eat comes from sources outside the United States. About 44 percent of fruit is imported, while 16 percent of vegetables cross the nation's borders to reach your local supermarket.[295] Support your health as well as your local economy by purchasing from local farmers.

Soil quality also appears to be a casualty of modern farming practices. Soils are largely depleted of selenium, zinc, magnesium, calcium, and other minerals. While chemical fertilizers contain the proper elements for rapid plant growth, they lack the nutrients essential to human health. Therefore, plant needs are being provided for, while human health needs are largely being ignored. When soil is depleted of nutrients, plants have no source from which they can draw elements essential to human health. The result is less nutritious food.

Combine lack of nutrients with an all-out assault on the body from pollution, chemicals, and environmental toxins and you have an optimal environment for disease to flourish. We live in a time when the assault on our body is tremendous. Besides pesticides in our produce, we also have to combat preservatives, artificial colors and flavors, excessive use of antibiotics and hormones in animal products, and a plethora of chemicals; all creating a smorgasbord of toxins for our bodies to process and eliminate. Without the use of supplements, our bodies simply can't handle this lethal overload.

The older you get the greater your requirement for nutrients to remain healthy. This is largely due to the fact that as you age your body's ability to absorb and utilize vitamins, minerals, and other nutrients (known as bioavailability) diminishes. In other words, your body uses the nutrients it receives from food and supplementation less efficiently as you age. This is one of the reasons we see more chronic illness among the elderly. Their bodies simply don't absorb and assimilate as many vitamins and minerals to ward off illness and disease.

Recent research even indicates that if you take a daily multivitamin it may slow the aging process and increase the number of healthy years in your life. Normal cells do not grow indefinitely; they have a limited number of times they can divide, which is referred to as the Hayflick limit. In humans, cellular division usually occurs about fifty times, creating a finite life span. This is because telomeres (protective fragments of DNA attached to the end of chromosomes) shorten with each cell division to prevent fusion or rearrangement of chromosomes. Without this protection by telomeres, DNA damage would occur. Once the telomeres are critically expended the cell is destroyed. A study found that women who take a daily multivitamin had longer leukocyte telomeres,[296] which suggest that the cell's life was extended, and likely the host's longevity as well. While more research is necessary to confirm these findings, it does appear multivitamins play an important role in the number of healthy years a person can enjoy and the prevention of chronic illnesses.

All of these factors offer convincing and compelling evidence to support the use of a dietary supplement. While some research has suggested that taking a multivitamin may increase your risk of cancer, these studies are significantly flawed. These poor studies are often based on questionnaires, which do not consider the form, dose, or quality of the supplement the person took. In addition, it is possible that the cancer risk could be related to fillers, excipients, or added sugars contained in particular brands. Whenever possible seek a multinutrient that contains no added sugar or artificial sweeteners. Most multivitamin and mineral formulas cost pennies per day to take. Isn't it better to err on the side of caution and give your body some added protection against illness and disease?

Because the Recommended Dietary Allowances (RDA) are established as a single standard for everyone, assuming a healthy adult and a healthy diet, many experts suggest taking larger quantities of vitamins and minerals. Much larger doses are likely required for optimum well-being, healthy aging, and disease prevention. In general, the elderly will need greater quantities of nutrients from supplements than the young. This dosage is indicated as the optimal range* to look for in a multivitamin and mineral supplement. In general, the body will decrease absorption and utilization of high doses of some vitamins, so they are best taken in divided doses throughout the day. To maximize the effectiveness of your supplement:

- **Individualize your supplement.** You need to determine what your optimal intake is, usually within the suggested optimal range; based on the nutrient density of what you eat, how active you are, your age, and your current health status—those with chronic illnesses usually need higher doses. Each of us is biochemically unique and has different nutrient requirements. Ideally everyone would undergo nutrient testing to determine deficiencies and optimum nutrient ranges, then have a personal supplement created for them based on these results. This type of supplement does exist; however, this approach can be cost prohibitive for many.
- **Take vitamins with food**. Vitamins are generally better absorbed when taken with food, particularly the fat-soluble vitamins that require fat for optimal absorption. Taking multivitamin and mineral supplements with food will help to reduce stomach upset that may be experienced when taking them on an empty stomach.
- **Take them in divided doses.** Your body can and will only absorb a certain amount of a vitamin or mineral at one time. Take your supplement in divided doses to enhance absorption and reduce excretion of excess nutrients. Preferably take supplements in three divided doses, one with each meal.
- **Take them at approximately the same time each day.** This allows the body to maintain a healthy supply of nutrients to promote optimal system and body function.

Optimal intake of vitamins and minerals encourages a healthy life span, peak vitality, and may support your body in its effort to combat the onslaught of environmental pollution, chemicals, and environmental toxins to prevent disease.

*Parents should always consult their pediatrician before giving their children supplements. Women who are pregnant or nursing should consult their OB-GYN before using supplements. It is important that you consult a qualified health care professional before taking any dietary supplement, particularly if you have been diagnosed with or believe you have a chronic illness or disease. Consult with a qualified health care professional before taking any supplement to avoid adverse reactions or interactions with medications or other supplements. Every person is biochemically unique and requires different amounts of vitamins and minerals based on individual circumstances.

EVALUATING SUPPLEMENTS: ARE YOUR SUPPLEMENTS BIOAVAILABLE AND BENEFICIAL?

There are so many different dietary supplement brands it is difficult to select an effective multivitamin and mineral supplement. Price, potency, additional ingredients (fillers, excipients, etc.), and form are all different among the countless manufacturers. The following suggestions may help guide your decision in selecting quality dietary supplements:

1. Choose a manufacturer that follows the international **Good Manufacturing Practices (GMP)**. These are guidelines of practices and procedures for manufacturers to follow in order to ensure composition, identity, potency, and purity of supplements. In short, it means what is on the supplement label is more likely to be what you are getting in the bottle, at the dosage listed, and without impurities.

2. **Disintegration and dissolution—It is important that your supplement is able to dissolve or breakup easily.** The supplement is useless if it will not disintegrate or dissolve. This is of real concern with pressed tablets. Many nurses will tell you they have found complete pressed tablets in patients' bedpans or ileostomy bags, which means it didn't dissolve at all. The same is true of finding undissolved supplements in sewage treatment plants. To test your supplement, you can use the vinegar dissolution test. Heat one cup of vinegar in a small bowl until it reaches 98°F, then place this bowl in a larger bowl filled with warm water to help maintain the 98°F temperature. Place your supplement in the vinegar and swirl or gently shake it about every five minutes. The tablet should ideally dissolve within thirty minutes. If it hasn't dissolved in one hour, choose another brand.

3. Look for products with the **preferred supplement forms** listed in this book. These forms have been selected for bioavailability, absorption, effectiveness, and safety.

4. Purchase **products that provide dosages at or near the optimal range** recommended for each nutrient listed in this book. This will ensure you are getting the optimal amounts of each nutrient to promote optimum health and help prevent disease.

5. Generally purchase a **name brand** dietary supplement from a well-known company that has been established for years. This

doesn't mean that all new companies or lesser known brands are inferior, but the name brand supplements normally have higher quality ingredients. You may also ask a health care provider knowledgeable in vitamins, minerals, and supplements if they prefer a particular brand.

6. Choose supplements that specify **non-GMO** whenever possible. Too many ingredients in supplements are derived from genetically modified sources and may have long-term adverse health effects.

VITAMINS

Vitamins are organic compounds that function as activators or catalysts in the chemical reactions that take place within the body. They are fundamental in normal body functions and essential to growth and to maintain good health. They are divided into two categories. Fat soluble (A, D, E, K) vitamins are stored in the liver and adipose (fat) tissue. Vitamin D is truly a steroid hormone because it can be manufactured by the body but for classification purposes we will include it with the fat soluble vitamins. Water soluble (B complex vitamins and vitamin C) dissolve in water and are not stored by the body. Because they are eliminated in the urine, they require regular replenishment. Upper limits are established by the Institutes of Medicine (IOM) and represent the maximum amount of a nutrient that should be taken daily by an adult to avoid adverse events or toxicity.

Vitamin A, also known as retinol, was the first vitamin officially named. It is predominantly stored in the liver until needed and principally absorbed in the small intestine. Alcohol use reduces the absorption of Vitamin A, while stress and illness reduce the amount stored. Vitamin A is divided into retinol and carotenoids. Carotenoids are a group of naturally occurring pigments, some of which can convert into a form of vitamin A. Those that can be converted into a form of vitamin A after ingestion, such as beta-carotene, are considered provitamin A. The retinol form of the vitamin is primarily acquired from animal sources such as liver, egg yolks, and milk products. Carotenoids are from plant sources such as yellow and orange colored fruits and vegetables and green leafy vegetables.

Vitamin A is crucial for healthy vision, growth and development, normal immune function, red blood cell production, reproductive health, and healthy skin. It also acts as an antioxidant and helps cells reproduce normally. Vitamin A is known as retinol because of its role in the production of pigments in the retina of the eye. It may help slow down damage to the retina. Beta-carotene is the most commonly known carotenoid. It is provitamin A and can be taken in large amounts because its conversion to vitamin A is decreased when the body has sufficient vitamin A already stored within the body.[297] Since beta-carotene supplements are not associated with major adverse effects, it is preferred to supplement with higher levels of carotenoids rather than substantial doses of retinol.

Vitamin A has been used during infections to help promote a speedy recovery. Because it supports the health of the eye, it is used for a variety of eye problems, including night blindness. Many skin conditions are treated, orally and topically, with vitamin A. It is very beneficial to help wounds heal, used to treat acne, and applied topically to rashes and other skin conditions.

Companions:	Vitamin E, Zinc, Vitamin C
Preferred Form(s):	Vitamin A—Retinol; Carotenoids—Natural Mixed Carotenoids
Adult RDA:	Vitamin A—Men 3,000 IU; Women 2,300 IU; Carotenoids—Not established
Adult Optimal Range:	Vitamin A—2,500–3,000 IU; Beta-Carotene—5,000–15,000 IU
Tolerable Upper Limit:	10,000 IU (Vitamin A)
Safety Concerns:	Toxicity can occur with excessive amounts of vitamin A. Women of child-bearing age should avoid retinol supplementation and substitute beta-carotene instead to avoid potential birth defects.

Vitamin D can actually be considered a hormone as well as a vitamin because our bodies can produce this vitamin when exposed to direct sunlight. This ability of the body appears to decrease as we age, particularly after age fifty, therefore greater quantities are required. Lack of sunshine reduces production of vitamin D so those living in northern latitudes may require more supplementation.

Vitamin D is extremely important in the maintenance of bone density because of its role in mineral absorption, particularly calcium. Many calcium supplements are combined with vitamin D for this reason. It also assists the body with phosphorus utilization, another mineral that makes up our bones. Vitamin D is important to build and maintain healthy teeth. Other research suggests Vitamin D may help prevent cancer,[298] and mildly prevents high blood pressure[299] and autoimmune disorders.[300] It is estimated that vitamin D controls up to 5 percent of the human genome[301,302] which is the complete set of genetic material that makes up the human organism. Remarkably, higher blood levels of vitamin D significantly alters the activity of 291 genes and more than 160 biological pathways linked to cancer, cardiovascular disease, and autoimmune disorders.[303] This suggests that vitamin D works at the genetic level to reduce the risk of a number of diseases, including the two top killers of Americans—cardiovascular disease and cancer. Another study determined that lower serum vitamin D levels are associated with premature death. The study considered low levels of vitamin D to be 30 ng/ml or lower—a level found in about two-thirds of Americans.[304] Low serum levels of vitamin D have also been associated with age-related macular degeneration[305]—a leading cause of vision loss in Americans sixty years and older.

Mood and cognitive fitness are significantly affected by vitamin D, and pioneering physicians and psychologists have used it successfully to improve depressive symptoms, neurological disorders, and behavioral disorders. One study concluded that the effectiveness of vitamin D supplementation was comparable to antidepressant medications.[306] According to scientific research, elderly adults with low vitamin D levels experience greater cognitive decline, especially over time, than those who maintain higher levels.[307] Some emerging evidence suggests that even children can benefit from higher vitamin D blood levels, particularly those with behavioral disorders like attention-deficit-hyperactivity disorder.[308,309]

Vitamin D is used to prevent or cure rickets and osteomalacia, a vitamin D deficiency disease that causes bone mineral loss and weak and soft bones. Vitamin D is used to prevent tooth decay and gum problems. Psoriasis has also been safely treated with vitamin D.

Vitamin D is such a critical nutrient that the American Academy of Pediatrics and the Institute of Medicine both suggest administering 400 IU of liquid vitamin D to your baby beginning within the first few days of birth if you are breastfeeding. Schoolchildren may benefit from 1,000 IU, whereas teens may be able to follow adult recommendations.

Companions:	Calcium, Boron, Vitamin K
Preferred Form(s):	Cholecalciferol D3
Adult RDA:	600 IU (Age 18–70); 800 IU (Age 71+)
Adult Optimal Range:	1,000–10,000 IU
Tolerable Upper Limit:	4,000 IU
Safety Concerns:	Vitamin D is generally considered very safe. Hypercalcemia (excess calcium in the blood) may occur with prolonged supplementation of 40,000 IU or greater daily.[310] The IOM's upper limit of 4,000 IU is severely

outdated and needs to be updated as many physicians prescribe 10,000 IU daily to their patients without serious side effects.

Special Circumstances: Osteoporosis sufferers and the elderly should dose at the higher range.

Vitamin E is actually made up of eight compounds: alpha-, beta-, delta-, and gamma-tocopherol, and alpha-, beta-, delta-, and gamma-tocotrienol. Alpha-tocopherol is considered the most common and active form. Vitamin E is not stored as readily as the other fat soluble vitamins, so it requires regular replenishment. The best sources of vitamin E are the oil contained in grains, seeds, and nuts, and from cold-pressed vegetable oils. Wheat germ oil is an excellent source, as are whole wheat products that have not had the germ part of the grain removed, as is the case with refined grains.

The primary function of vitamin E is as an antioxidant, where it protects the cell membrane from damage. An intact and permeable cell membrane is vital to allow nutrients in and cellular waste to exit the cell. It also prevents the infection of the cell by harmful substances. Vitamin E also protects the tissue of the skin, eyes, liver, and sexual organs. It essentially works to protect virtually the entire body from oxidative damage. It also supports a healthy immune system and stimulates (or enhances) the production and activity of immune cells.[311] This bolsters your body's natural protection against illness and disease. Its cellular protective nature may also help prevent a whole list of degenerative diseases, such as cardiovascular disease and neurodegenerative diseases. Additionally, vitamin E helps form red blood cells, muscles, and other tissues.

Since vitamin E acts in the protection of so many tissues and body systems it has been used for the treatment and prevention of a multiplicity of ailments from cancer to premenstrual syndrome. It can be used topically for wound healing, dermatitis, rashes, and even helps reduce the appearance of scarring and stretch marks.

Companions:	Selenium, Vitamin C
Preferred Form(s):	Natural Mixed Tocopherols and Tocotrienols or d-alpha Tocopherol
Adult RDA:	22–33 IU
Adult Optimal Range:	200–600 IU
Tolerable Upper Limit:	1,100 to 1,500 IU
Safety Concerns:	Although fat soluble, Vitamin E has an excellent safety record. Dosages greater than 1,000 IU may

result in reduced blood clotting ability, and very high doses (over 1,500 IU) may result in adverse effects such as nausea, headache, fainting, and heart palpitations.

Vitamin K is primarily known for its role in coagulation, or blood clotting, but not as recognized is vitamin K's importance when it comes to calcium utilization. It is well-known that vitamin D helps the body absorb calcium; however, vitamin K is required to conduct calcium into the skeleton and prevent its accumulation in organs, arteries, and joint openings.[312,313,314] Dark leafy green vegetables, asparagus, broccoli, olives, soybeans, spinach, and cabbage are excellent food sources. Vitamin K deficiency is very rare and so it is often overlooked or ignored in multivitamin supplements.

Vitamin K stabilizes the effect of blood coagulation medications, particularly in cases where a person experiences unexplained fluctuations in coagulation when taking medications.[315] It has been used to counteract excess thinning of the blood caused by Coumadin, also known as Warfarin. Blood thinning is the most common side effect of Coumadin. The American Academy of Pediatrics recommends giving all newborns a single intramuscular injection of Vitamin K1 to avoid the risk of vitamin K deficiency bleeding.[316] People who bruise easily or whose blood does not clot properly may benefit from vitamin K supplementation.

Companions:	Calcium
Preferred Form(s):	K2 menaquinone; K1 Phylloquinone
Adult RDA:	Males—120 mcg; Females—90 mcg
Adult Optimal Range:	50–150 mcg
Tolerable Upper Limit:	Not established
Safety Concerns:	Only the synthetic form, K3, is known to have any degree of toxicity.

The **B-complex vitamins** each have unique functions and properties. The B-complex vitamins include: thiamin, riboflavin, niacin, pantothenic acid, pyridoxine, folic acid, cobalamin, biotin, choline, inositol, and para-aminobenzoic acid.

The B vitamins are necessary for the production of energy and the metabolism of carbohydrates, fats, and proteins. B vitamins compete with each other for absorption within the intestines, which makes it very important to take them in the proper ratio. The general rule of thumb is to take them in equal amounts (1:1 ratio), with the exception of biotin, cobalamin, and folic acid, which are measured in micrograms unlike the other B vitamins that are measured in milligrams. The B vitamins act as coenzymes (a substance that catalyzes or enhances the action of an enzyme) and are essential for many body functions. They are all water soluble (with the exception of a few fat soluble forms of particular B vitamins) and require daily replenishment because they are not stored well.

Vitamin B1 (Thiamin, or Thiamine) was the first of the B vitamins to be discovered, isolated, and characterized, in the 1920s. It plays an essential part in the metabolism of carbohydrates and glucose, which helps produce energy. Deficiency of this vitamin may result in a condition called beriberi, with symptoms such as mental confusion, muscle cramps, gastrointestinal problems, and high blood pressure. This disease is now very rare in the United States, and is predominantly restricted to alcoholics. This important vitamin is depleted by consuming alcohol, nicotine, sugar, coffee, and black teas. Thiamin aids the production of hydrochloric acid, the acid found in the stomach that is necessary for proper digestion. It also aids in proper nervous system and muscular function.

Thiamin is primarily used for the treatment of beriberi. However, it is also beneficial in conditions such as certain metabolic disorders, depression, fatigue, and in the prevention of motion sickness. Thiamin may support normal cognition, and may be beneficial for Alzheimer's disease, due to its effects on the brain, particularly memory.[317]

Allithiamine is obtained from garlic and contains a fat-soluble form of B1 and other nutritional substances essential for biologic activity. It is considered more stable and more readily absorbed than the water-soluble form,[318] which may benefit those who are deficient. Benfotiamine is a synthetic, fat-soluble form of thiamine that may be useful for the prevention of diabetic complications like damage to the peripheral nerves (polyneuropathy) and eyes (retinopathy).[319,320]

Companions:	Riboflavin, Pyridoxine
Preferred Form(s):	Allithiamine, Benfotiamine
Adult RDA:	Males—1.2 mg; Females—1.1 mg; Pregnancy/ Lactation—1.4 mg
Adult Optimal Range:	25–100 mg
Tolerable Upper Limit:	Not established
Safety Concerns:	Currently no known toxicity.

Vitamin B2 (Riboflavin) got its name from its yellowish color (the word *flavus* in Latin means yellow). In fact, excess intake of this vitamin will result in a fluorescent yellow tint to urine. It plays a vital role in the production of energy through carbohydrate metabolism. It is also necessary for the proper function of the heart and nervous system.

Riboflavin is rarely used in the treatment of diseases. However, it is beneficial in the treatment of neonatal jaundice,[321] eye fatigue,[322] cataracts,[323] migraine headaches,[324] and as an adjunctive treatment for iron-deficient or sickle-cell anemia.[325]

Companions:	Thiamin
Preferred Form(s):	Riboflavin-5-phosphate
Adult RDA:	Males—1.3 mg; Females—1.1 mg; Pregnancy—1.4 mg; Lactation—1.6 mg
Adult Optimal Range:	25–100 mg
Tolerable Upper Limit:	Not established
Safety Concerns:	Currently no known toxicity.

Vitamin B3 (Niacin) can actually be produced by the body if sufficient tryptophan exists. It is found in three distinct forms: niacinamide (nicotinamide), nicotinic acid, and inositol hexanicotinate. Nicotinic acid should not be confused with nicotine, the active drug in cigarettes—there is no relation. As with the other B vitamins, niacin functions in the production of energy through the metabolism of fat, cholesterol, and carbohydrates. It is also involved in the synthesis of the sex and adrenal hormones. It is considered a vasodilator (a substance able to relax and widen the blood vessels).

Niacin is often used as an agent to lower LDL cholesterol—high LDL levels are associated with clogged arteries and cardiovascular disease. It also helps lower triglyceride levels—a type of fat found in your blood and used to store unused calories as energy, which may be a contributing factor to clogged arteries. Last, it helps raise HDL cholesterol levels—the good cholesterol that transports excess LDL cholesterol back to the liver for removal from the bloodstream.[326,327] All of these actions may help reduce the risk of cardiovascular disease. When niacin is taken at therapeutic dosage levels—1,200 to 3,000 mg or greater—to achieve balanced cholesterol levels and reduced triglycerides, you may experience a "niacin flush." A niacin flush produces a generally harmless redness, warmth, and sometimes itching of the skin. Some people will experience a flush with as little as 30 mg, but generally this only occurs at greater doses. To avoid this unintended reaction, other forms of niacin, inositol hexanicotinate or nicotinamide ribose, should be used. These forms do not cause flushing, but they still effectively reduce cholesterol and triglycerides, though possibly not as dramatically as nicotinic acid.[328] Because of its lipid modifying effect, niacin is considered helpful for reducing the risk of atherosclerosis—hardening of the arteries with plaque, which increases the risk of stroke and heart attack.

Niacin has also been used to benefit those with diabetes. Though further research is necessary to understand its role among diabetics, limited research suggests it may help control cholesterol levels and delay the need for insulin.[329] For the treatment of menstrual cramps, a high dose of niacin (100 mg twice daily, and every two to three hours while pain is experienced) has been used for decades and has demonstrated an impressive effectiveness. However, high doses of niacin have been associated with elevated blood homocysteine levels, a predictor of heart disease.

Preferred Form(s):	Nicotinamide Riboside, Inositol Hexanicotinate, or Niacinamide
Adult RDA:	Males—16 mg; Females—14 mg; Pregnancy—18 mg; Lactation—17 mg
Adult Optimal Range:	25–100 mg; limit the nicotinic acid form to 40 mg daily unless using it for high cholesterol.
Tolerable Upper Limit:	35 mg
Safety Concerns:	Some are not able to tolerate the niacin flush effect of nicotinic acid. High doses of the sustained release form has been associated with liver toxicity, and may be best not used at all.[330] The inositol form appears to be much safer. Liver function tests are recommended periodically with any form of niacin when taking at high doses. Those with ulcers, gout, or diabetes should use caution and consult a qualified health care practitioner before taking niacin.

Vitamin B5 (Pantothenic Acid) is extremely important to many bodily functions, including the metabolism of fats, carbohydrates, and proteins. It helps the body to synthesize the stress-related hormones, which may aid the body's response to stress. It is also involved in the production of the sex hormones (estrogen, androgen, and progestin). Pantothenic acid helps the body synthesize cholesterol, which is also used to form hormones, and helps form and maintain cellular membranes. Imbalanced hormone levels can dramatically alter the function of myriad body systems. B5 is a component of coenzyme A, a coenzyme present in all living cells and required for a variety of chemical reactions necessary to sustain life such as transferring fatty acids into mitochondria and the metabolism of amino acids. Pantothenic acid was investigated in the 1950s and 1960s for its use in autoimmune disorders, lupus and rheumatoid arthritis. Because of its role in the multiplication of cells, it is critical to a properly functioning immune system. In fact, it supports immune activity involved in healing. Pantothenic acid is also effective in relieving stress and anxiety.

Preferred Form(s):	Pantethine
Adult RDA:	Males/Females—5 mg; Pregnancy—6 mg; Lactation—7 mg
Adult Optimal Range:	25–100 mg
Tolerable Upper Limit:	3.5 mg
Safety Concerns:	No adverse or toxic effects presently known.

Vitamin B6 (Pyridoxine) is necessary for the optimum health and function of virtually all body structures and processes. It is essential for amino acid metabolism as well as the manufacture of neurotransmitters. Neurotransmitters play distinct roles in the brain, where they either excite or inhibit brain activity. It is vital for the conversion of tryptophan into the neurotransmitter serotonin, which supports mood, promotes relaxation, and improves depressive symptoms. Pyridoxine helps form red blood cells that are important in carrying fresh oxygen throughout the body. It is also involved in the manufacture of antibodies, which help neutralize pathogenic organisms to avoid damage to healthy cells. Vitamin B6 is required for the proper functioning of dozens of enzymes involved in essential functions such as the synthesis of hemoglobin and amino acids, fatty acid metabolism, and protein metabolism. This vitamin is critical during pregnancy because it helps maintain the mother's hormone balance and is important for the development of the baby's nervous system.

Pyridoxine has been used to alleviate the symptoms of premenstrual syndrome,[331] and it is beneficial in managing nausea and morning sickness during pregnancy.[332] It may also be a beneficial adjunct option in the treatment of ADHD and autism.[333] Infant seizures are often controlled with intravenous injections of pyridoxine.[334]

Companions:	Riboflavin; Magnesium
Preferred Form(s):	Pyridoxal-5-phosphate
Adult RDA:	Males/Females, age 19–50—1.3 mg; Males, age 51+—1.7 mg; Females, age 51+—1.5 mg; Pregnancy—1.9 mg; Lactation—2.0 mg
Adult Optimal Range:	25–100 mg
Tolerable Upper Limit:	100 mg

| Safety Concerns: | High daily doses and extreme acute doses (very large doses taken at one time) may cause toxicity and possibly the destruction of peripheral nerves, which promotes inflammation, irritation, pain, and loss of strength and sensation also known as neuronopathy.[335] |

Vitamin B7 (Biotin), also called vitamin H, is a relatively new B vitamin that is very difficult to obtain from diet alone. Luckily the body is able to recycle much of the biotin it has already used. Biotin comes from the Greek word *bios,* meaning "life," because without it many enzymes will not work. It is manufactured by intestinal bacteria and therefore not a true vitamin. It is necessary for the metabolism of fats, carbohydrates, and protein. In addition it is required for fat production and utilization of fatty acids. It also plays a role in DNA replication (a process essential to all living organisms that creates an exact copy of an original DNA molecule) and gene expression (which determines the function of the cell).

Biotin promotes healthy hair and nails. It is also useful for seborrheic dermatitis or cradle cap (the scalp becomes scaly, itchy, and red, often creating stubborn dandruff) that infants get. Biotin is useful for diabetics and those who are insulin resistant since it helps improve insulin sensitivity and glucose tolerance.[336] It is beneficial in restoring normal metabolism as well.

Companions:	Other B Vitamins
Preferred Form(s):	Biotin; Biocytin
Adult RDA:	Males—550 mcg; Females—425 mcg; Pregnancy—45 mcg; Lactation—550 mcg
Adult Optimal Range:	400–800 mcg
Tolerable Upper Limit:	Not established
Safety Concerns:	Biotin is extremely safe at very high levels. No known toxicity or adverse effects have been reported.

Vitamin B9 (Folate) is better known as folic acid, its synthetic form. Folate is the form of this vitamin naturally found in foods. It is necessary for the synthesis of DNA (the copying of genetic material in the cell), because without biotin cells do not divide properly. It is well-known for its essential role in preventing pregnancy complications like birth defects and anemia. Folate plays a critical role in the development of the fetus, particularly the nervous system. It assists in red blood cell production where it forms and carries the iron-containing portion of hemoglobin, known as heme. Sufficient levels of folate help to reduce excessive production of homocysteine—an amino acid and breakdown product of protein metabolism that may increase the risk of cardiovascular disorders when present in high levels.[337]

Folate is used to help prevent deficiency symptoms during pregnancy, lactation, and when taking oral contraceptives. Of course it is very effective when treating anemia due to folic acid deficiency. Folate is important for those who take the drug methotrexate because it helps prevent the toxicity and side effects that are associated with long-term, low-dose treatment.[338,339] It is often used in conjunction with other B vitamins to combat stress, anxiety, and depression. It is valuable in such conditions as atherosclerosis, osteoporosis, and cervical dysplasia (abnormal growth of cells on the surface of the cervix) as well.

It has been estimated that up to 50 percent of the world population has a disruption in the regular function of the methylenetetrahydrofolate reductase (MTHFR) gene. Known as MTHFR polymorphism, it is a growing diagnosis and problem worldwide, but remains a hotly debated and controversial subject. When this dysfunction occurs, the individual is not able to convert folic acid to its more active form in the body. Several symptoms arise, such as decreased production of S-adenosylmethionine (SAMe). SAMe is an abundant compound naturally found within the body that is involved in liver function, immune function, brain chemical balance, and cell membrane integrity. Neurotransmitter production declines, and other dysfunctions become more common. This cascade of events increases the risk of neurological disorders, cardiovascular disease, cancer, depression, neural tube defects, and miscarriage to name a few. Some researchers suspect that the sharp increase in this disorder is due to unhealthy food choices, increased exposure to toxins and pollution, lifestyle behaviors, and the way Western medicine attacks disease as a symptom-based medicine. In the case of MTHFR polymorphism, individuals should avoid folic acid and use natural methylated folate (L-methylfolate) instead.

Companions:	Cobalamin; Pyridoxine
Preferred Form(s):	Folate; L-methylfolate, Folinic Acid
Adult RDA:	Male/Females—400 mcg; Pregnancy—600 mcg; Lactation—500 mcg
Adult Optimal Range:	400–1000 mcg
Tolerable Upper Limit:	1,000 mcg
Safety Concerns:	No known toxicity of folic acid.
Special Circumstances:	Alcohol consumption depletes folate levels in the body. Women who are pregnant or nursing may need higher doses, particularly those with a history of

neural tube defects, where 4,000 mcg are taken daily under the guidance of a health care professional.

Vitamin B12 (Cobalamin) is essential for the production of red blood cells. Cobalamin is primarily used to treat anemia, both the cobalamin deficient and pernicious types; without sufficient levels of B12 your body will not produce enough red blood cells. B12 helps protect and maintain neurons. Neurons are specialized cells of the nervous system that process information, direct muscle actions, and sense external and internal stimuli. Since it protects neurons, it is appropriate for those with Alzheimer's or impaired cognitive function. Low B12 levels among the elderly is associated with neurocognitive disorders.[340] It helps produce myelin, which is the protective coating that surrounds the nerves. If this defensive coating is damaged, nerves are left unprotected and their ability to conduct signals from the brain to other parts of the body diminishes. Low levels and deficiencies in vitamin B12 are associated with elevated homocysteine levels.[341] Elevated homocysteine levels may be a contributing factor to both cardiovascular disease and chromosome damage. Chromosome damage alters gene activation; this may result in an increase in the number of and spread of cancer cells. Vitamin B12 is often referred to as an energy vitamin because it is frequently added to energy-boosting products or used by those with chronic fatigue. It is added to energy-boosting products because it helps convert carbohydrates to glucose (which is used for energy). But, clinical evidence suggests it will not boost energy levels unless you are deficient in B12. Cobalamin is only found in significant quantities in animal foods, therefore vegetarians and vegans are encouraged to supplement with this important nutrient. There is debate whether oral ingestion of cobalamin is effective or if administration by intravenous injection is the only effective method. However, the evidence suggests that oral ingestion of cobalamin does result in increased blood levels,[342-345] particularly when taken sublingually. Not only is oral cobalamin less expensive, but the cost of administering an injection also makes the oral form preferable when it comes to economic decisions.

Companions:	Folate
Preferred Form(s):	Methylcobalamin
Adult RDA:	Males/Females—2.4 mcg; Pregnancy—2.6 mcg; Lactation—2.8 mcg
Adult Optimal Range:	200–400 mcg
Tolerable Upper Limit:	Not established
Safety Concerns:	No known toxicity exists with cobalamin.

Choline is an essential nutrient involved in the manufacture of the primary components of our cell membranes. Healthy cell membranes efficiently move substances in and out of cells and protect the cell from harmful substances in its surroundings. Choline helps metabolize and transport fats and cholesterol. It is also required for the manufacture of the neurotransmitter acetylcholine, a chemical that carries nerve impulses and stimulates muscle tissue. Choline is a major building block of lecithin, a lipid that helps regulate the nutrients that exit and enter cells. Choline is not a true vitamin because humans can produce it within the body in small amounts, but adequate dietary intake is necessary to maintain proper levels. Choline helps the liver and gallbladder function properly and is also involved in detoxification.

Research suggests that choline may effectively reduce the severity and number of symptom days in asthma sufferers.[346,347] Because of its association with liver function, it is also used in the treatment of hepatic steatosis:[348] a condition characterized by the collection of excessive fat and triglycerides in the liver. It is normal to have fat in the liver, but excess fat disrupts the ability of the liver to filter and detoxify everything we eat and drink. Choline is also used in other liver disorders such as acute viral hepatitis, alcohol-induced fatty liver, and chronic hepatitis. It may also be beneficial for poor memory, delayed development, and nerve impulse problems.

Inositol is closely associated with choline and is also required to produce lecithin in the body. Like choline it is a lipotropic agent—a substance that promotes the removal of fat from the liver. Inositol has been used to treat eczema, anxiety, depression, and obsessive-compulsive disorder.

Companions:	Folate, Inositol
Preferred Form(s):	Phosphatidylcholine
Adult RDA:	Males—550 mg; Females—425 mg; Pregnancy—450 mg; Lactation—550 mg
Adult Optimal Range:	25–600 mg
Tolerable Upper Limit:	3.5 g
Safety Concerns:	Choline is generally considered safe, but high doses (5 grams or greater) may cause low blood pressure, nausea, dizziness, and vomiting.

Vitamin C is probably the most well-researched and well-known vitamin. Linus Pauling's research on its use against infectious diseases and cancer attracted much of this attention. Vitamin C is generally used by the body quickly and just as rapidly excreted from the body. This makes it important to take this vitamin in frequent divided doses. It is very unstable and easily destroyed with cooking.

Vitamin C plays an essential role in the production and maintenance of collagen, the structural protein that holds our bodies together. Without adequate collagen, skin would lose elasticity and have more wrinkles, bones would become brittle, and joints would be poorly supported. Vitamin C is also necessary to help heal wounds and maintain healthy blood vessels. It helps stimulate adrenal function and the release of the stress hormones (epinephrine and norepinephrine). This release of hormones directly affects the cardiovascular system. Chronic stress depletes vitamin C supplies. Large doses of vitamin C may also trigger the release of thyroid stimulating hormones and subsequently triiodothyronine (T3) and thyroxine (T4) hormones.[349] This is useful for those who are hypothyroid and produce insufficient thyroid hormones. Vitamin C is an immune system stimulant and enhances white blood cell function, triggers the production of lymphocytes (the immune cells that create antibodies and attack foreign invaders), and inactivates a variety of viruses and bacteria. All of these actions strengthen your body's defenses against harmful substances.

Vitamin C is one of the body's most important antioxidants. It has been used for the prevention and treatment of upper respiratory infections and urinary tract infections. It also encourages wounds to heal, may reduce atherosclerosis, helps lower high blood pressure, and is used to both prevent and treat cancer. It prevents free-radical damage as well as protects other antioxidant vitamins from being oxidized. It partners with other antioxidant nutrients like vitamin E and the carotenoids to maintain the body's internal antioxidant defenses. Those who take at least 500 mg of vitamin C daily may significantly lower both LDL cholesterol and triglyceride levels.[350]

Vitamin C is available in many forms. The most common form is ascorbic acid, but it is also available in its buffered forms as potassium, sodium, magnesium, or calcium ascorbate. These latter forms have an advantage because they are gentler on the stomach and aren't prone to tooth enamel erosion that can occur when ascorbic acid is chewed. Vitamin C also comes in different types such as powder, crystal, capsule, tablet, and timed-release. The camu berry contains remarkably high vitamin C levels—more than fifty times the levels found in an average orange. Camu berry is ideal for a whole food source of vitamin C.

Bioflavonoids, or flavonoids, are natural compounds found in plants that possess beneficial healing properties and work synergistically with vitamin C. Bioflavonoids are often added to vitamin C supplements because they improve vitamin C absorption. They are used therapeutically for such health conditions as hemorrhoids, cancer, and for those who bruise easily. Bioflavonoids should be taken in a 5:1 or 1:1 ratio with vitamin C (i.e., 1,000 mg vitamin C with 500 mg bioflavonoids) to increase absorption.[351]

Companions:	Vitamin E, Beta-carotene, Selenium, Iron
Preferred Form(s):	From Camu Berry; Magnesium or Calcium Ascorbate; other buffered forms that are combined with minerals to reduce acidity.
Adult RDA:	Males—90 mg; Females—75 mg; Pregnancy—85 mg; Lactation—120 mg
Adult Optimal Range:	500–2,500 mg
Tolerable Upper Limit:	2,000 mg
Safety Concerns:	There is no known toxicity of vitamin C. However, diarrhea may occur in some individuals at doses of 5,000–10,000 mg per day. Your individual upper limit for vitamin C may be determined according to the bowel tolerance level. Bowel tolerance level means this is the amount required to cause loose stools. The maximum daily dose (upper limit) for an individual is slightly below this level. For example, if you experience loose stools when you take 6,000 mg of vitamin C, your upper limit would be about 5,500 mg daily.

MINERALS

Minerals are chemicals or elements that originate in the earth and are required by living organisms to stay healthy. They are the basic constituents of matter. There are two primary types of minerals: macro minerals—those the body needs in large quantities, such as calcium, phosphorus, magnesium, sodium, potassium, chloride, and sulfur—and trace minerals (or micro minerals)—those the body needs in small or trace amounts. Our bodies require certain dietary minerals, called essential minerals, for the proper function of bodily processes and for proper development. We get our minerals from the soil, meaning that as a plant grows it uptakes whatever minerals are in the soil it is growing in, and then when we eat the plant we acquire the minerals.

Chelated minerals are minerals attached to other compounds—frequently amino acids. Evidence suggests that mineral chelation improves absorption in the body. Many minerals compete with one another for absorption, so it is important to take them in the proper ratios. The following are guidelines for ideal mineral ratios to maximize bioavailability and effectiveness:

- Calcium: phosphorus—1:1
- Magnesium: calcium—1:2
- Zinc: copper—10:1
- Manganese: zinc—1:3

The minerals that are essential (those required from the diet because the body can't produce them) is debatable, but there are sixteen that have important roles in human health. They are boron, calcium, chloride, chromium, copper, iodine, iron, manganese, magnesium, molybdenum, phosphorus, potassium, selenium, sodium, sulfur, and zinc. The typical American diet supplies more than enough sodium and phosphorus to meet bodily requirements; and if you eat enough fruits and vegetables chances are you are getting enough potassium. The other minerals must be obtained by supplementation or through the consumption of foods that contain sufficient quantities.

Boron is a trace mineral that may help prevent bone loss and demineralization, which is important for the maintenance of bone health as well as the prevention of osteoporosis. It naturally balances sex hormone levels in the body, particularly estrogen and testosterone.[352,353] The research suggests that boron increases free testosterone and decreases estradiol in men. In post-menopausal women, it caused both testosterone and estrogen to be elevated. This is desirable because postmenopausal women experience a steep decline in hormone production. Boron may help prevent osteoporosis by markedly reducing the excretion of calcium and magnesium. Both minerals are required to maintain bone mineral density and therefore bone strength. Boron is thought to be associated with longevity and considered an anti-aging nutrient, though no significant research has been conducted to confirm this theory yet. Some animal research has indicated that boron may help the body utilize vitamin D. By enhancing the utilization of vitamin D, boron may encourage strong bones.[354,355] Human studies do suggest that boron increases vitamin D levels in the body so this indicates boron and vitamin D work in tandem. Boron has also been researched for its ability to reduce inflammation.[356] This fact suggests boron may promote healthy aging because excess inflammation is linked to a whole host of chronic diseases and accelerates the aging process. Studies indicate that boron may reduce the risk of prostate cancer through the selective inhibition of the spread of prostate cancer cells (without affecting health prostate cells).[357,358]

Companions:	Calcium, Magnesium, Copper, Vitamin D
Preferred Form(s):	Boronamino Acid Chelate
Adult RDA:	Not established

Adult Optimal Range:	3–5 mg
Tolerable Upper Limit:	Not established
Safety Concerns:	Boron is generally safe and no toxicity has been reported at doses of 3–6 mg. High doses could potentially cause acute toxicity so caution should be used at doses above 6 mg daily.

Calcium is a macro mineral that is widely known for its role in maintaining strong bones and teeth, but the functions of this mineral go beyond this benefit. Calcium is essential for important tasks such as proper muscle contraction and regulation of the heartbeat. Calcium is the most abundant mineral in the body and accounts for approximately 2 percent of body weight. The bones contain almost 99 percent of the body's calcium supply.[359]

One study indicated calcium may be beneficial for symptoms of PMS.[360] This may be because many women who report PMS symptoms have an imbalance of calcium. Because of its role in the constriction and relaxation of blood vessels, calcium may affect blood pressure.[361,362] Calcium, in its carbonate form, is used as an over-the-counter antacid, but it is also the form of calcium most likely to be contaminated with lead.[363] Since lead is a toxic heavy metal, supplements that contain calcium carbonate should generally be avoided.

Calcium chloride is very important for the strength of heart contractions. It may be injected intravenously during cardiac arrest to stimulate cardiac tissue and stabilize the heartbeat when epinephrine fails to improve cardiac function. Although calcium is important in the prevention and treatment of osteoporosis, it is not effective without regular exercise and a reduction of phosphorus in the diet. In addition, it must be taken in tandem with vitamins D and K to encourage absorption and skeletal deposition of calcium.

Companions:	Vitamin D, Vitamin A, Vitamin C, Vitamin K
Preferred Form(s):	Calcium Citrate
Adult RDA:	Males/Females, age 18–50—1,000 mg; Males/Females, age 51+—1,200 mg
Adult Optimal Range:	250–1,200 mg
Tolerable Upper Limit:	2,500 mg
Safety Concerns:	Calcium is generally well tolerated (or won't cause side effects) up to 2,000 mg daily. Taking large quantities (1,400 mg or more daily) without vitamin D and K is ill-advised as it may increase the risk of cardiovascular disease mortality.[364,365]

Chloride is a trace mineral essential for the maintenance of proper body fluid balance. It helps regulate the amount of fluid inside and outside your cells, something that is very important because imbalance in cellular fluid will cause cells to shrink or swell. Chloride helps regulate the body's acid-base balance, maintains proper blood volume and pressure, improves nerve impulse transmission, and helps conduct electricity—important for heart, muscle, and digestive function. It is also important to the production of hydrochloric acid (digestive juices) in the stomach. If your body has insufficient levels of chloride, it may not produce adequate levels of hydrochloric acid, which could cause indigestion. Excessive sweating, vomiting, diarrhea, and certain medications can cause low chloride levels, but the majority of Americans get ample chloride in their diet from table salt. Chloride is often combined with sodium (sodium chloride) to help replace chloride lost during perspiration. Calcium chloride is used for the treatment of low blood calcium, magnesium sulfate overdose. It also reduces negative effects of excess potassium in the body and restores cardiac function following defibrillation. You don't need to look for a multinutrient that contains chloride; it can easily be obtained in healthy foods.

Preferred Form(s):	Food Sources
Adult RDA:	Males/Females, age 18–50—2.3 g; Males/Females, age 51–70—2.0 g; Males/Females, age 71+—1.8 g
Adult Optimal Range:	Acquire from food sources only, such as sea salt, rye, tomatoes, lettuce, celery, and olives; normally no need for supplementation.
Tolerable Upper Limit:	Not established
Safety Concerns:	Chloride is generally considered safe.

Chromium is a trace mineral with profound effects on blood sugar control mechanisms, namely glucose uptake by cells. It is integral for the improvement of your body's response to sugar and works closely with insulin to increase cellular usage of blood sugar.[366] This fact makes it ideal for diabetics, though you should never take it without consulting a qualified health care professional because it may reduce insulin injection requirements. Chromium also helps reduce high LDL cholesterol levels in the blood, while simultaneously raising HDL levels. Higher HDL levels help to reduce the risk of cardiovascular disease.[367] Some health care professionals also recommend chromium as part of a weight loss program because it is associated with an increase in lean body mass and reduced body fat. However, there is very little scientific evidence to support this benefit currently.[368,369]

Companions:	Biotin
Preferred Form(s):	Chromium Picolinate; Chromium Polynicotinate
Adult RDA:	Males, age 19–50—35 mcg; Females, age 19–50—25 mcg; Males/Females, age 50+—20 mcg; Pregnancy— 30 mcg; Lactation—45 mcg
Adult Optimal Range:	200–400 mcg; 600–1,000 mcg in divided doses for diabetics
Tolerable Upper Limit:	Not established
Safety Concerns:	Chromium has no known toxicity in supplement form.

Copper is a trace mineral that is essential for the function of many enzymes. It works with other minerals in the maintenance and formation of bones. It has a mild anti-inflammatory effect and is often used as part of arthritis formulas. Copper works with Vitamin C in the formation of collagen. It helps maintain skin elasticity, bone health, and joint stability. It also facilitates the absorption of iron and assists in the formation of hemoglobin. Hemoglobin is the protein in red blood cells that carries oxygen. Copper is often deficient in humans because of high zinc intake. Zinc competes with copper for absorption and thus it is very important to achieve the appropriate 10:1 ratio of zinc to copper.

Companions:	Vitamin C, Iron
Preferred Form(s):	No form seems to be better absorbed than the other, though copper gluconate may be gentler on the stomach.
Adult RDA:	Males/Females—900 mcg; Pregnancy—1,000 mcg; Lactation—1,300 mcg
Adult Optimal Range:	1.5 mg–3 mg
Tolerable Upper Limit:	Not established
Safety Concerns:	Copper can be toxic in doses of 10 mg or greater.

Iodine is a trace mineral closely associated with the proper function of the thyroid gland and the production of thyroid hormones. It requires a delicate balance of iodine to avoid thyroid dysfunction because intake levels above and below recommended amounts can be problematic.[370] Iodine deficiency can cause goiter—enlargement of the thyroid gland. Table salt is often iodized to reduce iodine deficiency and the risk of goiter. Deficiency of iodine is also the leading cause of brain damage and mental retardation in children worldwide.[371] Research suggests that an average loss of ten to fifteen IQ points occurs when insufficient iodine is consumed during pregnancy.[372] Iodine is necessary for cellular metabolism—the process of converting food into energy.

Preferred Form(s):	Iodine Derived from Kelp, Iodine Caseinate
Adult RDA:	Males/Females—150 mcg; Pregnancy—220 mcg; Lactation—290 mcg
Adult Optimal Range:	100–300 mcg
Tolerable Upper Limit:	1,100 mcg
Safety Concerns:	Iodine appears safe except in very high dosages of 1,500 mcg or higher.

Iron is essential to human life and is found in every cell in the body. Because iron is so important the body guards and conserves this mineral determinedly. Iron is central to hemoglobin formation and the transport of oxygen from the lungs to all other parts of the body. Iron provides strength to the body and helps produce energy. Non-heme iron from plant sources is much more difficult for the body to absorb than heme iron from animal sources. Despite this fact, most supplements contain non-heme iron because it is much easier to take higher quantities of it. Sufficient quantities of non-heme iron can provide the same net amount of heme iron absorbed. Ribonucleotide reductase, the enzyme responsible for DNA synthesis, is dependent on sufficient iron levels to function properly. Iron is also important in the synthesis of the neurotransmitters dopamine, norepinephrine, and serotonin. Each of these neurotransmitters plays a vital role in mood and focus. Dopamine improves focus, relieves depression, and can encourage both a relaxed and excited state. Norepinephrine is stimulating. Low levels cause decreased energy and focus whereas high levels may cause anxious feelings. Serotonin induces a relaxed state, it stabilizes the mood and balances excess excitability.

Iron is helpful for anemia, a condition where the body does not have enough healthy red blood cells that leads to fatigue and shortness of breath. The World Health Organization considers iron deficiency to be the most common international nutrition malady. Men have lesser requirements for iron than women, particularly menstruating women. Men have a daily requirement for iron of about 8 mg—taking more than this can result in excessive free-radical production and increased risk of heart disease.[373] During their reproductive years, women lose approximately 2 mg of iron daily during heavy menstruation and therefore require greater quantities to replenish lost stores. Men and postmenopausal women seldom require supplemental iron unless a known deficiency exists. Iron should be taken with vitamin C to enhance absorption. Iron deficiency can lead to anemia, depression, fatigue, learning disabilities, and increased susceptibility to illness. Iron supplements may promote gastrointestinal problems in some people, including nausea, diarrhea, dark stools, or constipation. Women who are pregnant are more susceptible to constipation from taking iron supplements.

Companions:	Vitamin C
Preferred Form(s):	Ferrous Succinate, Ferrous Fumarate
Adult RDA:	Males—8 mg; Females, age 19–50—18 mg; Females, age 51+—8 mg; Pregnancy—27 mg; Lactation—9 mg
Adult Optimal Range:	Women who are still menstruating 15–18 mg; Men and postmenopausal women should obtain iron from dietary sources only, unless a deficiency exists.
Tolerable Upper Limit:	45 mg
Safety Concerns:	Children under the age of six are extremely susceptible to iron toxicity, which may cause death. Except in children, iron is generally considered safe even at high doses because the body has a prevention mechanism set up to prevent excess and toxicity.

Magnesium is involved in over 300 enzymatic reactions within the body. It is required for strong bones and teeth, where it plays a critical role in bone growth and in the prevention of tooth decay. In fact, magnesium is especially critical for the health and strength of spongy bone found within the body, like in the spine, vertebrae, and ends of long bones. As you age, magnesium exits the bone at a faster rate, which increases the risk of osteoporosis.[374] It may be that the body removes magnesium from the bone to meet the magnesium needs of the cardiovascular system because as magnesium is removed from the bone, greater accumulation occurs in the arteries. Research suggests that an oral magnesium supplement can reduce this magnesium loss from the bone, and reduce the risk of age-related osteoporosis.[375,376]

Magnesium helps the muscles relax and appears to be beneficial in the relief of stress also. Magnesium may help prevent cardiovascular disease due to its ability to tone the blood vessels as well as its critical role in the optimal functioning of the entire cardiovascular system. It is beneficial if administered intravenously to patients experiencing a heart attack.[377,378] Additionally, magnesium may be valuable in the treatment of cardiac arrhythmias[379,380]—disturbances in the normal rhythm of the heartbeat.

Magnesium has proven effective in the treatment of preeclampsia (a condition characterized by high blood pressure and excess protein in the urine after the twentieth week of pregnancy).[381] In fact, a review of the literature determined that magnesium sulfate provides comparable, if not better results than diazepam, a common drug used to treat symptoms of preeclampsia.[382] Magnesium is nature's calcium channel blocker (helps lower blood pressure), but is much less powerful than drugs manufactured to carry out the same purpose. It is also important in the secretion and action of insulin, making it important for diabetics. Magnesium is associated with a reduction in occupational hearing loss. There was a study that included 300 young, healthy men who were exposed to high levels of impulse noises while attending basic military training. One group received 167 mg of magnesium in a drink, while a control group received a placebo. The men who received the magnesium experienced a reduction in hearing damage when compared to the placebo group.[383] Magnesium deficiency is often seen in migraine sufferers.[384] The deficiency is thought to be related to a genetic inability to absorb magnesium or excessive magnesium excretion among those who experience frequent migraines. Based on this fact, those who experience migraines regularly may benefit from a daily magnesium supplement.[385] It is often combined with the feverfew herb to reduce migraine occurrence and intensity.

Companions:	Pyridoxine, Calcium, Phosphorus
Preferred Form(s):	Magnesium Citrate
Adult RDA:	Males, age 19–30—400 mg; Males. Age 30+—350 mg; Females, age 19–30—310 mg; Females, age 30+—320 mg; Pregnancy, age 19–30—350 mg; Pregnancy, age 31+—360 mg; Lactation, age 19–30—310 mg; Lactation, age 31+—320 mg
Adult Optimal Range:	500–600 mg
Tolerable Upper Limit:	350 mg
Safety Concerns:	Magnesium is generally safe although those with kidney disease should avoid supplementation except by a physician's orders. The sulfate, hydroxide, or chloride forms may cause loose stools.

Manganese is found in the body in very small amounts; however, it has many important uses. Manganese is essential to the function of many enzyme systems including playing a critical role as part of the enzyme superoxide dismutase (SOD). SOD acts as an antioxidant, protects and repairs cells, encourages a healthy life span, and helps decrease inflammation and pain associated with arthritis. It also works with other enzymes in the metabolism of protein, fat, and carbohydrates. Manganese is important for the repair of bones and connective tissue, as well as healthy joint membranes. It also activates the enzyme that functions in collagen production and helps wounds heal.

Preferred Form(s):	Manganese Gluconate, Manganese Picolinate
Adult RDA:	Males 2.3 mg; Females—1.8 mg; Pregnancy—2 mg; Lactation—2.6 mg
Adult Optimal Range:	5 mg–7 mg
Tolerable Upper Limit:	11 mg
Safety Concerns:	Manganese ingested in the form of foods or supplements is very safe. Toxicity occurs with the inhalation of manganese as a result of pollution or mining.

Molybdenum is an essential trace mineral vital to the enzyme systems responsible for the detoxification of alcohol, uric acid metabolism, iron utilization, and carbohydrate metabolism. Excess uric acid in the blood can lead to deposits of it in the spaces between joints, such as gout. It is found in many foods, including whole grains, green leafy vegetables, and legumes. Molybdenum deficiency is rare but has been implicated in some cancers, particularly esophageal cancer.[386] It is also thought to play a role in the prevention of tooth decay and dental cavities.[387]

Preferred Form(s):	Molybdenum Amino Acid Chelate
Adult RDA:	Males/Females—45 mcg; Pregnancy/Lactation— 50 mcg
Adult Optimal Range:	100–300 mcg
Tolerable Upper Limit:	2,000 mcg
Safety Concerns:	Molybdenum is generally considered non-toxic. One study indicated gout-like symptoms may be experienced at daily intake levels of 10–15 mg because of increased uric acid production.[388]

Phosphorus is vital for energy storage, metabolism, and regulation, and aids fat, protein and carbohydrate utilization. It is important in the formation of bones and teeth. Phosphorus is essential to muscle contraction, nerve function, kidney function, and the regularity of the heartbeat. It is also necessary for the utilization of some of the B-complex vitamins. Better use of B vitamins can equal more energy. It can be found in pumpkin and squash seeds, salmon, Brazil nuts, beef, pork, veal, and beans. The typical American diet contains excessive phosphorus, particularly from soft drinks that provide excess phosphorus but no calcium to maintain the proper balance of these minerals in the body.

Most people would actually benefit from a reduction of phosphates in their diet. Several studies suggest that excess intake of phosphorus can increase the risk of cardiovascular disease and chronic kidney disease.[389,390,391,392] A fragile balance of phosphorus and calcium must be maintained because too much phosphorus can create an imbalance in bone mineral density and increase the risk of osteoporosis.[393,394] The more phosphorus you obtain from your diet, the greater your need for calcium. Phosphorus has few clinical uses, but it is an effective treatment for hypercalcemia (excessive calcium in the blood).[395] If too much calcium is present in the blood, nausea, abdominal, bone, and kidney pain may occur, as well as frequent urination, muscle weakness or twitches, and mood disorders. Phosphates can be used as a laxative for constipation and to promote bowel regularity after surgery. Potassium and sodium phosphate are used in the prevention of calcium oxalate kidney stones.

Preferred Form(s):	Food Sources
Adult RDA:	Males/Females—700 mg
Adult Optimal Range:	Phosphorus is usually easily obtained from diet alone.
Tolerable Upper Limit:	Age 19–70—4g; age 70+—3 g
Safety Concerns:	Phosphorus is generally considered safe at recommended levels. Excessive intake can lead to increased excretion of calcium as well as hyperphosphatemia (excessive blood phosphorus levels), which can lead to serious adverse effects including death.

Potassium is an essential mineral and electrolyte (mineral salts that carry a tiny electrical charge when dissolved in water) that regulates the water balance and acid-base balance of blood and tissues. It is critical for proper muscle, nerve, heart, kidney, and adrenal function. An increased intake of dietary potassium may be a more effective way to reduce blood pressure than reduced sodium intake alone.[396] It is often used clinically to reduce swelling caused by fluid trapped in tissues (edema) and high blood pressure and in the prevention of stroke and osteoporosis.

Preferred Form(s):	Potassium-rich Foods Like Fruits and Vegetables
Adult RDA:	Males/Females—4.7 g; Lactation—5.1 g
Adult Optimal Range:	From food sources. Deficiency cases—99 mg
Tolerable Upper Limit:	Not established
Safety Concerns:	Potassium is best when derived from food sources. Potassium supplementation is not recommended

unless under the supervision of a qualified health care professional, particularly among those with impaired kidney function or who are taking certain prescription medications.

Selenium is a powerful antioxidant trace mineral that protects cells from free-radical damage. Selenium works synergistically with vitamin E, which enhances the antioxidant effect of selenium. Selenium helps prevent cancer, particularly when taken regularly early in life and when supplementation is maintained over the entire life span.[397] Research has been mixed, but some studies suggest that selenium is effective in the prevention of cancer and/or the reduction of mortality from prostate, gastrointestinal, gynecological, lung, and colon cancers.[398-403] It also appears to protect the body from the toxic effects of environmental pollution, smoking, and heavy metals. Selenium is particularly beneficial to males, where it protects the prostate, and may increase fertility, sperm production and sperm motility.[404] Next to iodine, selenium is perhaps the most important nutrient for optimum thyroid function, and selenium deficiency is often seen in those with thyroid disorders.[405] It protects the thyroid from oxidative damage[406] and is essential to increase the production of thyroid hormones,[407] metabolism,[408] and activation of thyroid hormones.[409]

Selenium increases immune system activity,[410] particularly the activity of white blood cells.[411] Though research is mixed and somewhat controversial, selenium appears to provide protection against heart disease,[412] stroke mortality,[413] and mildly improves cholesterol levels and ratios.[414]

Companions:	Vitamin E, Copper, Iron, Zinc
Preferred Form(s):	Selenomethionine; Seleniumamino acid chelate
Adult RDA:	Males/Females—55 mcg; Pregnancy—60 mcg; Lactation—70 mcg
Adult Optimal Range:	50–200 mcg
Tolerable Upper Limit:	400 mcg
Safety Concerns:	Selenium toxicity may occur with prolonged usage of higher doses and with very large single doses. It is suggested to limit selenium intake to no more than 200 mcg daily unless advised otherwise by a qualified health care practitioner.

Sodium is the predominant positive ion in the blood and body fluids and helps control blood pressure and blood volume. Sodium works with potassium to regulate the balance of fluids in the body. Additionally, it helps maintain the proper acid-base balance of blood and tissues. Sodium helps transmit nerve impulses and aids muscle contraction and relaxation. Excess sodium in the typical American diet is a major contributing factor to high blood pressure—the primary risk factor for heart disease, and resulted in almost 2.3 million cardiovascular-related deaths worldwide in 2010.[415,416] While no actual RDA is set for sodium, many organizations recommend limiting sodium intake to less than 2,300 mg daily. This recommendation may actually be too low, based on research that the optimum range of sodium intake is between 2,645 to 4,945 mg.[417]

Preferred Form(s):	Food Sources Such as Sea Salt
Adult RDA:	Not established
Adult Optimal Range:	2,645–4,945 mg from food sources only
Tolerable Upper Limit:	Based on the latest research individuals should strive to stay within a range of 2,645 to 4,945 mg of sodium per day. The current guidelines from the US Centers for Disease Control and Prevention remains no more than 2,300 mg daily for adults and no more than 1,500 mg daily for those with high blood pressure.[418]
Safety Concerns:	Excessive sodium intake may contribute to high blood pressure—a key risk factor for heart disease—and possibly other adverse health effects.

Zinc is found in every cell in the body and is essential for the proper function of over three hundred different enzymes. Zinc is required for reproduction, growth, and development because of its important role in the production and duplication of our genetic blueprints and basic building blocks of cells (RNA and DNA). It is necessary for the maturation of sperm (the increased ability of sperm to fertilize an egg) and proper development of a fetus. Insufficient zinc during pregnancy hinders the rapid cell growth that occurs during pregnancy. Zinc is an immune-stimulant that enhances the activities of white blood cells and regulates the immune system's inflammatory response to infections.[419,420] It is a part of the enzyme systems that detoxify alcohol and environmental toxins and chemicals. Topical zinc may help wounds heal, particularly burns, and helps to reduce the appearance of scars.[421] It is important to the senses of taste, smell, and sight. Zinc also helps regulate insulin and thyroid hormone activity—especially T3.[422,423] Balanced production of these hormones is vital for blood sugar control and metabolism.

A healthy prostate contains significantly more zinc than a diseased or enlarged prostate. This concentration of zinc in the prostate suggests zinc plays a critical role in prostate health. However, there appears to be a finite range before zinc may cause more harm than good to the prostate. Daily high doses of 80 mg or more may increase the progression of prostate enlargement.[424] Conversely, reasonable doses—less than 40 mg—of zinc may help to reduce the size of the prostate in benign prostate hypertrophy.[425] Zinc helps restore damage to the stomach mucosal lining after peptic ulcers.[426,427] It is a treatment for sickle cell anemia and used both topically and orally for acne. Zinc can also be effective for attention deficit hyperactive disorder (ADHD) because research suggests children with ADHD may have lower levels of zinc in relation to children without ADHD.[428] Other therapeutic uses of zinc include fungal infections of the scalp, herpes simplex virus,[429,430] and to foster oral health.[431]

Preferred Form(s):	Zinc Amino Acid Chelate
Adult RDA:	Males—11 mg; Females—8 mg; Pregnancy—11 mg; Lactation—12 mg
Adult Optimal Range:	15–20 mg
Tolerable Upper Limit:	40 mg
Safety Concerns:	Zinc is generally safe and non-toxic. Mild gastrointestinal upset has been reported at doses greater than 50 mg per day. Copper deficiency can also occur from excessive intake. Vomiting will often occur with single doses of 225 mg or greater.

ADDITIONAL ESSENTIAL NUTRIENTS

Sulfur deficiency may lead to pain and inflammation in the body, slow metabolism, brittle hair or nails, fatigue, blood sugar problems, and aggravation of allergies. Vegetarians and vegans are at greatest risk for sulfur deficiencies because major food sources of sulfur include eggs, meat, poultry, and fish—though cruciferous and allium vegetables are also good sources. Sulfur is essential to the body's detoxification systems, immune function, and the proper function of some enzymes. Sulfur helps the body detoxify through the elimination of environmental chemicals, food toxins, drugs, and the normal by-products of hormones. It is involved in collagen formation, thus the reason it is often combined with glucosamine and chondroitin in joint health formulas. Sulfur helps supports the permeability of cell membranes to allow nutrients to enter and waste to exit cells. Cell permeability also supports the uptake of oxygen into cells, something required for the healthy development and function of cells. It is an essential nutrient for healthy hair, nails, and skin.

Sulfur is used topically and/or orally (usually in amino acid form) for skin problems like eczema. One sulfur compound, methylsulfonylmethane (MSM) has anti-inflammatory effects and is often used as part of joint formulas. MSM also exhibits antioxidant properties, and is used topically to reduce the appearance of aging.

Preferred Form(s):	MSM (supplemental)
Adult RDA:	Not established
Adult Optimal Range:	Therapeutic dosages range from 1,500–10,000 mg daily in divided doses.
Tolerable Upper Limit:	Not established
Safety Concerns:	There is currently no known toxic level of sulfur, and it is considered very safe.

The importance of **Essential Fatty Acids (EFA)** was discussed in the chapter about eating better. As a review they are divided into three categories, omega-3, omega-6, and omega-9 fatty acids. An array of diseases and health conditions are benefited from sufficient intake of EFAs. Proper balance of omega-3 to omega-6 EFAs is critical to health. Most people do not consume enough cold-water fish (recommended twice per week), flaxseed, walnuts, and natural or organic eggs to get the proper amounts of these health promoting fats. In addition, much of today's fish is contaminated with heavy metals, pollutants, chemicals, and radiation from nuclear power plants. Therefore, an EFA supplement is even more important and an essential part of any plan to improve health and increase a healthy life span.

There is much debate regarding the best EFA supplement source. Some argue for fish oils, while others make a case for plant-based options like borage or flaxseed oil. The research suggests that marine sources of EFAs (DHA and EPA) are far superior to plant-based EFAs. Flaxseed oil is rich in alpha-linolenic acid (ALA), which must be converted to EPA and DHA in the body. By contrast, fish oils are rich in DHA and EPA, avoiding the extra step of conversion. To get an equivalent amount of DHA and EPA you need to consume two or three times as much flaxseed oil as fish oil. But, some studies suggest that conversion of ALA to DHA or EPA is inefficient and it is more practical to supplement with the desired fatty acid.[432]

One particularly promising EFA supplement is krill oil. Krill oil appears to be better absorbed and more effective than fish oil at equivalent doses when it comes to the control of cholesterol levels.[433] Many people who take a krill supplement report that they experience less unpleasant effects such as belching and a bad aftertaste. Additionally, krill oil contains the natural antioxidant astaxanthin that naturally protects the oil from rancidity and oxidation, as well as provides your body extra free-radical defense.

Though not as much a concern as in years past, it is still important that you choose a quality fish oil supplement to avoid many heavy metals, dioxins, pesticides, or PCBs (polychlorinated biphenyl). Choose a marine oil supplement that is molecularly distilled to reduce or eliminate harmful substances, and preferably pharmaceutical grade—the highest quality grade of vitamins that meet the highest standards for purity, absorption, and ability to dissolve. Molecular distillation naturally concentrates the DHA contained in marine oils, which is a highly desirable trait. It appears that the dietary supplement industry is doing a respectable job keeping contaminants out of supplements. According to an independent study completed by ConsumerLab.com,[434] no mercury and only traces of PCBs were found in the products tested. In fact, a serving of fish is more likely to be contaminated than a fish oil supplement. It is essential you purchase a fish oil product that contains antioxidants to prevent rancidity. Fish oils are very delicate and prone to rancidity so they require antioxidants to prevent this. Indeed, rancid fish oil supplements can be more harmful to your health than not taking one at all.[435,436]

Adult Optimal Range:	250–500 mg DHA; 250–500 mg EPA
Safety Concerns:	There are no known toxic effects of omega-3 fatty acids.
Special Circumstances:	Taking up to 1,000 mg each of EPA and DHA may be necessary for those with heart disease.

The **Coenzyme Q10 (CoQ10),** also known as ubiquinone or its more bioavailable form ubiquinol, is an excellent nutrient for cardiovascular health. It plays an essential role in energy production, and is an integral component of the mitochondria (the parts of our cells that produce energy). It is abundant in organs that require significant amounts of energy, like the heart, kidney, and liver.[437] CoQ10 is a powerful antioxidant that protects cells and lipids (fats) from free-radical oxidation. Oxidized cells are often injured and their DNA is damaged. This damage, can cause a number of degenerative diseases like cancer, Parkinson's, Alzheimer's, and cardiovascular disease. When lipids are oxidized, called peroxidation, it also damages DNA, disrupts cell function, and can increase the production of cancer-causing compounds.

CoQ10 is very important in cardiovascular function and disease, and provides optimal nutrition, at a cellular level, to the heart. It has a remarkable protective effect and prevents heart damage due to angina or heart attack if it is administered within three days of the attack.[438] It is also used in patients with congestive heart failure (inability of the heart to pump blood properly), cardiomyopathy (reduced force of heart contractions), arrhythmia (irregular heartbeat), and mitral valve prolapse (the valve that separates the upper and lower chambers on the left side of the heart doesn't close properly).[439-442] CoQ10 effectively reduces oxidative damage that occurs during heart surgery as well.

CoQ10 is one of the nutrients essential for the production of ATP. ATP is what the body draws from to create energy, kind of like your body's energy savings account. Because of its role in energy production, CoQ10 is thought to improve symptoms of chronic fatigue syndrome. Studies have indicated CoQ10 may help prevent periodontal disease, thus many natural toothpastes and oral care products include it as an ingredient.[443] It is also considered an immune system enhancer, particularly for the elderly who tend to have reduced immune function.[444] If you have a family history of cardiovascular disease, a current heart condition, or are over the age of fifty, CoQ10 would be an ideal supplement to include in your regimen.

Adult Optimal Range:	50–300 mg
Safety Concerns:	CoQ10 is considered safe even at high doses (3,000 mg for up to eight weeks). However, you should not take more than 300 mg without first consulting a health care professional.

Flavonoids (Bioflavonoids) are a group of compounds synthesized by plants that provide a wide variety of human health benefits.[445] Many flavonoids have antioxidant properties and help reduce the oxidation of LDL cholesterol.[446] They may protect against cardiovascular disease,[447] lower cholesterol,[448] reduce inflammation,[449] and possess anti-cancer properties.[450] Each unique flavonoid appears to have its own set of properties, functions, and uses so variety is important. Some of the most researched and well-known flavonoids include quercetin, hesperidin, and rutin.

Adult Optimal Range:	Varies by flavonoid. Take flavonoids in a 5:1 or 1:1 ratio with vitamin C.
Safety Concerns:	Most flavonoids are considered very safe. Large doses of tea polyphenol flavonoids are associated with liver toxicity and should be used with caution.[451]

Ginkgo Biloba extract originates from one of the oldest living tree species on earth. The trees are known to live as long as 1,000 years. Amazingly many ginkgo trees survived the atomic bomb dropped on Hiroshima in 1945, despite being near the epicenter of the destruction. This helped the ginkgo tree earn a reputation for hardiness and the extraordinary ability to survive in extremely harsh environments. This remarkable tree seems to provide similar effects when consumed by humans. It is considered an anti-aging nutrient, which promotes longevity and increases the quality of life, particularly among the elderly.[452] It very effectively improves blood and oxygen supply to tissues, especially to the brain. More oxygen to tissues and the brain means greater efficiency. Ginkgo is also an antioxidant.

Ginkgo is commonly used to improve memory and reduce the severity of cognitive disorders, such as Alzheimer's disease and dementia.[453,454] Other uses for gingko include sleep disturbance related to depression,[455] glaucoma,[456] erectile dysfunction,[457] and menopausal symptoms.[458]

Adult Optimal Range:	A maintenance dosage of 80–120 mg standardized to 24 percent flavone glycosides and 6 percent terpine lactones. 240 mg is normally the therapeutic dosage.
Safety Concerns:	Ginkgo is considered safe and side effects are rare and generally mild. Caution is advised in persons with bleeding disorders. Do not take with drugs that increase the risk of bleeding. Stop taking ginkgo two weeks before undergoing surgery. The fresh seeds are considered toxic and deadly.

Probiotics (Intestinal Flora) are live organisms that aid digestion and elimination and help maintain the health of the gastrointestinal system. They are "friendly" or "good" bacteria that inhabit the mouth, digestive tract, and vagina. The greater quantity of probiotics in these locations, the more they crowd out harmful bacteria and pathogenic organisms. Probiotics may halt the growth of unfriendly bacteria, yeast, parasites, and fungi, which helps to promote a healthy intestinal environment. Probiotics are extremely important in a person's nutritional status and aid in the absorption of calcium, fats, B vitamins, proteins, and phosphorus. They are often used for inflammatory bowel diseases, like Crohn's and ulcerative colitis. Indeed, the probiotic strain *Escherichia coli* Nissle 1917 has been shown to be as effective as the drug mesalazine—commonly used to treat ulcerative colitis—to keep ulcerative colitis in remission.[459] Beyond gastrointestinal support, probiotics are influential to the immune system. Up to

80 percent of your immune system is located in your gut and probiotics can profoundly influence the permeability of the intestines and help balance the immune system's inflammatory responses to infections.[460] In addition, probiotics improve biological measurements associated with depression,[461] reduce allergic disease,[462] and help maintain a normal inflammatory response throughout the body.[463,464]

Research suggests that even infants and children may benefit if they take a probiotic supplement. Children who receive a probiotic experience reduced incidence and duration of respiratory infections, and miss fewer school days (up to 31.8 percent fewer missed school days) than children who do not take a probiotic supplement.[465,466,467] Remarkably, infants who received the probiotic strain *Lactobacillus reuteri* DSM 17938 during the first 90 days of life significantly improved gastrointestinal health and decreased medical care costs about $119 per infant during the first few months of life. The study also reported that colic episodes were reduced—crying time was thirty-eight minutes compared to seventy-one minutes in the control group. The number of times the infant spit up per day was 2.9 times versus 4.6, bowel movements were more regular, and medical care expenses were reduced, all from the simple addition of probiotics during early life.[468]

Probiotics are often used as a treatment for diarrhea as well as other gastrointestinal disorders like irritable bowel syndrome, inflammatory bowel disease, and stomach infections. They are very important to take during and after antibiotic treatment because antibiotics do not distinguish between "friendly" and "unfriendly" bacteria and destroy both the good with the bad. Without probiotic supplementation this leaves areas normally inhabited by probiotics wide open for invasion from harmful organisms. Probiotic supplementation during and after antibiotics helps prevent antibiotic-induced diarrhea and Candida yeast overgrowth. Probiotics can retard the growth of the yeast *Candida albicans* and may help treat and prevent vaginal yeast infections when administered orally or directly in the vagina.[469,470] Most probiotic supplements must remain in the refrigerator to maintain potency and viability of bacteria unless the product specifies it is shelf-stable.

Adult Optimal Range:	At least 8 billion organisms containing multiple clinically proven strains.
Safety Concerns:	Probiotics are very safe and there is no known safety risks associated with them.

A high-quality, optimum potency multinutrient and other foundational nutrients are fundamental to good health. So, whether you want to improve your health, gain more energy throughout the day, feel better, or reduce your risk of disease, dietary supplements are a must. They can provide you with greater assurance that your body has the nutrients it needs for cells, organs, and systems to thrive. Do your body a favor and support its efforts to maintain homeostasis and achieve the best, healthy you it can.

4

Move and Move Often

Modern conveniences and sedentary lifestyles have made physical activity more important than ever. While these modern conveniences have made life easier and more comfortable, they have also made life less physically demanding. Our ancestors expended a great deal of energy in all aspects of their life, from work to play, and everyday experiences. We, on the other hand, expend very little energy at work because most of our jobs are sedentary in nature. We stand behind cash registers or sit at desks for long periods. Our play involves sitting in an easy chair and staring at a television or spending hours in front of a phone, tablet, or computer. These lifestyle factors all contribute to excess weight, obesity, and ultimately poor health.

The fact is the average American is growing larger, but this size increase is largely in the waistline. Each year thousands of people make a commitment, or "New Year's resolution," to join a gym, lose weight, or get in better shape, yet few actually succeed. More than half of Americans want to lose weight but only 25 percent claim they are actively trying to do so according to a 2013 Gallup poll.[471] Physical activity can't be a short-term fad; it has to be regular, consistent, and continued throughout your lifetime. In other words, sustainable weight loss must involve behavioral changes.

THE FAR-REACHING BENEFITS OF REGULAR MOVEMENT

Regular and appropriate physical activity is essential to good health. When participating in moderate activity, stress is placed upon the body. Your body responds and adapts to this stress, ultimately enriching and enhancing overall health and performance. Body functions are improved and many body systems benefit. The cardiovascular system works more efficiently because of increased blood circulation as well as the oxygen and nutrients that are delivered to tissues. Regular physical activity can reduce your blood pressure and resting heart rate, your heart rate while awake but relaxed. Regular physical activity enhances energy levels and may increase endurance. The musculoskeletal system gains stronger bones, more limber and flexible joints, and increased muscle strength; all leading to decreased likelihood of injury.

In the most simplistic view, you need to expend more energy (calories) than you consume to lose weight, and consume and burn equal amounts of energy to maintain a weight. Regular physical activity expends energy, thus helping to maintain a healthy weight and reduce the risk of obesity. The greater the intensity of your exercise the more energy you will burn. In fact, research suggests that those who participate in high-intensity interval training expend energy up to nine times faster than those who participate in steady state cardio exercise—and your metabolism remains elevated for up to seventy-two hours following the activity.[472-475] Regular physical activity that includes strength training increases lean muscle mass, preserves bone and muscle density and mass, and helps you burn more energy while you aren't at the gym. The more lean muscle mass you have, the more calories you burn while at rest (increasing your basal metabolic rate, or BMR). Your BMR (metabolism) is the amount of energy your body requires to sustain normal function at rest. One pound of muscle will burn about six calories per day at rest, compared to only two calories per day with fat.

When you consume less energy than you expend, your body turns to stored fat for its energy requirements. In order to lose one pound of fat per week you must decrease your energy intake by about 3,500 calories, increase the amount of energy you burn by about 3,500 calories, or a combination of both. Regular physical activity helps your body use stored fat for energy rather than muscle. When weight loss occurs without the use of exercise, much of the weight lost is from excess water stores and muscle rather than fat.

Besides transporting oxygen and nutrients to cells, physical activity accelerates the body's natural detoxification process, to help remove accumulated waste products, poisons, and toxins. The lymph system's primary function is to circulate lymph fluid throughout the body to filters (lymph nodes and glands) that help eliminate these undesirable materials and foreign invaders. Unlike the heart, which pumps blood throughout the body, the lymph system has no pump and therefore requires movement in order to circulate and perform its vital function. So, if you aren't moving, your lymph system is functioning less than optimally and you may be accumulating a large store of toxins and waste.

Regular physical activity stimulates peristalsis—the rhythmic contraction of the bowel, moving bowel waste more quickly through the intestines. Deeper breathing during exercise improves cellular function, tissue oxygenation, and waste removal. Upon exhalation carbon dioxide is eliminated from tissues. Don't forget to shower to wash away any toxins you have removed through perspiration! Fatty tissues are a storage location for toxins and exercise helps reduce the amount of fatty tissue in the body, which diminishes storage space and releases toxins for elimination. In fact, regular physical activity temporarily increases the amount of toxins and free radicals within the body. Your body can increase oxygen utilization up to twenty times greater than while resting in response to intense physical activity. This breakdown and utilization of oxygen significantly increases the production of free radicals that can damage DNA, cells, and tissues. Fortunately your body has a built-in mechanism to defend against exercise-released free radicals. When free radicals are released during exercise your body adapts and increases growth factors and the production of enzymes that defend the cells against damage.[476,477] In other words, intense physical activity stimulates the body's innate antioxidant defense system. In addition, intense movement improves circulation, which in turn carries mobilized toxins to the elimination channels. Small amounts of toxins can exit through the skin via perspiration during intense movement. So it is important to drink plenty of water to assist the elimination channels in excreting toxins.

Physical activity will also release a flood of neurotransmitters and feel good endorphins—which are similar in structure to opiates like morphine. The release of endorphins may balance and enhance one's mood, as well as temporarily increase your pain threshold. This suggests that physical activity could possibly be utilized to assist those with chronic conditions that cause pain. The endorphins interact with receptors in the brain and block pain signals from nociceptors, specialized neurons that initiate the sensation of pain.

Physical activity decreases stress and helps maintain cognitive fitness. Cognitive fitness is an often overlooked aspect of well-being. But, your brain needs "exercise" to maintain optimal functioning just as much as your musculoskeletal, cardiovascular, and respiratory systems all need physical activity to work efficiently. Moderate to high intensity physical activity reduces blood cortisol levels, which may be the reason it helps relieve stress.[478] Moreover, physical activity relaxes tense muscles, which helps promote psychological relaxation and helps reduce anxiety. Experts suggest that regular physical activity may calm anxiety by elevating body temperature and increasing the number of neurons that release gamma-aminobutyric acid (GABA), a neurotransmitter involved in the regulation of anxiety. Physical activity has even demonstrated therapeutic effects for persons with mild to moderate depression.[479] We know physical activity releases endorphins, which can trigger sensations of joy and relaxation, but it also increases tryptophan levels.[480] Tryptophan is essential for the production of serotonin—a calming neurotransmitter that affects mood and social behavior, and is often deficient in depressed patients. Scientists attribute the antidepressant activity of regular physical activity to an increase in both tryptophan and serotonin.[481] Additionally, increased oxygen and blood flow exerts a positive effect on the central nervous system—the system that processes thoughts and emotions.

A growing body of evidence now suggests that those who engage in regular physical activity experience improved cognitive fitness and a reduced risk of Alzheimer's disease, even among those who have an increased genetic risk.[482-485] Researchers have discovered that participating in regular physical activity increases neurogenesis, the growth of new brain cells (neurons).[486,487] Brain neurons are responsible for thought and memory as well as myriad body functions that keep humans alive.

Regular physical activity improves not only quality, but quantity of life. Yes, being active can help you live longer! Research indicates that for every hour spent being active, life expectancy increases two hours—doubling your return on investment. Those who are physically active and are a normal weight may live 7.2 years longer than those who are inactive and obese.[488] A Swedish study indicated that men who routinely participated in physical activity decreased mortality rates.[489] Another study revealed women who utilized walking or cycling as transportation increased their average life span and quality of life.[490] So, again, you don't have to expend your energy in a gym, it can be as simple as walking. The research makes sense, as regular physical activity significantly enhances several key body systems, which encourages a healthy life span.

Moderate physical activity enhances immune system function by elevating hormone levels and immune cell activity. In fact, decreased incidence of illness and infection frequently is the result of moderate and regular physical activity. When we work our body at a greater intensity than usual our immune system is stimulated, actually making us feel better when we are sick. This may be why many believe they should "sweat out a cold." There is some truth to this belief because the heightened activity of the immune system, coupled with increased hormone levels, does make you feel better during and immediately following physical activity. However, following the physical activity, the immune system returns to a normal level and then slightly below normal. With the immune system mildly suppressed infectious agents may have an increased opportunity to cause illness. It is a good idea to avoid intense physical activity when you feel sick, though mild to moderate physical activity may be safe as long as you do not have a fever, severe chest congestion, extreme tiredness, or shortness of breath.

MAKE PHYSICAL ACTIVITY A WAY OF LIFE

All of these benefits can be yours without ever setting foot in a gym if you make physical activity a way of life. Adding regular activity throughout the day as you do everyday tasks—even if the tasks only get you active for one to two minutes at a time—is beneficial according to research. In fact, evidence suggests that the cumulative effect of short periods of activity as a part of routine daily behaviors can produce similar health effects to going to the gym for similar or greater amounts of time.[491] The key is to incorporate enough one- to two-minute regular daily activities to equal thirty minutes per day.

Many adults perceive that they don't have time to go to the gym, nor spend thirty or more consecutive minutes to be active each day. Going to a gym or track is not absolutely necessary to get your daily allotment of physical activity, and certainly most people can carve out a few minutes here and there throughout the day to be active. In fact, people are more likely to achieve the goals set forth in The Physical Activity Guidelines for Americans this way as opposed to those who attempt to meet the guidelines at a gym. Instead, seek out opportunities to be active throughout the day, such as:

- Walk around while talking on the phone.
- Do pushups and/or sit-ups during TV commercials.
- Take several breaks throughout the day to walk or run up and down stairs for a few minutes at a time.
- Walk the dog.
- Park in the farthest parking spot from the entrance to the grocery store.
- Choose the stairs instead of the elevator.
- Go to the bathroom at a restroom that is farther away from your office.
- Play with your children.
- Don't stay seated for more than thirty to sixty minutes.

When comparing sporadic activity accumulated throughout the day with sustained periods of physical activity, similar health benefits can be achieved,[492] including improved cardiovascular fitness,[493-495] reduced risk of metabolic syndrome,[496] weight reduction,[497,498] improved oxygen uptake,[499] and improved fatty acid profiles.[500] The evidence for accumulated activity is strong enough that in 2007 the American College of Sports Medicine and the American Heart Association updated their recommendations for physical activity to "Moderate-intensity aerobic activity...can be accumulated toward the thirty-minute minimum by performing bouts lasting ten or more minutes."[501] What we learn from these studies is that every minute of activity counts, and the key is to move and move often no matter how you do it.

THE POSSIBLE DANGERS OF ULTRA-ENDURANCE ACTIVITIES

While moderate physical activity may increase immune system activity both temporarily and long term, extreme or ultra-endurance activities can actually decrease immune system function over time.[502,503] Extreme physical activity causes the sustained release of significant levels of cortisol and adrenaline, the so-called "stress hormones." In addition significant numbers of free-radicals are released. Not only do these factors decrease immune system activity, they increase the risk for degenerative and chronic diseases.

Research suggests that ultra-endurance runners have an increased susceptibility to infection following competitive races and during intense training. A study of 2,311 Los Angeles marathon runners in 1987 revealed that almost 15 percent of the runners became ill after the race.[504] This is a rate five times higher than those who trained for but did not run the marathon. Another study that compared elite athletes, recreationally competitive athletes, and inactive persons as control subjects indicated that the recreationally competitive athletes were the least susceptible to upper respiratory infections. Of those participating in the study, 65.6 percent of the elite athletes experienced an upper respiratory infection compared to only 22.6 percent of recreationally competitive athletes.[505] Even the sedentary control group fared better with a 45 percent incidence of upper respiratory infections. Even more alarming, studies suggest that ultra-endurance athletes may experience temporary cardiac dysfunction following a competition. What researchers discovered is that the excess stress placed on the heart during these competitions can cause long-term abnormalities of right ventricle diastolic function, which is when the heart is in a period of relaxation and expansion.[506,507] It is obvious from these studies that athletes who routinely participate in ultra-endurance training and competitions are at greater risk for a dramatically impaired immune system and potential cardiac dysfunction. It can take up to seventy-two hours for the immune system to recover after ultra-endurance competitions, which leaves the immune system in an impaired state and the body more susceptible to illness during that period.

The three key types of physical activity are endurance, strength, and flexibility/balance. Because each has a unique set of benefits, all three are important for the maintenance of optimal health and should be incorporated into your life. The most important factor is that you choose one or several activities you enjoy and are willing to stick with. A variety of activities can make physical activity more interesting, not to mention successful.

GET YOUR HEART PUMPING WITH ENDURANCE ACTIVITIES

Endurance (also known as aerobic or cardio) activities are cardiovascular in nature, which means they involve the heart and blood vessels and increase the amount of oxygen in the blood. Endurance activities involve the repeated movement of large muscles for an extended period of time. Endurance activities provide the most benefit when participating in them for at least twenty to thirty continuous minutes and should be moderate to vigorous in nature to be most effective. A good way to know if you are working hard enough is to calculate your "target heart rate." To determine your target heart rate, first calculate your maximum heart rate, which is roughly 220 minus your age. Your target heart rate is the range between 60 and 85 percent of your maximum heart rate. For example if you are thirty years old, your maximum heart rate is 190 (220 − 30 = 190). Your target heart rate would be 114 to 161 (190 × .60 = 114 and 190 × .85 = 161.5). You should aim for two to three days a week of activity that is endurance in nature. Endurance activities include vigorous walking, swimming, running, elliptical, and cycling.

Endurance activities have many benefits. They increase stamina, reduce fatigue, stimulate immune system function—helping to ward off illnesses such as colds and flu—and reduce the risk of cardiovascular disease. The cardiovascular benefits are likely due to a reduction in blood pressure and LDL cholesterol in the arteries, combined with an increase in HDL cholesterol levels.[508,509] Through endurance activities, the heart becomes stronger and functions more efficiently. Endurance exercise promotes greater blood flow and widens the capillaries, which allows more oxygen to reach the muscles. Hearts that are conditioned to vigorous endurance activities have increased size and mass, after all the heart is a muscle too. The risk of chronic health conditions such as obesity, diabetes, and stroke may be reduced with participation in consistent endurance activity. Indeed, endurance activities have even been linked to reduced cancer risk in scientific research.[510,511,512] The Diabetes Prevention Program study demonstrated that walking five days per week for about thirty minutes decreased diabetes risk by 58 percent and improved insulin response, which suggests regular physical activity may reduce diabetes risk.[513] When combined with modest weight loss regular physical activity may reduce the risk of type 2 diabetes up to 58 percent among high-risk populations.[514]

STRENGTH TRAINING IS NOT JUST FOR BODYBUILDERS

Strength training, also called resistance or anaerobic activity, conditions the musculoskeletal system. Strength training improves tone and physical appearance as well as muscle endurance. Regular strength training increases muscle strength and size, improves bone health and density, and increases the strength of tendons and ligaments. Your muscles and bones will only give what you ask of them and if you allow them to be idle for too long muscles begin to atrophy[515] (partial or complete wasting away of muscles) and bones lose density (the amount of minerals stored in a section of bone).[516] In other words, your muscles adapt to the demands that are placed upon them and either become less capable and weak or stronger and more efficient. Strength training is a preventive measure against osteoporosis (a bone disease characterized by low bone strength and density and increased risk of fracture). At the very least it may help slow the rate at which bone density is lost.[517]

Many women are afraid of strength training because they mistakenly believe they will look too muscular if they participate. This is a myth and the reality is that strength training may be more important for women than men because they are at a greater risk for osteoporosis. Women and men don't need to follow different strength training programs either. An appropriate strength training program should be designed based on body size, ability, and strength level, not gender. Strength training has something for virtually everyone.

Physically inactive individuals may lose up to 8 percent of their muscle mass every decade after age thirty, whereas those who remain active may lose up to about 3 percent of muscle mass during the same time period—a conservation of 5 percent of muscle each year.[518] Over time this can lead to muscle wasting, poor stamina, muscle dysfunction (inability to contract), and loss of physical strength. In addition to strength training, consuming 25 to 30 g of high-quality protein per meal—about four ounces of chicken, three eggs, or six ounces of tuna—may reduce or eliminate this muscle loss.[519] You must strength train consistently to combat this trend. If you don't, you could potentially lose a significant amount of muscle by age fifty, leading to a reduction in the number of calories you burn each day.

Muscles are the force behind bodily movements and utilize energy to produce action. Sadly, we have come to accept the fact that at a certain age we should stop being active, almost as if we have earned the right to lounge in an easy chair. It is as if many choose to yield to old age rather than continue to enjoy life to its fullest. This notion is entirely false, with the very rare exception of physical challenges that may make movement more difficult. There are few reasons a person can't remain active and healthy through the so called "golden years," and many individuals choose to remain active well into their eighties and nineties. They may reduce the duration and intensity of the physical activity they engaged in when younger, but they remain active according to their capabilities and fitness level.

An important element in staying healthy throughout your life is strength training. If you don't regularly participate in strength training exercises, your muscles will slowly waste away and become weaker. Additionally, your metabolism will decrease, increasing your risk of carrying excess weight and becoming obese. So don't believe the myth that because you are increasing in age, you have to slow down completely. You should aim to maintain an active lifestyle throughout your entire life.

Besides the physical benefits of strength training there are also psychological benefits. A person who participates in strength training will generally be more physically fit resulting in a more appealing physical appearance. This can promote increased self-esteem and confidence. Why do you think gyms install so many mirrors on the walls? For example, a man who weighs 180 pounds with a body fat percentage of twenty-five is carrying forty-five pounds of fat. This will obviously show in his physique. In contrast, if he weighed the same but only had a body fat percentage of 15 percent he would only be carrying twenty-seven pounds of fat. Although his weight hasn't changed, his muscle tone, strength, metabolism, physical appearance, and overall well-being would all likely improve.

Most people think of and gravitate toward endurance activities when trying to lose weight. But anyone who has the desire to lose weight would be wise to investigate the benefits of strength training for weight loss. The evidence suggests that strength training combined with better eating is more effective than endurance activities combined with better eating when it comes to losing weight. Again, the more muscle one has, the more calories a person will burn while at rest. In addition, body fat percentage will decrease as muscle mass increases and metabolism is improved.

It is also detrimental to one's health to limit calorie intake without exercise. This attempt to lose weight by calorie cutting alone often results in muscle loss in addition to any fat that is lost. The end result is the person's metabolism is diminished and greater caloric restriction is necessary to maintain a desired weight. Simply stated, regular physical activity coupled with eating better is the healthiest way to lose weight.

An important aspect of strength training is to build up all the major muscle groups. Men like to show off a bulging chest and large biceps, but if efforts are only focused on these muscles it creates imbalance and increases the risk of injury. Each muscle has an opposing muscle that needs to be equally trained to create or maintain balance. When a muscle contracts, the opposing muscle lengthens and vice versa. Well-balanced muscles will be developed if the opposing muscle groups are trained. For example, the biceps, and triceps muscles are opposing muscles. If you train your biceps, you should also train your triceps.

When strength training is mentioned, most people will conjure up images of bodybuilders who spend hours in the gym. While this type of strength training is effective, you can strengthen and tone your muscles without any special equipment and in the comfort of your own home with only your body weight as resistance. For instance, to strengthen your calf muscles you can place the balls of your feet on stairs or a thick book, slowly raise your toes and then lower them as far as you can. Repeat this procedure until your calf muscles are fatigued. Go on to a different exercise and then eventually come back to the calf raises. One of the best strength training exercises for upper body tone and strength is push-ups. Push-ups strengthen the muscles in your arms, shoulders, upper back, and chest all in one movement. Planks, sit-ups, or leg raises are all great movements to improve core strength and tone your belly area. Therefore, you can't use the excuse that you can't afford a gym anymore. You have free strength training activities available in the comfort and convenience of your own home.

Another advantage of strength training is that it doesn't require significant time. You can effectively strengthen your muscles with metabolic resistance (or strength) training (MRT) in as little as twenty minutes, two to three times per week. MRT is designed to optimize your workout for fat loss, calorie burn, muscle gain, and improved tone in a minimal amount of time. Strengthening exercises that challenge multiple muscles at once are performed in a circuit at or near maximum effort with little rest between sets. When you participate in any strength training program, your muscles need time to rest and recover after each workout, so it is best to avoid working the same muscles on consecutive days.

Here are a few tips to properly strengthen your body:

■ Consult a health care professional and ensure you are in good health before you start any exercise program. It wouldn't hurt to receive some formal strength training instruction from a certified personal trainer to make certain you perform each movement or activity correctly.

■ Warm up and stretch before strength training.

■ Perform activities with a weight that fatigues your muscles after eight to twelve repetitions (called a set), but that you can perform three sets of. Gradually increase your weight as you progress.

■ Work all the major muscle groups to maintain proper muscle balance. Start your workout with your large muscles—quads, chest, glutes, hamstrings, back—and finish with smaller muscle groups—triceps, biceps, calves.

- Don't hold your breath while strength training. Doing so can increase blood pressure. Inhale when the muscle is resting and exhale when the muscle is working during each repetition.
- Stop immediately if you feel pain.
- Remember to drink moderate amounts of water to maintain hydration during your workout.
- Cool down after the session. This can be accomplished through stretching, which will also help prevent muscle soreness.

STRETCHING, FLEXIBILITY, AND BALANCE

Stretching is often thought of as an adjunct to other exercise routines, rather than a beneficial physical activity in and of itself. While it is important to stretch before and after a rigorous activity or an athletic competition, flexibility/balance activities carry their own list of benefits. Stretching increases the elasticity of tendons[520] and ligaments and enhances muscle flexibility, which improves the range of motion in your joints. This improves your balance and decreases your risk of injury. Stretching your muscles increases blood flow and circulation, which speeds muscle recovery. After a workout, muscles are fatigued and shortened. Stretching lengthens muscles and relaxes contracted muscles. Flexibility activities also relieve built-up muscle tension, promoting stress relief and relaxation.

Some experts estimate that up to 80 percent of the population suffers from low back pain. Stretching the muscles of the back may help provide much needed relief to lower back pain. Additionally, stretching increases the strength of the back muscles, which decreases the likelihood of injury. Don't forget to stretch the hamstrings, because they are attached to bones associated with back pain. An exercise ball is an excellent way to stretch and strengthen back muscles.

Some techniques to be aware of as you take part in flexibility exercises:

- Walk or jog in place to warm your muscles before stretching to avoid injury to cold muscles.
- Stretch and strengthen muscles you commonly use during everyday activities.
- Hold your stretches for at least thirty seconds and up to sixty seconds for problematic or tight areas.
- Work joints in a full range of motion but avoid painful stretches. If a stretch hurts, you are going too far.

- Don't bounce during stretches. Maintain a constant stretch on the muscle. Bouncing can create small tears in muscles and promotes scar tissue buildup and tight muscles.
- Strive to maintain equal flexibility on both sides of your body to promote balance.
- Remember to breathe.

When it comes to flexibility and balancing exercises, yoga is one of the most beneficial activities one can participate in. Originating in India about 5,000 years ago, Yoga involves learning physical poses, called asanas, which promote balance, proper breathing, increased strength and endurance, and flexibility. Yoga involves many styles, each with a specific focus, including relaxation and meditation, strength or power, endurance, and flexibility. Yoga is a complete exercise meaning it encompasses working the mind and body as one.

There are many benefits to yoga physically, emotionally, and mentally. Yoga increases flexibility and range of motion in joints. It stretches all soft tissues (tissues that connect, support, or surround structures and organs of the body, such as ligaments, tendons, and fascia, which surrounds muscles) of the body. Yoga is particularly beneficial for spinal pain and may even reduce the amount of medication required to relieve back pain.[521-523] Interestingly, yoga appears to affect mood and anxiety levels more than other forms of physical activity. Yoga stimulates specific areas of the brain, which results in an increased release of GABA, improved mood, and reduced anxious feelings.[524] Emerging research also suggests that yoga may be beneficial for sleep disorders and depression.[525]

Yoga improves muscle tone and strength. As you begin yoga, you will notice it requires great muscle strength and coordination to maintain balance. Yoga often engages muscles you don't normally use, or maybe didn't even know existed until they felt sore. Power yoga, called Ashtanga, is a form of yoga that focuses on muscle strength and improved stamina, and it may help improve athletic performance.

Yoga synchronizes breathing with movement, which promotes long and steady inhalations and exhalations through the nose. Yoga breathing is called pranayama, which literally means "life force control." Yoga breaths carry more oxygen to tissues and cells in the body and enhances their function and efficiency. As lung capacity improves, the respiratory system is strengthened, and sports performance is enhanced with deep, diaphragmatic breathing. Additionally, yoga breathing soothes the nervous system, calms the mind, and promotes relaxation. It may even help with respiratory conditions like asthma.[526,527]

Yoga is an anti-stress activity. Yoga decreases the production of stress hormones created by the adrenal glands, which increases relaxation and peace and reduces stress and depressive symptoms.[528] The meditation techniques used during yoga help clear the mind of stressful and worrisome thoughts and circumstances and may even improve concentration and focus. Many people report feeling happier and more satisfied after yoga. Yoga may also help you sleep better at night. Aging is associated with physiological changes that can result in changes in sleep patterns, including less sleep, decreased sleep quality, and interrupted sleep. Poor quality sleep later in life has been linked to the development of cognitive decline,[529] which makes quality and duration of sleep very important for the elderly. Adults over the age of sixty who participated in yoga twice per week for twelve weeks experienced improved overall sleep quality and duration, as well as decreased fatigue, depression, stress, anxiety, anger, and tension.[530] Based on these findings, yoga may be an excellent exercise for care centers to implement, particularly those that care for patients with neurological disorders, like dementia, Alzheimer's disease, and Parkinson's disease that are prone to sleep disturbances.

Proper posture is very important to avoid unnecessary strain on joints and muscles. The increased strength and flexibility achieved from regular participation in yoga improves posture—many asanas are aimed at strengthening your core, which is vital for good posture. Additionally, you will gain heightened body awareness, and avoid that slouchy posture common to the average person.

Physical activity is more effective and enjoyable when you take part in a variety of activities, instead of focusing on just one. It takes commitment and effort but the benefits are worth it. One way to stay committed is to find a partner to enjoy physical activity with. You can motivate each other as you work toward your goal to become more fit and improve overall well-being. You may also set yourself a goal with a reward for reaching that goal, be it a new dress, a new electronic gadget, or whatever you will find motivating. It is also important to choose activities that you enjoy and are willing to take part in—it's hard to participate in a physical activity if you dread it. You may wish to refer to the following information for typical energy/calorie expenditure per hour.

Activity	Energy/Calorie Costs/Hour*
Aerobic Dancing	546
Basketball (recreational)	450
Bicycling (5 mph)	174
Bicycling (13 mph)	612
Dancing (ballroom)	210
Football (touch, vigorous)	498

Activity	Energy/Calorie Costs/Hour*
Jogging (10 minute mile, 6 mph)	654
Racquetball	588
Sitting Quietly	84
Sleeping	90
Swimming crawl (20 yards/minute)	288
Swimming crawl (45 yards/minute)	522
Volleyball (recreational)	264
Walking (2 mph)	198

*Hourly estimates are based on values calculated for calories burned per minute for a 150-pound person.

Sources: William D. McArdle, Frank I. Katch, Victor L. Katch. *Exercise Physiology: Energy, Nutrition, and Human Performance* (2nd Edition). Lea & Febiger: Philadelphia, 1986.

Melvin H. Williams. *Nutrition for fitness and Sport.* William C. Brown Company Publishers: Dubuque, 1983.

5

Detoxification:
Your Body's Natural Housekeeper

Detoxification is an often ignored and overlooked essential step in health and healing. Detoxification is in reality a normal part of your body's daily routine. Every day your body eliminates or neutralizes toxins through the body's eliminative channels: the intestines, kidneys, liver, lungs, lymph, and skin. These eliminative channels work cooperatively and if any one system is working less than optimally, the others are forced to work harder to pick up the slack. When these systems are overloaded, detoxification may not operate efficiently. The notion of cleansing and detoxifying is not new but is one of the oldest traditions practiced throughout the ages and among all cultures. The only difference now is that it is more critical than ever before.

Detoxification should be an integral part of a health plan. A short detoxification is important at least twice per year, more often if necessary. It is common for people to cleanse with the seasons—spring, summer, fall, and winter. Others cleanse when they experience flare-ups in chronic illness symptoms, or when they feel their body needs to. Some indications that your body requires detoxification are:

- Excess mucous or congestion
- You become exhausted easily
- Frequent headaches
- Abnormal body odor
- Chemical or environmental sensitivities

- Digestive disorders
- Skin rashes

Never in recorded history has humankind been exposed to so many chemicals and harmful substances as now. The body must detoxify industrial chemicals and pollutants, pesticides, food additives, heavy metals, and drugs, just to name a few. Humans are exposed to a plethora of toxins every day through water, air, personal care products, household cleaners, and more. Unfortunately, research is indicating these chemicals are more influential in disease, especially cancer, than previously thought.[531] Accumulated toxins can disrupt hormone production, encourage genetic alterations, and disturb the cells from organizing into healthy tissues. The superfluity of toxins we are exposed to is having a severe detrimental impact on our health. Our bodies are simply being overloaded with toxins, which makes the eliminative organs struggle to maintain normal detoxification processes.

When your body is exposed to a toxic or harmful substance, it attempts to protect itself by flushing it out through the urine or feces. If the body is unable to expel the substance, the body will surround it with fatty tissue or mucous and store it in fatty deposits. This is likely a major factor in the increased cancer mortality rates among overweight and obese individuals—52 percent higher for overweight men and 62 percent higher for overweight women.[532] When your body burns or releases fat for energy or during physical activity, these toxins can be released for expulsion from the body. This is why those who go on a diet or exercise after a long hiatus often experience feelings of sickness. Another way these toxins are released is through deep tissue massage, which makes it very important to drink large quantities of water immediately after a massage to flush these toxins out of the body quickly.

The body's internal detoxification mechanism is designed to remove toxins before they have a chance to make us sick. Unfortunately, the body's systems of elimination are heavily burdened and overloaded, which make it difficult for them to properly protect us from toxins. Detoxification should be performed a few times per year. This practice may well be one of the most critical steps in disease prevention and health promotion.

THE LIVER: THE PRIMARY DETOXIFIER

The liver is the primary organ of detoxification and the largest internal organ of the body. Substances absorbed by the intestines pass through the liver before they enter general circulation. Our health largely depends on the optimal functioning of this critical organ. The liver filters the blood to remove bacteria, endotoxins, immune system by-products, and various other substances. Caffeine, alcohol, hormones, histamine, drugs, and other chemicals are neutralized by the liver's enzymatic processes. The liver also manufactures bile, which serves as a transportation system to neutralize and eliminate cholesterol and other fat-soluble toxins.

The liver works in two phases. Phase I neutralizes or modifies the toxins in preparation for removal from the body through a series of enzymatic reactions. The enzymes involved in this process are collectively known as cytochrome P450 pathway. Cytochrome P450 uses free radicals in order to neutralize harmful substances. If this system becomes overactive, it can produce excess free radicals, which can result in harmful health effects. Sufficient antioxidants are very important during Phase I detoxification to offset the production of free radicals. Phase II detoxification binds these neutralized or modified toxins and makes them less harmful and prepares them for excretion. This process is called conjugation.

Fat-soluble toxins like heavy metals and pesticides are very difficult for the body to remove. Fat soluble toxins are primarily excreted through the bile, but a significant portion of the bile and the toxins it contains are reabsorbed. For this reason the body uses glutathione to help convert fat-soluble toxins into water-soluble ones, for easier excretion through the kidneys and urine.

ELIMINATION OF TOXINS THROUGH THE BOWEL

The intestines include the small and large intestine (or bowel). The bowel's primary purpose in detoxification is to receive the bile acids and toxin mixture for elimination. The intestines and bile require sufficient fiber and water to perform optimally and eliminate efficiently. Without adequate fiber most of the bile will be reabsorbed, including the toxins bound to it. Adequate fiber also helps the intestines perform their other responsibility, which is to remove mucous. If mucous is not removed, it provides an excellent breeding ground for bacteria to cultivate. A healthy bowel will produce at least one bowel movement per day, two to three is even better.

Another way to assist the removal of toxins through bowel movements is with bentonite clay. Bentonite clay is edible clay that supports the intestinal system by absorbing water and toxins to create a gel like substance that is then carried out of the colon. It is believed that forms of clay have been used for thousands of years by indigenous societies around the world for eliminative purposes.

THE KIDNEYS: ESSENTIAL FILTERS

The kidneys are two fist-sized, bean-shaped organs that sit below the rib cage, one on each side of the spine. They filter almost 200 quarts of blood each day, of which approximately two quarts of waste products and water are removed to be excreted in the urine. The kidneys neutralize many toxins after they are made water soluble by the liver, through filtration and urine excretion. Just as adequate water is essential to proper intestinal function, adequate water is critical to proper kidney function. The kidneys provide hormones and enzymes to regulate blood cell production (erythropoietin), blood pressure (renin) and regulate blood pH.

THE SKIN: THE LARGEST ORGAN OF DETOXIFICATION

The skin is the largest organ of detoxification. Just as toxins can enter through the skin, they can also exit through it in small quantities. Heavy metals, phthalates, and fat-soluble toxins are released via perspiration.[533,534] One method to stimulate the skin's detoxification process is by skin brushing. This process removes old skin cells and opens up pores for enhanced detoxification through the skin. Skin brushing is also thought to stimulate blood and lymph circulation. All you need to do is use a natural bristle skin brush on dry skin and brush your skin in a circular motion so that all brush strokes move toward the center of your chest. Regular physical activity and alternating hot and cold showers stimulates perspiration and boosts detoxification through the skin. Saunas do increase perspiration, though there is debate whether this helps release toxins through the skin or only mobilizes toxins from fat cells and into the bloodstream.

EXPULSION OF TOXINS THROUGH THE LUNGS

Our lungs don't just provide us the oxygen we need for life. They are also a critical organ of detoxification because they are the first organs exposed to harmful substances through inhalation. The lungs help discard the waste that occurs through normal metabolic processes. Deep breathing, breathing that raises your diaphragm, promotes optimal lung function and efficient use of your air supply. When you inhale large quantities of oxygen, it supplies oxygen to the blood and tissues, which promotes healing and displaces harmful gases. Deep breathing should be practiced daily (preferably in a non-polluted environment) for optimal lung health and detoxification.

The lymph system is an important part of your body's immune system that consists of a network of nodes (glands), ducts, vessels, and organs. The lymph system includes the tonsils, spleen, adenoids, and thymus. The tonsils and adenoids act as filters to remove debris and antigens that have entered the body. Unfortunately, the tonsils and adenoids are frequently removed. This removal leaves the individual with a less than whole immune system. The lymph nodes are located throughout the body and also act as filters for debris, abnormal cells, and harmful organisms. Behind the sternum is the thymus gland, which is larger in infants than adults because it shrinks as we age. Its primary function is to process and store special immune cells called T-lymphocytes. These specialized immune cells regulate the immune system's response to cells that have been affected or damaged by harmful substances. The spleen acts as a quality control center for red blood cells and also filters blood and houses lymphocytes that attempt to destroy pathogens that pass through.

THE LYMPH SYSTEM: AN OVERLOOKED DEBRIS FILTER

As was mentioned earlier, the lymph system does not have a pump and therefore requires stimulation for effective function. Movement and physical activity stimulate the lymph system and help it to work more efficiently. Another way to stimulate the lymph system is through lymphatic massage, a technique intended to encourage the natural drainage of the lymph.

It is possible to restrict lymph flow through wearing tight underwear, pants, or bras because of the location of nodes and ducts within the armpit, between the breasts, and in the groin. Some research has indicated that women who wear their bras twenty-four hours a day are significantly more likely to develop breast cancer than those who don't wear them at all.[535] This is likely the result of improper fitment, not just wearing a bra. It is very important to wear a proper fitting bra and it wouldn't hurt to consider lymphatic breast massage to promote breast health. Lymphatic breast massage is a technique designed to move lymph out of the breast so that toxins can be filtered through the lymph system for removal. This practice is believed to help reduce the risk of breast cancer.

The four main types of toxins that the elimination channels must defend us against are heavy metals, chemical toxins, microbial compounds, and the breakdown products of protein metabolism. A toxin is defined as any harmful substance that has a detrimental effect on the functioning and viability of living organisms. While some toxins have negligible effects, others can lead to a wide range of symptoms including death.

HEAVY METALS

The accumulation of the heavy metals, including aluminum, arsenic, cadmium, lead, mercury, and nickel, can lead to serious illness and in some cases death. The industrialized world has increased the presence of these toxins in our air, soil, and even drinking water. They are so prevalent that it is virtually impossible to avoid exposure to them. Few statistics are available to accurately portray just how widespread heavy metal poisoning is; however, it is likely that a significant number of the world's population has accumulated enough of these toxins to have detrimental effects on health.

The best solution to reduce the ill health effects of heavy metals is to limit exposure to them as much as possible. Avoid mercury dental amalgams and fish that contain high levels of mercury (or limit their consumption to twice weekly). Drink clean filtered water. Drinking lots of water helps provide sufficient urine for harmful substances to be eliminated more efficiently, as well as promotes frequent bowel movements. Avoid industrial areas and inhalation of industrial pollution when possible. Eat organic produce. In addition, a high-potency multivitamin and mineral will help your body deal with this onslaught of heavy metals by supplying nutrients and antioxidants for your body's detoxification systems to work more efficiently.

THE HARMFUL EFFECTS OF HEAVY METALS EXPOSURE

Aluminum exposure is widespread and a significant threat to human health. We are exposed to aluminum in our canned foods and beverages, processed foods, cookware, antiperspirants, and antacids. Aluminum can enter the body through ingestion, inhalation, and even skin contact. It appears that aluminum must be retained in the body in greater quantities than other heavy metals to have toxic effects; though accumulation through repeated, long-term exposure to small amounts is also a concern. Aluminum exposure can cause skeletal and neuromuscular problems[536] as well as brain degeneration.[537,538] High levels of aluminum can leach calcium from bones and make them more susceptible to fracture.

Arsenic is a naturally occurring compound found throughout the environment. Meat, fish, and poultry account for 80 percent of all arsenic exposure from food—one more reason to limit meat consumption. Exposure is possible in drinking water and secondhand smoke as well. It is known to cause cancer in humans, including lung, skin, bladder, liver, and kidney cancer. Once ingested, arsenic accumulates in almost all organs of the body. Acute poisoning—poisoning caused by a single exposure or multiple exposures during a short period of time—is a medical emergency because it can result in internal bleeding, inflammation of the heart, and kidney failure. It has been shown to cause diarrhea, nausea, abdominal pain, central and peripheral nervous system disorders, skin and mucous membrane irritation, anemia, peripheral neuropathy, skin lesions, and kidney and liver damage.[539]

Cadmium is an extremely poisonous element commonly found in manufacturing facilities where car batteries are made or where ore is smelted and processed. Low levels of this element are found in many foods, with the highest concentration being found in shellfish, kidney, and liver meats. Exposure also occurs from smoking, through some drinking waters, and from living in close proximity to industries that process cadmium. Even trace amounts of this metal can produce unhealthy effects. Acute inhalation may result in long lasting impairment of lung function, while chronic exposure can result in kidney, lung, liver, bone, immune system, blood, and nervous system damage.[540] Cadmium is also a known human carcinogen.

Lead is naturally found in the earth's crust. It is abundant in the environment due to the burning of fossil fuels, mining, and the manufacture of batteries, ammunition, and other lead products. Individuals who live in older homes are often exposed to lead in their drinking water (from the lead solder in their water pipes) and lead-based paints used during that time period. Lead exposure also occurs through contaminated soil, some metal jewelry, lead dust, food additives, and some imported foods sealed in cans with lead solder. Virtually every organ in the body is affected by lead poisoning, the nervous system being the most significantly affected. High levels of lead can lead to severe kidney and brain damage and even death. Lead can result in miscarriage and is detrimental to newborns. Lead is more harmful to young children than adults and can cause arrested development and learning difficulties in children. It may also result in damage to the male sex organs.

Mercury is widespread in the environment and predominantly comes in three forms: organic (contaminated fish, thiomersal, fumes from burning coal), inorganic (batteries, some disinfectants, chemistry labs), and elemental (thermometers, dental fillings, fluorescent bulbs). All mercury is toxic, though some forms are more dangerous than others. Mercury is frequently injected in our children through the use of thiomersal and other mercury containing preservatives in vaccines. It is commonly consumed from marine life—tuna, swordfish, king mackerel, tilefish, shark, and shellfish. Mercury containing dental amalgams and some medical devices and treatments are other sources of human exposure. The brain and nervous system are both very susceptible to the detrimental effects of mercury. High levels of mercury can cause irreversible brain and kidney damage. Acute exposure to high levels may result in lung damage, nausea, increased blood pressure, and eye irritation.

Nickel is an abundant odorless and tasteless natural element. Nickel exposure can occur from smoking, drinking water, skin contact, nickel jewelry, and foods that contain traces of nickel (beer, figs, tea, coffee, and some nuts). Many people are sensitive to or have allergic reactions when exposed to nickel, which may result in a skin rash or an asthma attack. Respiratory difficulty and increased lung and nasal cancers have also been reported from nickel exposure.

CHEMICAL TOXINS

Chemical toxins are primarily processed by the liver. They include toxic chemicals, solvents, cleaning materials, drugs, alcohol, pesticides, herbicides, formaldehyde, and food additives. There are literally thousands of these chemicals making it almost impossible to avoid exposure. Humans are exposed to these chemicals through skin absorption, ingestion, or inhalation of fumes. Given this long list, the liver has an awesome burden to detoxify an overabundance of harmful chemicals.

Long-term and repeated exposure to chemicals may cause the body to become overwhelmed and unable to eliminate them all. When this overload occurs acute and chronic illness may emerge. Unfortunately, of the thousands of chemicals currently in use, few have been tested for the possible adverse health effects they may cause. Symptoms of chemical overload include headache, mental illness or confusion, and impaired nervous system function. Many chemical toxins suppress immune function allowing harmful microorganisms to infest the body. Some of these chemicals, called endocrine-disrupting chemicals, have been implicated in reduced fertility in both men and women, decreased thyroid function, and suspected as contributors to breast and prostate cancer.[541] Some of these chemicals are even more harmful when combined together.

To reduce exposure to chemicals:

- Choose organic foods.
- Rinse produce thoroughly before consumption, or clean with a natural produce wash.
- Use natural cleaning agents like baking soda, lemon juice, essential oils, and vinegar in place of chemical-laced household cleaners.
- Reduce aerosol product usage.
- Don't consume alcohol or consume it sparingly to reduce the load on the liver.
- Avoid warming or cooking foods in the microwave in plastic containers or with plastic wrap over the container (use a plate with a paper towel as a cover instead).
- Use non-chlorine bleach.
- Use borax and washing soda instead of chemical laundry detergents.

MICROBIAL COMPOUNDS

Microbial compounds are toxins produced by bacteria and yeast inside the gut. These compounds have been implicated in numerous diseases including cancer. One way to reduce exposure is to eat plenty of fiber, which increases peristalsis—the rhythmic contractions of the bowel to promote a bowel movement. When peristalsis is increased, toxins are moved through the bowel more quickly so that harmful substances are in contact with the intestinal wall for shorter periods of time and absorption of these substances is reduced. Fiber also helps promote a healthy intestinal bacteria environment, and encourages the growth of healthy bacteria.

Common microbial compounds include:

- Endotoxins (a toxin present in the outer membranes of bacterial cell walls that is released when the cell dies).
- Exotoxins (a toxin formed and secreted by a microorganism).
- Toxic amines.
- Toxic derivatives of bile.
- Carcinogenic (cancer causing) substances.

HOW TO AID YOUR BODY'S NATURAL DETOXIFICATION PROCESSES

Detoxification provides many benefits besides the obvious benefit of removing harmful substances from the body. It may improve certain health conditions aggravated or initiated by toxins. It helps clear the digestive tract of accumulated waste and harmful substances within the waste. Immune system function may be restored or enhanced. Detoxification can reduce congestion, fermentation, and excess mucous. The eliminative organs of the body have their heavy burdens lightened. Last, detoxification removes accumulated toxins and waste that may help prevent future disease and illness from occurring.

Detoxification is often performed by simply consuming only fresh fruit and vegetable juices for one to three days (called a juice fast). Serious health problems may require longer cleanses. Add plant foods that contain rich sources of nutrients like spirulina, chlorella, and wheat grass during a cleanse to provide the body ample nutrients. There are also various herbs that support the elimination systems and organs as well as promote urination and bowel elimination, such as garlic, dandelion, mullein, hawthorn berry, psyllium, ginger, yarrow, celery seed, burdock root, and red clover. Additional methods of detoxification that are beneficial include:

- Colonic irrigation cleanses the large intestine with purified water, herbs, or other cleansing agents. In addition to its action on body detoxification, this practice is intended to improve metabolism, prevent diseases of the colon, improve gastrointestinal system function, aid peristalsis, and encourage weight loss.

- Chelation therapy involves the use of binding agents, orally or intravenously, to bind to toxins and flush them out. Chelation therapy provides a number of benefits like reduced free radical damage, improved cardiovascular function through the removal of calcium and plaque in the arteries, enhanced energy levels, balanced hormone levels, and improved psychological well-being.

- Hydrotherapy is commonly used to aid detoxification. It involves the external use of hot and/or alternating cold water to stimulate the release of toxins through the elimination systems. The release of toxins by hydrotherapy can be enhanced through the addition of Epsom salts. Hydrotherapy dramatically enhances elimination of toxins, encourages relaxation of tense muscles, helps hydrate the cells, improves metabolism, and increases blood supply to the organs, which helps them function more efficiently.

- Physical activity helps your body detoxify through increased perspiration and blood circulation. It also promotes regular bowel function and waste elimination. Movement transports lymph throughout the body to help remove debris through the lymph nodes. Last, toxins are often stored in fatty tissue within the body. Regular physical activity helps reduce fatty tissue and the amount of real estate for toxins to be stored in.

6

Optimizing Mental, Spiritual, and Emotional Health

The mind, emotions, body, and spirit are intimately interconnected, and optimal health cannot be achieved without a focus on all four aspects. The primary problem with Western medicine is that each of these aspects of health are treated by different practitioners. The body is treated by a physician, the mind by a therapist, and the spirit through an ecclesiastical leader. The spirit, mind, and emotions are largely ignored, but a keen focus on these aspects is required to realize optimal health and wellness. In fact, our emotions affect our physical, mental, and spiritual aspects of well-being so profoundly it may be the foundation of overall wellness.

More and more evidence suggests that emotions and spirituality are a significant factor in, and powerful influencer of health and wellness. When we feel happy, have a positive attitude, and positive self-esteem we establish an environment where health and wellness can thrive. Conversely, if we are unhappy, pessimistic, and think of ourselves poorly, we create an atmosphere for ill health to flourish. It is simply unwise to overlook the affect both emotional and spiritual well-being has on physical health.

A physical cause of death such as invasion by a microorganism or clogged arteries may be detected; however, there may also be a secondary cause that is psychological or mind oriented. There have been numerous cases of someone staying alive "on their death bed" or on the brink of death because of an important upcoming event such as a birthday, holiday, or anniversary. This is one side of the psychological effect, where someone appears to be willing themselves alive.

The other side of the psychological effect results in death or illness. A study conducted by UC Irvine demonstrated that those who experienced acute stress after the 9/11 attacks on the United States had a 53 percent increase in the incidence of cardiovascular ailments during the three years following the event.[542] This was true despite the fact that the study excluded other cardiovascular disease risk factors such as smoking. Another example is the Iraqi Scud missile attacks on Israel during the Gulf War (1990 to 1991). Approximately one dozen Israeli citizens died not from the physical missile strikes but from fear of being killed by a missile. Hundreds of others were admitted to the emergency room for various complaints and listed as "psychological casualties." Meaning, they had not been exposed to any missile fragments or chemical agents, they simply were stressed and frightened into physical symptoms.

Physical symptoms and illness such as digestive disturbances, sleep troubles, decreased immune system activity, and cardiovascular problems can all have an emotional connection. A person may be predisposed to a health problem, but the catalyst of the disease may be an emotional stimuli. Did you ever wonder why so many people were sick around final exams in high school or college? Stress actually makes you more susceptible to whatever virus is going around because it suppresses the immune system. Ever wonder why people who always seem to be happy, tend to be healthier? They have learned that a positive attitude and including joy in life promotes health.

If you want to achieve optimal health and wellness, you can't overlook the power of the human mind. Because the mind, body, and spirit are interconnected they must all be a focus of a suitable health and wellness plan. Indeed, the brain (or mind) is the governor and regulator of all body functions. If you don't nourish your mind, you may just lose control. You can't achieve optimal physical health without optimal spiritual and emotional health, and vice versa. The following are valuable strategies to establish mental, emotional, and spiritual wellness:

1. Reduce and learn to manage stress.
2. Participate in relaxation techniques.
3. Maintain an optimistic attitude.
4. Maintain high self-esteem and a positive self-image.
5. Learn to laugh.
6. Maintain meaningful relationship(s).
7. Get adequate sleep.

REDUCE AND LEARN TO MANAGE STRESS

Stress is unavoidable, an almost daily occurrence. Everyone faces challenges and situations that have the potential to create a stress response each day. The difference is how people react to these situations. Some thrive and learn from stressful experiences, while others experience a multitude of physical and emotional effects. The American Psychological Association estimates that up to 90 percent of doctors' office visits are stress related.[543] This is an amazing and eye-opening statistic that further bolsters the unequivocal connection between all four areas of health. To achieve optimal health, stress must be reduced and managed appropriately.

Stress is defined as a state when an organism perceives the demands placed on it are greater than it can handle. A stressor is any stimulus that causes stress to an organism. The organism's response to the stressor is the stress response. Eustress is positive stress (not all stress is bad). Eustress allows us to adapt to challenging situations and provides opportunities for growth.

Dr. Hans Selye pioneered stress research and described our response to stress, whether negative or positive, as the general adaptation syndrome (GAS). He also identified three stages of the GAS. First is the alarm stage, where the body prepares to fight or run. Stress hormones (adrenaline, noradrenaline, and cortisol) are released by the adrenal glands during the alarm stage to prepare the body for fight-or-flight. In response to elevated hormone levels, heart rate and blood pressure increase, the respiratory capacity and rate may increase, the eyes dilate, nutrient stores are released and broken down for energy, and muscle tone and performance is elevated. In addition, the body shuts down or limits certain body functions that are not considered necessary to respond to the threat, such as the immune, digestive, and reproductive systems; and all growth processes are suppressed. The resistance stage is next, where the body continues in a state of readiness, but to a lesser extent than during the alarm stage. Finally, the body reaches the exhaustion stage in which the body is no longer able to maintain the constant state of readiness.

Once a threat is neutralized the body should reverse this process and return all body systems and functions to a normal state. Conversely, if the body remains in a constantly elevated stress response the body is set up in a perfect biochemical and biological environment for disease and ill health to take place. The stress response is an innate function, the purpose of which is to enable us to protect ourselves from harm. However, our bodies can't continue efficient function under the constant demand of stress.

Short-term (acute) stress results in the body's immediate responses mentioned above. Long-term (chronic) stress can exacerbate or generate a plethora of health effects. Stress is involved in arrhythmia, high-blood pressure, headache, nausea, diarrhea, fatigue, heart attack, tightness in the back or neck, irritability, excess anger, anxiety, ulcer, irritable bowel disorder, decreased fertility, poor sleep, propensity to alcohol or drugs, asthma, acne, forgetfulness, substandard judgment, poor productivity, and carelessness just to name several. It is also associated with cancer, cardiovascular disease, premature aging, and autoimmune disorders. Stress not only makes you more susceptible to illness, it can also make the symptoms of chronic illnesses worse.

It should be clear by now how important it is to limit and manage stress effectively. It may just save your life!

Stress reduction and management techniques include:

1. **Identify your sources of stress.** Determine your stressors so you can deal with them more appropriately. It helps you to understand what causes your stress so you can avert or reduce these events as much as possible. You can also determine better solutions to cope with these situations when they arise before you are faced with them.

2. **Change the situation or change your response.** Find positive ways to deal with stress. Smoking, drinking alcohol, and overeating are all unhealthy ways to deal with stress. Try healthy techniques like avoiding the person or situation when possible, or change the way you respond. Look for the positive in stressful situations to avoid self-inflicted stress. View challenges as opportunities for growth.

3. **Accept the things you can't control or change.** There is no sense in stressing over situations or events that are out of your control. Focus instead on what you can control and discover better ways to cope with those events or situations. Avoid perfectionism. As an alternative focus on your good qualities.

4. **Know your limits.** Don't "bite off more than you can chew." If you over-commit, you invite unnecessary stress. Learn to accept your limits. Don't compare yourself with others or create competition, instead compare yourself only against yourself. Manage your time better to avoid self-inflicted schedule stress. Make sure you take the time to do something you enjoy every day even if it's only for ten to fifteen minutes.

5. **Express and acknowledge your emotions.** Keeping all of your emotions stowed away builds up pressure that eventually will explode, usually in a time and manner we don't wish. Find someone you can talk with openly and share your feelings with regularly. Forgive others and yourself. Eliminate grudges and don't harbor unkind feelings because ultimately this only hurts you.

6. **Relax.** Find ways to unwind and relax, have fun, or do something you enjoy. This should be a daily activity.
7. **Maintain a healthy lifestyle.** Eat a healthy diet. Drink plenty of water. Regularly participate in physical activity—you need the endorphins! Avoid stimulants. Get adequate rest.
8. **Set realistic goals and priorities.** If you set goals you can't achieve, you add a great deal of stress to your life. Set challenging goals that you have to stretch to reach, but that you are confident you can achieve. People often get stressed when things don't turn out the way they intended. If you have a setback, reset the goal and don't dwell on it. Everyone "fails." It is reported that Thomas Edison failed to invent the light bulb thousands of times before he finally achieved success. The difference was that he looked at these "failures" as learning experiences. He didn't give up when he failed; he remained focused on his goal. If your results are different than your desires, you did not fail, you permitted yourself a learning experience. Don't let the fear of failure blind your ability to realize your dreams and steal your victory. Instead, claw, fight, battle, and use every ounce of your strength and desire to defend your dreams, seize your success, and release the amazing potential you have within. Only if you give up, do you truly fail.
9. **Take anti-stress supplements.** Your daily high-potency multivitamin and mineral is a good place to start to avoid stress-caused nutrient depletion. The B vitamins are regularly depleted in individuals who experience chronic stress, so take ample amounts (those in the optimum range) to keep them replenished. Other supportive supplements include kava, lemon balm, lavender essential oil, and L-theanine.

JUST RELAX

Relaxation techniques include a wide variety of calming methods and practices. It is deliberately letting go of tension and stored negative emotions with the intent to create peace and inner tranquility. These techniques can be used to relieve anxiety, stress, depression, and create a sense of emotional well-being. The effects of relaxation are both physiological and psychological in nature.

A person who is relaxed will generally have reduced blood pressure, normal heart and breathing rates, and eased muscle tension. The relaxation response is the exact opposite of the stress response. It slows heart rate, lowers blood pressure, and balances stress hormone levels. Many physiological conditions can be improved or alleviated through relaxation, including chronic pain, headache, cardiovascular disease, premenstrual syndrome symptoms, and digestive disorders. Some research even indicates relaxation may help ward off illness—particularly those strongly associated with stress like anxiety, asthma, depression, cardiovascular disease, and menopausal symptoms.

Mental clarity, improved concentration, and reduced negative emotions can all be achieved through proper relaxation techniques. A clear mind can help one focus on what is important at that very moment, instead of past trauma or future trials. It is possible to retrain the brain and eliminate bad habits using relaxation techniques. Emotions can also be tempered to decrease anger, anxiety, and frustration.

Relaxation is an essential part of any optimal health and wellness plan. Some of the easiest techniques to learn and implement without the assistance of others are prayer, meditation, breathing exercises, visualization, and progressive muscle relaxation.

Prayer is a very personal and powerful experience practiced in some form by virtually all organized religions. It is the act of reverent communication with God. According to a 2013 Pew Research survey more than half (55 percent) of Americans pray on a daily basis.[544] Praying to our Creator is a wonderful experience and can often grant us peace and comfort. Prayer requires faith, hope, concentration, and sometimes persistence.

Scientific efforts to determine the actual power of prayer have proved inconclusive for decades. However, research suggests that prayer helps reduce blood pressure, heart rate, and anxiety levels in cancer patients,[545] and improves depression and anxiety overall.[546,547] Prayer creates focus on a desired outcome or objective. It can be on behalf of someone else (known as distant healing) or a personal petition. The reality is, communication with God can elicit a relaxation response, provide comfort, and has proven an effective remedy for numerous illnesses whether as an adjunct or single-handedly. Whether you are a member of an organized religion, or not, the power of daily prayer should not be underestimated or overlooked.

Meditation has been practiced for thousands of years as a relaxation technique. It is often associated with Buddhism, though it is practiced regardless of religious affiliation by thousands of people. Science has explored the connection between meditation and stress and discovered that meditation decreases cortisol levels in the blood,[548] and thus is useful for stress reduction. In fact, one study reported that the more meditation training a person participated in the greater the influence on the endocrine system and cortisol levels.[549] It also profoundly affects the brain. Meditation has been linked to an increase in alpha brain waves—which are associated with a relaxed state—and improved ability to concentrate.[550] Meditation has also been associated with increased creativity.[551] Meditation involves focused attention to produce a deep state of relaxation and a tranquil mind. It allows one to focus on the present and eliminate the clutter of thoughts and pressures that exist in our daily lives. It helps reduce destructive emotions and creates a sense of balance and self-awareness.

The six steps to meditation:

1. Choose a quiet and tranquil spot where you can be alone and undisturbed. Yes, this means you have to turn off your cell phone and unplug from other distracting electronic devices.
2. Sit in a comfortable position.
3. Close your eyes and breathe deeply.
4. Focus your attention on your breathing. Become aware of your abdomen rising and falling.
5. Clear all thoughts and emotions from your mind and continue your breathing awareness. Don't allow anything or anyone to distract your attention. If you begin to be distracted, refocus on your breathing.
6. Continue this until you feel deeply relaxed.

Deep breathing may actually be the fastest way to achieve a relaxed state of mind and body. You can ensure you breathe deeply by doing the following: Place your hand on your abdomen and ensure that it rises and falls with each breath. If not, you are breathing too shallow and mostly from your chest.

Breathing should be predominantly accomplished through the nose, not the mouth. The nose has defense mechanisms in place (hairs and glands) to prevent the entrance of foreign invaders when you breathe. Breathing through the nose also helps maintain the correct balance of oxygen and carbon dioxide. Breathing through the mouth tends to be quick and shallow, while nasal breathing can be more controlled.

Each deep breath allows oxygen to reach all the cells of the body. Oxygen purifies the blood stream and stimulates cognitive function (the brain uses and requires the greatest amount of oxygen). More oxygen enhances the function of digestion, the nervous system, glands, and organs. Deep breathing is essential and should be practiced every day for at least three to five minutes.

Basic Deep Breathing Steps:

1. Breathe in deeply through your nose with your mouth closed until your lungs are filled to capacity.
2. Exhale through your nose slowly.

3. Repeat the process, consciously raise your abdomen on inhale and pull your abdomen in toward your spine on exhale.

Left and Right Brain Balance Breathing Technique:

1. Place your right thumb over your right nostril and your right pointer finger over your left nostril.
2. Close your right nostril with your thumb and inhale deeply and slowly.
3. At the peak of your inhalation, release your right thumb to reopen your right nostril as you simultaneously close your left nostril with your pointer finger and exhale through your right nostril slowly.
4. On the next inhalation, keep your left nostril closed and inhale through your right nostril.
5. Release your pointer finger as you seal your right nostril with your thumb (again at the peak of the inhalation) and exhale through your left nostril
6. Repeat this process three to ten times.
7. Then complete the basic deep breathing technique three times.

Visualization is an experience of guided thoughts to lead your body and mind to a relaxed and contemplative state. You can direct your thoughts through a recorded voice, a script, or a live person. The intent is to create images and thoughts that appear real, not imaginary. As you focus your attention on the picture being painted in your mind, you draw further into the scene and become more relaxed. Your body physically responds to the mental imagery being portrayed.

Visualization involves creating a mental image of a calm, peaceful, and safe place. Images and words are used to promote a deep sense of relaxation and well-being. It is an excellent anti-stress tool. At first you will require help to practice visualization (also known as guided imagery). This can be accomplished through recordings of trained professionals. Once you become comfortable with the process, you will be able to reach deep relaxation much more quickly and may even be able to create your own recording to practice this important process.

Visualization is often united with positive affirmations. Once people reach a state of complete relaxation and focus, they state positive beliefs or desires. This can be used to help achieve goals, break bad habits, increase self-esteem, or promote healing. Visualization has even been used in cancer treatment, where patients imagine the attack and destruction of cancer cells within the body by white blood cells. Indeed studies have confirmed that visualization can enhance immune system activities, particularly natural killer cell function.[552]

Progressive muscle relaxation (PMR) was developed by Dr. Edmund Jacobsen. It involves moving sequentially from one major muscle group to another, consciously tensing and relaxing muscles. A group of muscles is tensed tightly. While the muscles are contracted as tightly as possible, the person inhales and holds this for five to ten seconds. Finally the person exhales and the muscles are relaxed to their prior state. This process is completed progressively from head to toe until the body is deeply relaxed. Take care not to hurt yourself by creating too much tension on the muscles.

Besides the achievement of the relaxation response and its associated benefits, PMR has been shown to reduce anxiety, reduce stress, improve cognitive abilities, and improve the symptoms of many health conditions. This may be because of the reduction of cortisol levels seen in those who practice brief PMR exercises.[553] The evidence suggests that PMR is as effective as cognitive behavioral therapy (CBT) for the relief of physiological disorders with physical symptoms of an unknown origin.[554] This is a significant finding since CBT is a technique employed to improve emotions, behaviors, and cognition. This technique is frequently suggested for insomnia, chronic pain, Parkinson's disease, and Alzheimer's disease.

PMR Technique:

1. Find a quiet location where you will not be interrupted.
2. Assume a comfortable position; preferably that supports all the muscles of your body, like a supportive sofa or a firm bed.
3. Give yourself permission and make a conscious effort to disregard all concerns and worries. Employ a passive attitude that focuses completely on you and the desired results of relaxation you hope to achieve.
4. Tense your muscles progressively by following the suggestions below. As you contract each muscle group, inhale deeply and hold for five to ten seconds. Then exhale and return the muscle group to its prior state and allow it to relax.
   - Forehead—raise your eyebrows as high as they can go.
   - Eyes and Nose—close your eyes and clench them tightly.
   - Mouth, Cheeks, and Jaw—open your mouth widely.
   - Neck—pull your head back as far as comfortably possible while being careful to avoid injury.
   - Shoulders—shrug your shoulders to your ears.
   - Biceps—draw your forearm up to your shoulder and make the typical muscle pose with both arms.
   - Triceps—straighten your right arm, locking your elbow. Repeat for the left arm.

- Forearms—extend your arms out straight in front of you as if pushing against a wall.
- Hands and fingers—make a fist with your right hand and squeeze tightly. Repeat with the left hand.
- Chest—consciously flex your pectoral muscles while taking in a deep breath to expand your chest.
- Upper Back—push your shoulder blades back as if you were going to touch them together.
- Lower Back—arch your back off the floor (omit if you are experiencing lower back pain).
- Stomach—tighten all of your abdominal muscles by sucking your stomach in back toward your spine.
- Buttocks—clench your buttocks tightly.
- Thighs—squeeze your upper legs together tightly.
- Calves—point your toes and flex your calve muscle in both legs.
- Feet and Toes—curl the toes of your right foot under tightly. Repeat with the left foot.

5. Inspect your body for any muscle tension that remains. If any tight muscles remain, tense and relax that muscle again as many times as is necessary to make it relax.

6. Imagine warm oil being poured over your body from your head to the tip of your toes, which allows the relaxation response to slowly spread throughout your entire body.

Other forms of relaxation worth considering are yoga, tai chi, hydrotherapy, and massage. Each applies a different strategy in promoting relaxation and calmness. Experiment with the different techniques until you find those that are most beneficial to your individual health and wellness.

Yoga is an ancient Indian practice that is considered a form of exercise, a relaxation technique, and a system of healing all in one. Yoga postures, called asanas, are designed to increase flexibility, and strengthen, tone, and align the body. It is beneficial for asthma, high blood pressure, anxiety, joint pain, depression, and heart disease.

Tai chi is a sequence of movements and positions intended to restore and/or maintain balance and harmony. It is a mind/body practice and martial art that originated in China. It improves flexibility, strength, and muscle definition. Tai chi is beneficial for and can improve the quality of life among the elderly, including improved balance and coordination, reduced chronic pain, and enhanced cardiovascular function.

EXUDE OPTIMISM

It is necessary to maintain an optimistic attitude to realize optimal health and wellness. The opposite of optimism, pessimism, is a detriment to health. Studies indicate that optimists enjoy better health, live longer, and have lower incidence of chronic illness than pessimists.[555] Research suggests that those who are positive realize a significant and consistent reduction in coronary heart disease as well.[556] The good news is if you aren't already optimistic by nature, optimism can be learned and you can still enjoy the benefit of improved health.[557]

Optimism can reduce fear, minimize pain, and influence quality of life.[558] Optimism protects against stress because it is associated with a reduction in the negative effects of cortisol, especially among those who experience high stress levels.[559,560] Being optimistic even helps you cope better with life.[561]

Optimism is differentiated from pessimism by outlook and point of view. The way in which a person views a situation as either bad or good determines whether they are optimistic or pessimistic. Optimists look on the bright side, they look for the good in all situations, and they are a "glass half full" kind of person. Optimists are hopeful in tragedy and learn from adversity. They realize that unfortunate events are the result of external circumstances, often which are beyond one's own control. Optimists believe life holds more good than bad.

Your temperament (optimism or pessimism) can often lead to a self-fulfilling prophecy. Meaning frequently your results (success or failure) are determined by your attitude. If you are optimistic, you believe you can reach your goal and give one hundred percent to achieve it. On the contrary, a pessimist believes he or she will fail and therefore doesn't strive to accomplish his or her goal. Thinking of it this way makes us realize how self-defeating pessimism really is.

If you are a pessimist, make a concerted effort now to learn optimism. This involves thinking positively and searching for good in all situations. We are all optimists from birth. We learned to be pessimists (if we are pessimistic) because of a skewed view of life; a belief that the world is innately painful and unpleasant, devoid of joyful experiences and success. If you learned to be pessimistic, you can certainly learn to be optimistic again.

SELF-ESTEEM AND SELF-IMAGE

Strive to maintain high self-esteem and a positive self-image, which go hand in hand with optimism. Self-talk (internal dialogue of thoughts that saturate our minds every day), whether positive or negative, makes an indelible impression on your subconscious. Wouldn't you prefer to supply your mind with positive rather than negative self-talk? Choose to praise and commend yourself, rather than belittle and criticize. The cells in your body are powerfully affected by your thoughts and self-talk. Positive self-talk results in positive mind and body effects, while negative self-talk results in the opposite. Positive affirmations are personal statements we make to ourselves, about ourselves. They both support and empower those who perform them regularly. Repeating the same affirmation again and again helps your cells "believe" what you are saying. The theory behind cellular memory is that memories, whether positive or negative, can be stored in cells. There is some credence to this theory based on the fact that organ transplant recipients often take on the characteristics or personality traits of their donor. Place positive remarks in conspicuous places (like the bathroom mirror, refrigerator, or in your car) where you can be reminded to guide your self-talk and make it more constructive.

You have a right and a vested interest to feel good about yourself. To build high self-esteem, start by listing all the things you like about yourself and your strengths. If you are really down on yourself, ask a close friend to help you create this list—you may be surprised with the list of qualities and virtues they recognize in you.

LAUGHTER IS THE BEST MEDICINE

"Laughter is the best medicine" is more than a catchy phrase. Laughter has both psychological and physiological effects on the body that can lead to dynamic psycho-physiological changes. Learning to laugh makes life more enjoyable. Laughing is contagious. It is almost impossible not to laugh and smile when you hear the raucous giggle of an infant. You may have a smile on your face right now with just the thought of it.

Psychologically, laughter helps eliminate anxious, angry, and gloomy emotions. It reduces stress and promotes a sense of relaxation. Laughter is a coping mechanism and strategy with the ability to promote confidence and create a feeling of optimism in difficult situations.

Laughter alleviates pain and discomfort. The subsequent surge of endorphins during a good laughing episode is like receiving a temporary morphine shot, and a study suggested that laughter actually increases your pain tolerance.[562] Endorphins not only naturally relieve pain, they promote an overall sense of well-being and euphoria. Remarkably, one study concluded that just the mere anticipation of a good laugh releases not only endorphins, but human growth hormone.[563] A good hardy laugh may also relieve tension by encouraging the muscles to relax.

Laughter enhances blood flow and improves the circulation of oxygen to tissues. A study conducted by the University of Maryland illustrated that laughter causes the inner lining of blood vessels, called the endothelium, to relax, expanding blood vessels and increasing blood flow.[564] This suggests that laughter is actually beneficial to the heart and brain because they require a continual flow of oxygen from the blood.

Laughter may stimulate immune system activity. Some research indicates laughter may raise antibody activity and reduce levels of stress hormones.[565,566] Norman Cousins famously battled his destructive disease, ankylosing spondylitis, with laughter and high doses of vitamin C. He contended that a good belly laugh provided him with two hours of pain-free sleep. Amazingly he actually recovered from his illness reportedly through mega-doses of vitamin C, laughter, and a positive attitude.

Laughter appears to have social benefits as well. Laughter is so contagious that when you hear laughter your brain is primed and prepared to laugh. Laughter positively effects relationships and can help two people grow closer together. Laughing together can forge a connecting link and bond. Finally, laughter is attractive, with a tendency to draw others in.

Research has also demonstrated the ability of laughing to reduce blood glucose levels following the consumption of a meal.[567] This makes laughter a supportive therapy for diabetics. Another reported benefit of laughter for diabetics is a possible reduction in the risk of heart disease—something diabetics have an elevated risk of. One study demonstrated the ability of laughter to reduce blood vessel inflammation and increase HDL cholesterol, thus lowering the risk of cardiovascular disease among diabetics.[568]

THE GENUINE NEED FOR MEANINGFUL RELATIONSHIPS

Men and women are not meant to be alone. This is why maintaining meaningful relationships is an important part of achieving optimal health and wellness. Just as an unhealthy relationship can cause both physical and emotional strain, healthy relationships can add pleasure and happiness to life. The number of relationships you experience each day (even those with the grocery store clerk, a restaurant waitress, coworkers, neighbors, or animals) definitely has an effect on your well-being. It has been reported time and time again that people who maintain meaningful relationships are healthier, happier, and live longer more fulfilling lives.[569,570]

Meaningful relationships provide a network of support and encouragement. They involve mutual trust, sharing, two-way communication, sincere caring, unconditional love, and a safe environment for all involved parties to thrive within. Harmful relationships do just the opposite. They incorporate suspicion, doubt, lack of communication, selfishness, constrained love, and a hostile environment that suppresses growth and progression.

Unfortunately some people stay in unhealthy relationships because they long for human contact or feel they have no other choice. They have convinced themselves that this type of relationship is normal or maybe that they can't obtain any better. This is a repressive and harmful belief, which injures the person who accepts it as true. Everyone deserves and is entitled to meaningful and healthy relationships and need not settle for the opposite.

Touch is an essential part of meaningful relationships. It can be as simple as a hand on the shoulder or an enthusiastic hug. Pleasant physical touch—even massage[571]—releases the bonding hormone oxytocin. Interestingly oxytocin induces feelings of optimism, euphoria, trust, generosity, and enhances the ability to maintain relationships with the person you share touch with. Physical intimacy with your spouse is a beautiful expression of love and endears the two participants as one. An infant lying on your chest is enjoyable and comfortable. A hug from a child can eradicate a bad day quickly. A gentle arm around a shoulder can elevate your mood during times of distress. All of these are examples of appropriate touch that occur in meaningful relationships.

Doctors in the early 1900s were puzzled by a condition labeled "failure to thrive syndrome" that was prevalent in orphanages and hospitals. This is a condition in which infants and toddlers fail to grow and develop properly mentally and or emotionally despite proper nourishment, a healthy environment, and adequate medical care. It was determined that these infants were not thriving because they did not receive enough physical touch, stimulation, and love necessary for proper growth and development. Regrettably, infants and toddlers who don't receive the touch and love they long for and require can die.

The same "failure to thrive" condition can hold true for adults, particularly the elderly. Loneliness and a lack of affectionate touch can slowly deteriorate the health of all human beings. Many elderly people die shortly after the death of their spouses. Loneliness, lack of affectionate touch, and inadequate meaningful relationships is likely a contributing factor in this phenomenon. The human body craves touch and needs it to remain healthy.

THE IMPORTANT BENEFITS OF A GOOD NIGHT'S SLEEP

Sleep is a fundamental and basic requirement of life. Sleep is more than a motionless, inactive state, it is a critical time the body uses to repair and restore balance internally. Think of it as your body's housecleaning time. Most adults require between six and eight hours of sleep, school-age children need about ten, toddlers need somewhere between ten and thirteen, while infants require at least fourteen to sixteen hours. The key is balance. Too much sleep is harmful and associated with increased death rates,[572] while too little sleep can encourage dysfunction the next day.

Memory consolidation is a process that helps us commit recently learned information to long-term memory storage. This process also happens unconsciously while we sleep, called sleep consolidation, and may enhance the retention of learned information.[573] Next time you need to take an important test, it may be advantageous to study right before going to bed—you may improve your test score.

We are all familiar with the grumpiness and irritability that occurs when someone doesn't get enough sleep. The immune system is particularly active and sends out natural killer cells to tag and destroy harmful microorganisms during sleep. The brain requires rest and the ability to regenerate after a period of wakefulness. This regeneration occurs during sleep. For those still growing, a significant amount of growth hormone is released while sleeping.

Some substances can either promote or reduce restful sleep. Avoid caffeine, alcohol, and heavy meals a few hours before sleep. If you still struggle to sleep comfortably, consider sleep supplements like melatonin, valerian, chamomile, skullcap, L-tryptophan, and L-theanine. Lavender and cedarwood essential oils are also great options to encourage a restful night's sleep. A few drops of either, or both, rubbed into the shoulders and a drop on the pillow can go a long way.

NATURAL REMEDIES FOR DEPRESSION

Anxiety and depression are two of the most common mental illnesses in the United States. Almost 7 percent of adults in the United States experience major depression each year,[574] while anxiety disorders affect more than 18 percent of the adult population.[575] Both disorders are triggered or related to a variety of factors including hormone levels, nutrient deficiencies, genetics, neurotransmitter levels, and psychological, emotional, spiritual, social, and environmental factors. While not the same, anxiety and depression often occur together and the management strategies for both conditions are interrelated. Antidepressants are the primary weapon employed by Western physicians against depression. Unfortunately, these medications often fail to work—only 31 percent of patients experienced remission of depressive symptoms after fourteen weeks and 65 percent after six months[576]—or cause serious side effects that cause the patient to quit taking them. Many of the recommendations throughout this book apply to the management of depression and anxiety, but there are further specific strategies that may offer hope. People who suffer from depression should consider natural remedies to manage symptoms. A number of natural remedies exist that can profoundly influence mood and emotions to benefit those who feel persistent sadness. Severe depression may be life threatening so you should seek medical attention if you suffer from it.

A variety of dietary supplements have proven effectiveness in the management of depression. St. John's wort has traditionally been used for the treatment and management of nervous disorders. Researchers believe that it helps those who are depressed because it influences hypothalamic-pituitary-adrenal (HPA) axis function. The HPA is commonly hyperactive in depressed individuals and can lead to imbalanced hormone levels. It also weakly inhibits monoamine oxidase A and B activity. MAOI drug therapies are used to modify neurotransmitter levels in depressed individuals and prevent the reuptake of serotonin. Serotonin strengthens brain cell communication and higher levels in the brain are associated with improved mood.[577] When all of these beneficial properties of St. John's wort are taken into account, it is no wonder taking it as a supplement regularly leads to mood enhancements and a reduction of depressive symptoms. Even better, all of this is accomplished without the serious side effects associated with antidepressant use.[578] British researchers concluded that it was as effective as the tricyclic antidepressant imipramine.[579] The adult therapeutic dosage of St. John's wort is 250 to 400 mg three times per day standardized to 0.2 percent or 0.3 percent hypericin. Extracts standardized to 5 percent hyperforin have also been used at a dosage of 300 mg three times a day. St. John's wort may interfere with a number of medications: frovatriptan (Frova), naratriptan (Amerge), rizatriptan (Maxalt), sumatriptan (Imitrex), zolmitriptan (Zomig), and benzodiazepines (psychoactive drugs). St. John's wort should not be taken with pharmaceutical antidepressants because it may increase serotonin levels to dangerous levels. St. John's wort may increase the sedative effects of barbiturates, enhance the effects of blood thinners, decrease the effectiveness of birth control pills, interfere with immunosuppressive medications, decrease the effectiveness of cardiac medications like digoxin, reduce effectiveness of antiviral drugs for HIV, AIDS, and hepatitis B, interfere with P-glycoprotein substrates, increase the risk of photosensitivity, and may interfere with cytochrome P450, which significantly influences the metabolism of myriad drugs.

5-hydroxytryptophan (5-HTP), a neurotransmitter, is able to cross the blood-brain barrier and stimulate the synthesis of serotonin by the central nervous system.[580] Serotonin is responsible for mood, hunger, and sleep. It isn't directly acquired from food, but the body can make it from tryptophan—an essential amino acid found in turkey, spirulina, spinach, and other foods. A study comparing the effectiveness of 5-HTP versus fluoxetine (better known as Prozac) determined that 5-HTP provided comparable reduction in depressive symptoms within two weeks of treatment.[581] This is noteworthy because St. John's wort typically takes multiple weeks to become effective. This was also accomplished with relatively few adverse side effects.[582] Normally adults take 150 to 300 mg of 5-HTP daily for depressive symptoms. 5-HTP should not be taken with medications that affect serotonin levels such as SSRIs (fluoxetine, paroxetine, sertraline, carbidopa), MAOIs, tricyclic antidepressants, atypical antidepressants (amitriptyline, clomipramine, imipramine), meperidine (Demerol), tramadol (Ultram), pentazocine (Talwin), and dextromethorphan (Robitussin DM, and Delsym) because interactions could occur that may cause serotonin syndrome. Serotonin syndrome is a potentially life threatening reaction from drug and/or supplement use that leads to excess serotonin levels. 5-HTP may increase the sedating effects of central nervous system depressant medications.

Another alternative therapy for depression, S-adenosylmethionine (SAMe), has long been prescribed in Europe and has demonstrated equivalent mood improvement results as some antidepressants. It is a naturally occurring compound produced in the body from the amino acid methionine and found in abundance throughout the body. Good food sources of methionine include Brazil nuts, eggs, sesame seeds, and fish. Like 5-HTP it crosses the blood brain barrier and influences serotonin and dopamine levels.[583] SAMe has been used in conjunction with SSRI medications to enhance the medications' activity.[584] It also effectively reduces depressive symptoms when taken alone. It is considered a very safe remedy except among people who have bipolar disorder because it may cause manic episodes among these people.[585] Dosages used in studies are typically 1,600 mg of SAMe daily for adults with depression, although the therapeutic range appears to be between 400 and 1,600 mg daily. SAMe is not recommended while taking antidepressant drugs because it may promote unsafe levels of serotonin. It may also reduce the effectiveness of levodopa, and interact with Demerol and Ultram.

There is a strong correlation between vitamin D deficiency and depression.[586-589] Whether the deficiency is a causal factor in depression or a result of the depression is yet to be determined, and the research regarding the use of vitamin D as a treatment for depression has been mixed.[590-592] Some of the negative results observed may largely be due to insignificant quantities of vitamin D used in the study, like 400 IU. Evidence suggests that it takes nearly 8,000 IU daily to reverse deficiencies. Nevertheless, clinical observations suggest that supplementation with vitamin D may have positive effects on depressive symptoms. Very large doses of vitamin D are generally required to produce therapeutic effects. Up to 100,000 IU weekly can be taken for one month and up to 40,000 IU weekly for one year without producing significant adverse effects. Large doses of vitamin D should only be taken for short periods of time—less than three months—and blood levels should be monitored to avoid toxicity. If more than 10,000 IU per day is taken for long periods (three months or more), it may cause toxic levels and symptoms such as excess calcium in the blood (hypercalcemia), nausea, vomiting, kidney problems, weakness, and poor appetite. If blood levels reach over 150 ng/ml, toxicity symptoms such as constipation, fatigue, irritability, muscle weakness, and vomiting may occur.

Essential oils simultaneously work on the emotional and physical aspects of depression. In 2004, Iranian researchers compared the effectiveness of citrus essential oils versus Prozac. They observed that those who received ten drops of a 2 percent dilution of citrus oil (orange) three times per day improved depressive symptoms more effectively than Prozac.[593] This is a very inexpensive means to improve depressive symptoms because citrus essential oils are inexpensive and a 3 percent dilution can be created with only four drops of citrus oil per teaspoon of carrier oil. Citrus oils can be photosensitizing, so they are best applied where the sun will not interact with them (such as the feet).

CALMING ANXIETY NATURALLY

Some of the most common natural remedies employed to manage anxiety include kava-kava, passionflower, lemon balm, lavender, and German chamomile essential oils.

Native to the South Pacific and used as part of ceremonies by Pacific Islanders for centuries, kava-kava, or just kava, is well-known for its relaxing qualities. Kava roots are ground into a pulp and mixed with water to make the ceremonial drink, which encourages relaxation, sedation, a balanced mood, and relieves pain. Kava has been successfully used to manage and treat anxiety disorders for years, with less risk for dependency and side effects than the typical drugs used. A double-blind, placebo-controlled, and randomized study that investigated the anti-anxiety effects of kava reported that after six weeks of taking a kava extract, 26 percent of people reported remission of their generalized anxiety disorder (GAD). Conversely, only 6 percent of the placebo group reported remission.[594] Even more importantly, no significant adverse reactions, withdrawal symptoms, or liver dysfunction was reported. This is significant because previous reports suggested that kava may adversely affect liver function. However, evidence suggests that the previous reports of liver toxicity were due to poor quality of raw materials.[595] Interestingly, the study authors observed that female participants in the study also reported an increase in libido. Another study investigating the safety of kava also reported that liver function remained normal with no adverse reactions reported from kava.[596] Again, the study shows that females experienced significant increases in their sex drive while they took kava. For anxiety, the typical dosage is 100 mg (standardized to 70 percent kavalactones) three times per day.[597] Kava should not be taken with central nervous system depressants (alcohol, barbiturates, benzodiazepines) or anxiety medications because it may increase the risk of drowsiness, lethargy, disorientation, and motor reflex depression.

Passionflower (*Passiflora incarnata*) has a long history of use in Europe and the Americas as a calming and relaxing herb. A small clinical trial that included thirty-six people with GAD compared the effectiveness of passionflower versus oxazepam, a common drug used to treat anxiety, and concluded that forty-five drops of passionflower daily reduced GAD as effectively as 30 mg of oxazepam daily, but without the side effect of impaired job performance.[598] Some situations, such as dental or medical procedures may increase anxiety. Research suggests that passionflower significantly reduces anxious feelings before these types of procedures.[599,600] Anxiety often interrupts sleep, which in turn can exacerbate anxiety and create a vicious cycle. Researchers discovered that passionflower increases sleep quality and reduces sleep disturbance.[601]

Lemon balm (*Melissa officinalis*) herb was used as a medicinal remedy by the ancient Greeks to reduce anxious feelings, agitation, balance mood, and improve sleep quality. It is a nervine herb—a substance that can calm the nerves. One challenge with research that examines the effectiveness of lemon balm for anxiety is it is rarely tested by itself. Instead, it is often combined with valerian or other anti-anxiety herbs in studies. For example, a study using a combination of valerian and lemon balm found that children with sleep disturbance and restlessness could receive relief by taking the two herbal remedies together.[602] In another study, when 600 mg of lemon balm was administered before a stressful incident, subjects experienced increased calm and a more balanced mood.[603] Long-term use of lemon balm appears to significantly reduce anxiety and improve sleep among those who suffer from mild- to moderate-anxiety and sleep disorders. Remarkably, 70 percent of people who were administered a standardized lemon balm extract, achieved full remission of anxiety and 85 percent reported improved sleep quality.[604] Lemon balm can be taken as a tea (1.5 to 4.5 g daily), in capsules (300 to 500 mg, three times daily), as a tincture (60 drops in divided doses daily), or as an essential oil (inhaled, applied topically, or orally) to relieve anxiety. It may interact with sedative medications and alcohol, and an animal study suggests that lemon balm essential oil may lower blood glucose levels, potentially interfering with diabetic medications.[605]

The amino acid L-theanine is a common supplement for anxiety, although usually it is combined with other herbs. Scientists have discovered that L-theanine modifies brain waves to transition a person to a more relaxed and alert state.[606] fifth-year pharmacy students who received 200 mg of L-theanine twice daily experienced decreased stress, anxious feelings, and salivary alpha-amylase activity,[607] an enzyme that is often hyperactive in sufferers of GAD.[608] L-theanine effectively reduces anxiety symptoms in persons with schizophrenia and schizoaffective disorder.[609] The common dosage of L-theanine for anxiety is 200 mg per day. L-theanine may increase the effects of stimulants (caffeine) and blood pressure medications.

Both lavender and German chamomile essential oils have been valued for their calming and relaxing properties for centuries. Inhalation of either essential oil alone can produce substantial calming effects, but their effects are intensified when used together. A lavender oil supplement, Silexan, used in Germany for those who suffer from anxiety disorders, has proven effective against anxiety in multiple studies.[610-612] Another study tested the effects of lavender for crying infants. The infants who received a lavender aromatherapy bath were more relaxed, had lower levels of stress, cried less, and slept better.[613] Interestingly, the study authors also observed that both the infant and the mother had lower cortisol levels. When patients in an intensive care unit inhaled a combination of lavender essential oil, neroli, and Roman chamomile they slept better and had lower anxiety levels.[614] German chamomile demonstrates similar effectiveness in patients with GAD.[615-617] One or two drops of each may be applied to a hanky or tissue to inhale as needed for anxiety. In addition, a few drops of each may be taken in a capsule to reduce anxious feelings.

By now you should realize the importance of spiritual, mental, and emotional health and their considerable effect on physical health. Because the mind, body, emotions, and spirit are interconnected you must support all four areas of health to achieve optimal health and wellness. This is akin to playing basketball without your brain. Yes, you have the physical ability to accomplish this but you don't have a brain to guide the physical body accordingly. Make a conscious effort today to implement a few changes to improve your mental, emotional, and spiritual wellness and watch your physical health rise up with them.

7

Reducing the Risk of America's Top Killers

According to the US Centers for Disease Control and Prevention, the most common causes of death in the United States are heart disease, cancer, stroke, chronic lower respiratory diseases, accidents and injuries, diabetes, Alzheimer's disease, and influenza and pneumonia. Although a healthy lifestyle does not guarantee you will live a life free from the diseases that kill the most Americans, you can reduce your risk of disease and untimely death through better lifestyle choices. In reality, so many people are affected just by heart disease, cancer, and diabetes that virtually everyone can benefit from taking some of the supplements that will follow to prevent their risks.

The foundation of your health and wellness plan includes eating better, regular physical activity, nutritional supplementation, detoxification, and being mindful of your mental, emotional, and spiritual wellness. All of these have been reasonably discussed throughout this book. The current chapter will provide more specific preventive measures to support your body and reduce your risk of the health-related leading causes of death in the United States. The subsequent recommendations assume that you have already incorporated or plan to integrate the first five areas of this book. Without them, the suggestions for a particular health condition will not be as effective.

NATURALLY REDUCING HEART DISEASE RISK

Heart disease accounts for one in every four deaths in the United States, claiming about 600,000 lives each year.[618] Heart disease is a broad term used to describe conditions that affect the heart or blood vessels such as arrhythmia, cardiomyopathy, congestive heart failure, coronary heart disease, heart attack, and mitral valve prolapse. Heart disease is largely preventable with proper nutrition, regular physical activity, and healthy lifestyle choices. The goal in the prevention of heart disease is to support the body by improving heart function and blood supply.

The risk factors for heart disease include: increased age in women (fifty-five or older), high blood pressure, high blood cholesterol, heredity, smoking, physical inactivity, and being overweight. In addition, having diabetes,[619] chronically elevated stress levels,[620] and excess alcohol use may be risk factors for heart disease.[621] Of these risk factors, all but two (age and heredity) can be modified or controlled.

If you implement healthy lifestyle choices such as reduce alcohol consumption, stay physically active, manage stress, and maintain a healthy weight for your age and build, you can reduce the risk of heart disease. You also should not smoke. Eating better may be the single most important factor to prevent heart disease. You should limit the amounts of trans and saturated fats and simultaneously increase omega-3s (DHA and EPA) as part of your campaign to reduce heart disease risk. If you consume an average of 566 mg each of DHA and EPA—from marine sources—every day, research suggests you may reduce your risk of coronary heart disease by 36 percent.[622] This helps to reduce the amount of cholesterol that will build up in your arteries and cause congestion. Eat lots and lots of fruits and vegetables, especially green leafy vegetables. Your goal should be at least five servings daily. Stay within the optimal range for salt intake (2,645 to 4,945 mg daily) and don't add salt to your food with the salt shaker. Reduce refined sugar intake, particularly high-fructose corn syrup obtained through sugar-sweetened beverages. Don't forget to drink plenty of purified water.

Physical activity should be balanced with calorie consumption to avoid gaining weight. Physical activity helps strengthen the heart muscle, increase blood flow, and reduce the risk of high blood pressure, high cholesterol, and diabetes. Aim for at least thirty minutes of moderate activity daily—sixty minutes is even better. You can more easily reach this total if you add physical activity into your daily routine, like taking the stairs instead of the elevator, parking in a space farther from the store, and by going for brisk walks.

There are many supplements that are supportive and beneficial to the cardiovascular system. Each may affect one or more of the risk factors for heart disease. The following supplements may be useful for your heart disease prevention plan. You don't necessarily need to take all of them. Several options are listed because each person is unique and reacts differently to different nutrients. If you are at high risk of heart disease, pick one or two. The supplements are listed in preferential order.

COENZYME Q_{10} (COQ$_{10}$)

The coenzyme Q_{10} has already been discussed and is a super nutrient for the heart. It is necessary for the basic function of cells and offers significant benefits to the cardiovascular system. If you have a primary risk factor for heart disease or a family history of heart disease, you should begin to take COQ$_{10}$ as early as the age of thirty. While rare, it is not unheard of for a person in his or her thirties to die of heart disease. A preventive dose should be in the range of 60–200 mg daily. If you already have heart disease, ask your doctor about therapeutic dosages that range from 3 mg/kg daily to 3,000 mg per day in divided doses. You will need to gradually work up to this amount. The dosage that is best for you will depend on lifestyle choices, nutrition, exercise, and other risk factors. CoQ$_{10}$ has been used therapeutically for various forms of heart disease such as congestive heart failure, mitral valve prolapse, cardiomyopathy, hypertension, angina, and heart attack.[623-631] But, it can also be taken to prevent heart disease because of its influence on blood pressure and the prevention of LDL cholesterol oxidation. Higher blood levels of CoQ$_{10}$ are associated with a decreased risk of coronary heart disease.[632] In fact, CoQ$_{10}$ has demonstrated the ability to prevent heart damage caused by the cancer drug Doxorubicin.[633] It is possible that CoQ$_{10}$ could interfere with high blood pressure and blood clotting medications, so you should check with your doctor or pharmacist before using them together.

It can be quite difficult to achieve optimal blood levels of CoQ$_{10}$ but scientific research suggests that ubiquinol, the active form of CoQ$_{10}$, is more bioavailable and more effective.[634,635] Once ingested, ubiquinone must be reduced in the body to its active metabolite ubiquinol for the body to use it. If you take ubiquinol it saves this conversion step. One drawback to ubiquinol is that it is highly unstable, but scientists have recently been able to stabilize it. This stabilized form of CoQ$_{10}$ is the preferred from.

Bottom Line: CoQ$_{10}$ reduces the risk of heart disease through enhancing the ability of the heart to pump enough blood (improved mitochondrial function), reduced blood pressure, enhanced antioxidant protection of the heart, and through prevention of LDL cholesterol oxidation.

MAGNESIUM

The ability of the heart to produce energy and beat properly is dependent on sufficient magnesium levels in the blood. Many people with heart disease are deficient in this essential mineral. In fact, according to research, people with a high risk of heart disease who eat a magnesium-rich diet reduce their risk of heart disease and risk of sudden cardiac death.[636] Similar reductions in heart disease risk have been observed when a magnesium supplement is taken.[637] Magnesium is beneficial for arrhythmia, cardiac arrest, cardiomyopathy, congestive heart failure, heart attack, hypertension, and mitral valve prolapse.[638-642] The amount of magnesium recommended in the daily multivitamin/mineral should provide sufficient levels for protection. However, if you already have heart disease or are deficient in magnesium your requirements may be greater.

Bottom Line: Magnesium helps reduce heart disease risk because it profoundly influences heartbeat, reduces blood pressure, and reduces the risk of coronary events (heart attack, heart-related deaths, and narrowing of the blood vessels).

INDIAN GOOSEBERRY

Indian gooseberry, also known as Amla, Amalaki, or the botanical name *Phyllanthus emblica*, is an antioxidant that supports the cardiovascular system. Studies suggest that Indian gooseberry protects the heart, influences cholesterol levels,[643-647] lowers triglyceride levels,[647,648] reduces C-reactive protein (a marker for inflammation),[645] improves endothelial function,[649-651] and inhibits platelet aggregation.[652,653] The therapeutic dosage appears to range from 250 mg to 1,000 mg daily. There are no currently known interactions with medications.

Bottom Line: Reduced heart disease risk may occur with Indian gooseberry because it influences cholesterol levels, decreases triglyceride levels, helps reduce cardiac inflammation, improves blood vessel lining function, and through reduced clumping of platelets (the reason a baby aspirin is often recommended to reduce heart disease).

RESVERATROL

The active form of the polyphenol resveratrol, trans-resveratrol, is an anti-aging antioxidant found in grapes, red wine, purple grape juice, and some berries. It is thought to protect the heart,[654-657] improve left ventricle diastolic function and endothelial function, improve cholesterol profile, preserve vascular function, reduce atherosclerosis, and inhibit platelet aggregation.[658-665] Dosages from 10 to 250 mg are typically used. Trans-resveratrol may inhibit cytochrome P450 enzymes, which could theoretically increase blood levels of drugs metabolized by these enzymes. It may also enhance the activity of anticoagulant and antiplatelet drugs, so caution is warranted.

Bottom Line: Resveratrol improves heart function, helps prevent plaque build-up in the arteries, and reduces clumping of platelets (the reason a baby aspirin is often recommended to reduce heart disease). All of these actions help reduce the risk of heart disease.

L-CARNITINE

L-carnitine is a compound required to transport long-chain fatty acids into the mitochondria for breakdown. L-carnitine helps protect and improve heart function in a number of heart conditions. These include angina, arrhythmia, congestive heart failure, and heart attack.[666-669] It reduces the risk of irregular heartbeat and significantly reduces chest pain symptoms, and therefore decreases the risk of heart disease.[670] Some research suggests that the molecular-bonded form of carnitine, glycine propionyl-L-carnitine (GPLC), is more effective to raise cellular L-carnitine levels, circulation, and fatty acid metabolism than L-carnitine.[671] Avoid the synthetic form, D-carnitine, that has undesirable side effects. A preventive dose to support heart health may be from 250 to 500 mg daily in three divided doses. Therapeutic doses range from 900 to 6,000 mg daily in divided doses. L-carnitine may interact with acenocoumarol, a fast-acting oral anticoagulant, and Coumadin. It may also inhibit entrance of thyroid hormones into cells.

Bottom Line: L-carnitine may help reduce the risk of heart disease through the promotion of heartbeat regularity, protection from oxidative damage, and reduced chest pain.

GARLIC

Garlic may help reduce heart disease risk because of its ability to improve lipid profiles and normalize blood pressure. Studies have indicated that garlic has the ability to mildly reduce total and LDL blood cholesterol levels.[672,673] This may be important to reduce the risk of atherosclerosis. Research has also indicated that garlic mildly lowers blood pressure.[674] There are various forms of garlic supplements, so take the amount listed on the label by the supplement manufacturer and this should be sufficient as a preventative dose. Those who take the following drugs should consult a physician or pharmacist before consuming garlic: antimycobacterial, drug contraceptives, non-nucleoside reverse transcriptase inhibitors, protease inhibitors, anticoagulants, antiplatelet medications, and cyclosporine.

Bottom Line: If you take garlic you may reduce your heart disease risk because it mildly reduces blood pressure and cholesterol levels.

HAWTHORN

Hawthorn has been traditionally used for heart disease for thousands of years. It is highly regarded in Europe where it has been used for a number of heart ailments. It strengthens the heart and enhances heart performance, strengthens heart cell metabolism,[675] and increases blood flow to the heart. It has been used therapeutically for heart failure,[676-678] angina,[679] high cholesterol,[680] hypertension,[681] and atherosclerosis—with a better reduction in LDL cholesterol when compared to the drug simvastatin.[682,683] Hawthorn is generally given in standardized form, being standardized for either oligomeric procyanidins or vitexin rhamnosides. Therapeutic doses vary from 160 to 1,800 mg three times per day based on the form used. Hawthorn may increase heart failure progression and risk of heart failure mortality, so it should not be used by heart failure patients without first consulting a physician.[684] Hawthorn should not be used concurrently with nitrates (nitroglycerin, isosorbide) or phosphodiesterase-5 inhibitors (Viagra, Cialis). It may also interact poorly with beta blockers, calcium channel blockers, and digoxin.

Bottom Line: Hawthorn is not only used for the treatment of heart disease, it also provides protective and preventive benefits. It strengthens the heart and increases circulation, which may be why it is still used as a drug in Brazil, China, Russia, and many European countries.[685]

PREVENTING CANCER NATURALLY

Cancer is the second most common cause of death in the United States and affects approximately one-third of American women and half of American men throughout their lifetime.[686] It is estimated that 585,720 American men and women will die of cancer in 2014, and the United States is certainly not alone in this crisis.[687] Almost 25 percent of men and about 20 percent of women will die of cancer.[687] Astonishingly, cancer takes the lives of 8 million people worldwide.[688] That is more than fifteen people who die from cancer every minute—or roughly one person every four seconds.

The most common cancers among men and women varies. For men, prostate cancer is the most common followed by lung and colorectal cancer.[689] The most commonly diagnosed cancer among women is breast cancer, with lung and colorectal cancer numbers two and three.[690] Lung cancer is the most common cause of cancer death among both sexes and also the most preventable.[690,691] Children most commonly suffer from leukemias, brain, and central nervous system cancers.[691]

Cancer does not discriminate against age, gender, or race. Most cancer research is geared toward genetics and familial inheritance, despite the fact that cancer occurs as a result of a single inherited factor less than 10 percent of the time.[692] One report determined that up to 80 percent of cancers diagnosed in the United States in 1981 could have been prevented by lifestyle changes.[693] This suggests that only about 20 percent of cancers are caused by other factors outside of diet, activity levels, smoking, and environmental factors. Some experts believe approximately 25 percent of all cancers are preventable through dietary and lifestyle behaviors alone.[694] Other cancers, for example colon cancer, are up to 70 percent preventable through diet and lifestyle modifications.[695] Cancer is preventable and therefore it is prudent to take defensive measures that include modifying lifestyle behaviors. Now, this doesn't mean that if you modify your lifestyle that you will never get cancer, the fact is some still get cancer despite living very healthy lives, but you are likely to reduce your risk of it.

Normal cells will only grow and divide a specified number of times, whereas cancer cells grow and divide uncontrollably. This uncontrolled growth—bypassing the telomere signal to self-destruct—is a result of damaged DNA within the cells. Under normal circumstances the body is able to repair damaged DNA but cancer cells seem to avoid this repair process. Damage to DNA is sometimes inherited, though this is uncommon. It generally occurs as a result of environmental exposure or an outside trigger. Most cancers form a tumor or growth, while some cancers circulate through other tissues where they develop. The most common human cancers are carcinomas (start in cells that surround tissues and organs), sarcomas (begin in the connective tissues of the body), leukemia (cancer of the blood cells), and lymphoma (cancer that develops in the lymph system).

According to the National Cancer Institute, the most common risk factors for cancer are: cigarette smoking or tobacco use, infections, radiation, immunosuppressive medicines, diet, alcohol, physical inactivity, obesity, and environmental risk factors.[696] Most of these risk factors can be minimized or modified. Though family history is a definite factor in cancer risk, a family history does not doom a person to get cancer. Normally other factors, such as those listed previously, also contribute to cancer development and are indeed the triggers for cancer initiation.

Tobacco use is the single most preventable cause of cancer and death. Tobacco use directly contributes to a plethora of cancers, diseases, illnesses, and deaths. At least 30 percent of all cancer deaths are tobacco-related.[697] The statistic is worse for lung cancer deaths, where tobacco is estimated to account for 87 and 70 percent of deaths among men and women respectively.[698] If you smoke, make a commitment to quit so you can reduce your risk of cancer. If you don't smoke, don't start, and avoid places where smokers are known to assemble to reduce your risk of environmental tobacco smoke.

It would be virtually impossible to avoid exposure to some amount of radiation, though exposure can be limited with a few easy steps. We are exposed to radiation every day from the sun, stars, radon, and radioactive materials in rocks and soil. Medical X-rays are the largest source of avoidable exposure. Do not forestall necessary X-rays, but don't involve yourself in needless X-rays. Two recent studies indicated physicians used CT scans too frequently (an astounding 68.8 percent of 655,613 enrollees in the study received an image procedure that incurred radiation exposure in a thirty-six-month period) and the exposure to radiation was greater than originally thought from CT scans.[698] The authors of the studies estimated that just one year of these scans would result in 29,000 occurrences of cancer, of which 14,500 would end in death.[699,700]

Another frequent exposure to radiation for women is mammography. Some physicians have questioned the need for the frequency of these exams, while others believe they are not beneficial and increase the likelihood of false positives. The value of mammography is a hotly debated and contentious subject, but some evidence does suggest that mammography does not reduce incidence or mortality of breast cancer.[701] Other studies assert that a reduction in breast cancer of 28 percent can be achieved with regular mammography.[702] Early detection of breast cancer is crucial to successful treatment and the risk versus reward should be carefully considered. One option that many women now choose is thermal breast imagery, or breast thermography. Breast thermography uses infrared cameras instead of radiation to detect abnormal breast tissue, but this method of detection is quite controversial, with inconclusive evidence about its effectiveness.[703,704] Women should discuss this option with their health care provider and consider all alternatives prudently.

Proper sun avoidance is necessary to reduce risk of skin cancers. And if you are like most people, the first thing you think of to avoid too much sun is to slather your body with sunscreen. Unfortunately, some limited evidence suggests sunscreen may accelerate skin cancer, not offer protection from it.[705,706] Some practical, non-sunscreen suggestions to limit UVA and UVB exposure from the sun include:

- Cover up and wear long-sleeved shirts and long pants.
- Wear a wide-brimmed hat to protect your head, face, and neck.
- Don't sunbathe or tan in tanning beds.
- Include plenty of carotenoids in your diet, which are associated with a reduction in UV damage.[707,708]

Strive to reduce your exposure to chemicals that may increase your risk of cancer as much as possible. Substitute natural household cleaners and detergents (i. e. borax, vinegar, and baking soda) for toxic chemicals. To reduce exposure to pesticides, eat as much organic food as possible. If you work in an environment that exposes you to chemicals, wear proper protective equipment to limit exposure. Use personal care products and makeup made from natural ingredients that are chemical-and toxin-free. The bottom line is to be aware of the chemicals you are exposed to every day and take steps to reduce or prevent exposure.

Synthetic hormones found in drug contraceptives and administered during hormone replacement therapy are strongly associated with increased risk of cancer. As a woman transitions from her fertility years to menopause unpleasant symptoms such as hot flashes, night sweats, and lack of libido, vaginal dryness, mood swings, and disturbed sleep may occur. A woman is considered in menopause if her last menstrual cycle occurred twelve months ago or longer. These symptoms are largely due to a reduction in the production of key reproductive hormones, particularly progesterone and estrogen. Conventional medicine attacks menopausal symptoms with hormone replacement therapy. Unfortunately several studies have concluded that hormone replacement therapy with synthetically derived hormones is associated with increased risk of certain cancers and cardiovascular disease.[709-712] Astonishingly, elevated risk may last several years after discontinuance of synthetic hormone replacement therapy.

There are viable options for menopausal symptoms outside of risky synthetic hormone replacement therapy. For example, frequent physical activity has been associated with a reduction of menopausal symptoms.[713,714,715] In addition, herbal remedies—dong quai, chasteberry,[716] black cohosh,[717] and naturally compounded progesterone cream derived from wild yams[718] have supported thousands of women through this transitory period. Wild yam is often used in natural menopausal formulas in the hopes that it will increase progesterone production within the body, but there is little evidence to support this belief. Wild yam contains a compound called diosgenin, which has a chemical structure very similar to progesterone. However, diosgenin is not readily converted to progesterone in the body. Instead diosgenin must be synthesized to progesterone outside the body in an experienced compounding facility.[719] On the other hand, wild yam may influence female health as it mimics progesterone and interacts with progesterone receptors on cells. To date, the jury is still out whether wild yam extract should only be used to extract diosgenin and create bioidentical progesterone or if it is beneficial alone.

Eating and physical activity has been discussed adequately in previous chapters and will help avoid excess weight that is associated with increased risk of cancer.[720] Eating and physical activity are the foundation of your health and this is true in your efforts to create an inhospitable environment for cancer. Psychological factors are also essential. Other important factors are appropriate self-checks such as regular testicular and breast exams. Learn how to properly perform self-examinations. If you aren't sure how to perform self-examinations, seek this information from a qualified health care practitioner. The American Cancer Society website has good information about the importance of regular self-exams and instructions for how to perform them. Early detection is essential in the success of cancer treatment, so regular screenings should also be integrated.

The following table is a list of the estimated deaths attributed to the top five most common cancer causes of death among men and women.[721]

MEN		WOMEN	
Lung & bronchus	28 percent	Lung & bronchus	26 percent
Prostate	10 percent	Breast	14 percent
Colon & rectum	9 percent	Colon & rectum	9 percent
Pancreas	6 percent	Pancreas	7 percent
Liver & intrahepatic bile duct	5 percent	Ovary	5 percent

Lung, breast, prostate, colon, and rectum cancer cause the most deaths among men and women so it is important to discuss specific ways to reduce the risk of these cancers.

LUNG CANCER

Lung cancer is the most lethal of all cancers and has the lowest survivability rates. Survival rates reduce with each stage of cancer. The five-year survival rate (patients usually survive at least five years after cancer diagnosis) is 49 percent with stage IA and only 1 percent with stage IV.[722] More people die from lung cancer than from the next three most common cancers combined (pancreas, breast, and colon cancers).[723] Though the statistics seem bleak for those who are diagnosed with lung cancer, many people do survive with proper treatment.

The single most important step to reduce lung cancer risk is to avoid tobacco use. Eighty-seven percent of lung cancer deaths in men and 70 percent in women are smoking related.[724] It can't be stressed enough how important it is to avoid this harmful and destructive product.

As with all disease, it is critical to eat better, participate in regular physical activity, and take an optimum-potency multivitamin and mineral. Make a concerted effort to get five to seven servings of fruits and vegetables, with a heavy focus on vegetables, each day. If you are at higher risk for lung cancer, have a superfood green drink, such as spirulina or chlorella, every day. Scientific research suggests both spirulina and chlorella may provide protection against cancer.[725-728]

Optimal lung health and function can be supported through daily deep-breathing exercises. Regular physical activity may also enhance lung and respiratory system function. Avoid polluted and industrial areas that are devoid of healthy clean air for you to breathe. One study indicated that those who live in heavy soot and sulfur dioxide pollution areas have an increased risk of lung cancer.[729] Quite simply the cleaner air you breathe the better for your lungs.

The World Health Organization considers radon a worldwide health risk. It is a good idea to have your home tested for radon levels. A good place to determine your relative exposure risk is through the EPA's website where a map of counties with the highest potential for radon exposure exists. The EPA recommends all homes be tested. Contact your local state radon agency to determine the availability of test kits within your area.

QUERCETIN

The research surrounding the flavonoid quercetin, found in apples, blueberries, onions, and white grapefruit, suggests it provides cancer-preventive benefits.[730] It appears quercetin has the ability to inhibit lung cancer cell growth.[731] If you are at high risk of lung cancer, you may want to take 300 to 750 mg quercetin daily in divided doses. It also helps resolve DNA damage, protects against chemical-caused cancer, and reduces other cancer pathways such as inflammation and obesity.[732,733] Quercetin may interact unfavorably with high blood pressure medications, cyclosporine, and drugs metabolized by the cytochrome P450 enzymes.

Lung Cancer Risk Reduction Role:	Repairs DNA damage that leads to cancer; protects against chemical-caused cancer, inhibits cancer cell growth, and reduces inflammation and obesity.

SILIBININ (MILK THISTLE)

Another potential botanical extract is silibinin, a water-soluble form of milk thistle silymarin—which has demonstrated promise against non-small-cell lung carcinoma cells.[734] Silibinin causes destruction of lung cancer cells, slows tumor growth, and reverses drug resistance so that chemotherapy is effective against lung cancer cells.[735,736] A therapeutic dosage of silibinin is commonly 70 to 140 mg three times per day. Caution is advised if you take Tamoxifen, glucuronidated drugs, or medications metabolized by the cytochrome P450 enzymes as milk thistle may interact with these drugs.

Lung Cancer Risk Reduction Role:	Slows the spread of and helps destroy lung cancer cells, reduces tumor growth, and improves the effectiveness of chemo-therapy agents.

PROSTATE CANCER

The prostate gland is a male reproductive organ about the size of a walnut positioned beneath the bladder and surrounding the urethra. The prostate cells grow uncontrollably and squeeze the urethra, making normal urination flow difficult. About one in every seven men will be diagnosed with prostate cancer at some point during his lifetime.[737] Prostate cancer is considered very treatable and survivable if detected early. Remarkably the relative five-year survival rate is almost 100 percent.[738]

Prostate cancer generally strikes men over age fifty. It is believed that the ratio of testosterone to estrogen, and conversion of testosterone to dihydrotestosterone (DHT) are factors in prostate enlargement. In some men, during their late forties, prostate cells grow more rapidly enlarging the prostate gland, called benign prostatic hyperplasia (BPH). The most common symptoms of an enlarged prostate are frequent urination, inability to urinate or interrupted urine flow, painful ejaculation, and difficulty having an erection. However, if the prostate is only slightly enlarged, no noticeable symptoms may be present. Prostate cancer is usually diagnosed through a prostate biopsy after an abnormal digital rectal examination (DRE) or abnormal prostate-specific antigen (PSA) test result.

Nutrition, smoking, and weight are the most controllable risk factors in regards to prostate cancer. Eating better will help maintain a healthy weight and reduce the risk of obesity, and therefore the risk for prostate cancer. Eating better should be coupled with regular moderate physical activity. Some research indicates eating processed food (just about anything in a can, bag, or box) and red meat (particularly cooked at high temperatures and well-done like on a grill) contributes to prostate cancer risk.[739-742] Men in Japan tend to have much lower incidence of prostate cancer and some experts contribute this to their higher intake of soy foods containing isoflavones.[743]

SELENIUM

Selenium has received mixed reviews in prostate cancer prevention studies. Studies that were controlled for body mass index, smoking, and alcohol use have indicated a positive reduction in prostate cancer development,[744] while recent research that suggests selenium was no more effective than a placebo may not have been as actively controlled for these factors.[745] Men diagnosed with prostate cancer generally have lower blood plasma levels of selenium,[746] which suggests increased blood plasma levels of selenium may reduce prostate cancer development. It is important to take selenium with its antioxidant partners vitamins E and C to avoid an increased risk of cancer observed when high doses of a single antioxidant are taken. To reduce the risk of prostate cancer, 200 mcg of selenium daily has been used.[747,748] Selenium may interact with anticoagulants, antiplatelet medications, barbiturates, statins, and blood pressure medications.

Prostate Cancer Risk Reduction Role: Protects against DNA damage that may cause uncontrolled growth of prostate cancer cells.

SAW PALMETTO

Saw palmetto is another herbal supplement worth considering. It is known to inhibit the enzyme responsible (5-alpha reductase) for the conversion of testosterone to DHT—a more potent form of testosterone. It has also been used traditionally to support male sexual vitality, libido, and normal urination. Saw palmetto may also slow prostate growth,[749] and support overall urinary health.[750,751] Commonly 160 mg twice daily or 320 mg once daily is recommended for benign prostatic hyperplasia (BPH).[752] Consult with a physician or pharmacist before using saw palmetto if you are taking anticoagulants, antiplatelet medications, contraceptive drugs, or estrogen hormone replacement therapy.

Prostate Cancer Risk Reduction Role: Protects against uncontrolled growth of prostate cancer cells.

PUMPKIN SEED EXTRACT

Pumpkin seed extract may influence hormone balance in men and subsequently reduces the risk of prostate cancer.[753] Clinical studies have demonstrated improvements in prostate function and health after taking 320 mg daily.[754] Theoretically, pumpkin seed extract could increase blood levels of lithium through decreased excretion.

Prostate Cancer Risk Reduction Role: Helps balance hormone levels to avoid prostate cancer and supports normal prostate function.

BREAST CANCER

Breast cancer occurs in both men and women, though very rarely in men. It is estimated that 12 percent of women will develop breast cancer during their lifetime and about 40,000 will die from it each year.[755] Some women are so fearful of this disease they choose to have their breasts removed, called a prophylactic mastectomy, to avoid it. The most controllable risk factors for breast cancer are contraceptive use (oral or injectable), synthetic HRT, being overweight or obese, physical inactivity, and chest radiation exposure. Other risk factors include gender, age, genetics, family history, dense breast tissue, some benign breast conditions, early menstruation (before age twelve), never having children, and never breastfeeding.[756] The most controllable risk factors include contraceptive use, HRT, weight management, and physical activity levels.

Estrogen is a female hormone produced by the ovaries that produces and maintains female sexual characteristics. One of the functions of estrogen is to stimulate production of breast cells, but excess estrogen encourages the abnormal development of breast tissue. Conversely, progesterone supports the normal development of breast tissue. The longer a female is exposed to estrogen (particularly synthetic estrogens) the more likely she is to develop breast cancer.

Early menses (before age twelve) and late menopause (after age fifty-five) results in greater estrogen exposure and a slightly increased risk of breast cancer.

Another source of estrogen exposure is hormone therapy, which is often used in traditional medicine for the treatment of menopause. Hormone replacement therapy may make tumors less visible during a mammogram and is associated with other risks like uterine cancer and increased cardiovascular disease. Progesterone is known to destroy breast cancer cells through encouraging apoptosis.[757] Remarkably, for every 0.1 g per day incremental increase of marine omega-3 fatty acid intake, women can receive a 5 percent reduction in their risk of breast cancer.[758] Unfortunately, plant-based omega-3, alpha linolenic acid, did not produce the same results, suggesting marine omega-3s provide greater protection from breast cancer. Frequent physical activity, foods that help balance female hormones (omega-3 fatty acids, coconut oil, avocados), raw green plants, and supplementary measures (black cohosh, chasteberry, dong quai, and natural progesterone) are safer natural alternatives to hormone replacement therapy

Drug contraceptives increase exposure to synthetic estrogens that are strongly associated with a slight increase in breast cancer risk. Remarkably, research also suggests that this elevated risk continues for ten years after discontinuance of oral contraceptives, meaning that if you are currently taking oral contraceptives and decide to stop today, your risk of breast cancer may remain elevated for the next ten years.[759] Before using oral contraceptives as a birth control method it is a good idea to weigh the risks versus the benefits and consider all other methods available (condoms or a copper intrauterine device).

Smoking and excess alcohol consumption increases breast cancer risk. Many carcinogenic chemicals in cigarettes are fat-soluble, resistant to metabolism, and often stored in breast tissue. Women should follow the American Cancer Society's recommendation to drink no more than one alcoholic beverage per day to help reduce breast cancer risk.

Being overweight or obese increases the risk of breast cancer, especially if the excess weight is in the waist. Obesity is associated with early menses,[760] reproductive organ abnormalities,[761] and breast cancer.[762] Excess weight is also a causative factor in late menopause. When you experience menopause after age fifty-five (considered late menopause), your exposure to estrogen and risk of reproductive cancers increase.[763] Risk increases further if excess weight is gained after menopause. During menopause the ovaries cease to produce estrogen and the body relies on estrogen stored in fat tissue. Increased fat tissue means more estrogen exposure and thus greater breast cancer risk. It is important to maintain a healthy weight based on your height and frame and particularly avoid weight gain in later life.

Women who have had no children or have them after age thirty have an increased risk of breast cancer and this risk increases with each year that childbirth is delayed.[764] This may be due to the decrease in the number of menstrual cycles a woman experiences during pregnancy due to several months of hiatus from menstruation. Women who breast feed experience a 4.3 percent reduction in breast cancer risk for every twelve months of breast feeding in addition to a 7 percent reduction for every birth.[765] This indicates that a mother of four that breast fed each child for twelve months could potentially reduce her breast cancer risk by an amazing 45.2 percent. This is good news for mothers.

Foods that contain phytosterols (rice bran, corn, wheat germ, flax seed, olives, soy products, and cashews) are also important for the reduction of breast cancer.[766] These cholesterol-like compounds help reduce serum cholesterol levels, including in the membrane of cancer cells, and are essential to apoptosis (programmed cell death), which helps reduce uncontrolled growth of cells, and reduces the risk of cancer development.[767,768] Another group of phytochemicals, glucosinolates, found in cruciferous vegetables (cabbage, broccoli, and cauliflower) may help prevent cancer.[769] Don't forget to eat at least five servings of fruits and vegetables a day for optimum health. Substitute fish and lean poultry for red meat and reduce total consumption of red meat and processed meats. DHA, found in fish or fish oil supplements, can prevent cancer genes from activating.[770] If you eat a significant number of vegetables and fruits, your body receives a superfluity of phytochemicals that supports your body's cancer and disease prevention efforts.

Breast health may be enhanced if you perform self-lymphatic breast massage. This promotes flow of lymph in the breast and nearby tissues and promotes the release of toxins from the breast. These techniques can be learned from the privacy of your home through instructional videos available on the Internet. Self-exams are essential to detect cancer early and the earlier the detection, the greater the possibility of successful treatment and cure. If you don't know how to properly examine your breasts, ask your health care provider at your next annual checkup, or search online. There are many resource tools available to learn proper self-exam techniques. As was previously mentioned, a proper fitting bra and reduced time wearing a bra may help promote breast health and reduce breast cancer risk.[771]

CONJUGATED LINOLEIC ACID (CLA)

Conjugated Linoleic Acid (CLA) supplements are worth considering if you are at a high risk for breast cancer. This supplement is often used for weight loss because of its ability to increase lean muscle mass and decrease fat without changing the way you eat;[772] but CLA research is stronger for its anticarcinogenic activity.[773,774] CLA possesses antiestrogenic properties as well as anti-tumor activities with breast cancer cells.[775,776] CLA dosage is generally 1 to 3 grams daily in fatty acid form. There are no known drug interactions with CLA currently.

Breast Cancer Risk Reduction Role: Helps balance hormones and reduce the negative effect of excess estrogen on breast tissue, protects against breast tumors, and promotes the destruction of breast cancer cells.

TURMERIC

Turmeric, or its active ingredient curcumin, is more than just a curry ingredient, it is considered by some experts to be the chief anti-cancer herb. Evidence suggests that turmeric is able to prevent cancer initiation, promotion, and progression.[777-779] Researchers at the MD Anderson Cancer Center of the University of Texas concluded that turmeric is effective in slowing and preventing breast cancer progression especially when combined with the drug Taxol.[780] The anti-cancer activity may be related to its antioxidant, anti-inflammatory, anti-bacterial, and DNA protective effects. Use this spice in your cooking and if you are at high risk for breast cancer or simply want to enhance your breast cancer prevention strategy. Studies with colon cancer have used therapeutic levels of 440 to 2,200 mg of turmeric in divided doses daily.[781] You may increase the absorption of curcumin, the active constituent in turmeric, if you take it with food. It is possible that turmeric or curcumin could interact with anticoagulant or antiplatelet medications (drugs used to prevent blood from clotting, prevent the enlargement of existing clots, or prevent cells and platelets from sticking together to form a clot).

Breast Cancer Risk Reduction Role: Protects DNA from damage that may lead to cancer, inhibits uncontrollable cancer cell spread, protects against factors that may promote cancer cell production, and aids chemotherapy agents.

COLON CANCER

Colon cancer occurs in the large intestine while rectal cancer occurs in the last several inches of the colon closest to the anus. They are often collectively referred to as colorectal cancer. Normally these cancers begin as benign clumps called polyps, which later grow into colorectal cancer. Only adenomas can become cancerous. The majority of people diagnosed with this type of cancer are over age fifty—an astonishing 90 percent of all cases. This is possibly due to the increased number of polyps seen in people over age fifty.

Colorectal cancer may be a disease of affluence, because the incidence of colorectal cancer is highest among developed countries and lowest in developing countries.[782] This is possibly due to the higher red meat consumption in developed countries, because of its availability and affordability as compared to undeveloped countries.[783] Risk factors for colorectal cancer include inflammatory bowel diseases (Crohn's, ulcerative colitis), family history of colorectal cancer or polyps, genetics, physical inactivity, low fruit and vegetable intake, not enough fiber in the diet, being overweight or obese, alcohol consumption, and tobacco use.[784]

Poor eating habits are thought to cause the majority of colon cancers, meaning it is highly preventable by eating better.[785] This makes eating the right foods the most crucial aspect of a colorectal cancer prevention plan—particularly fruits and vegetables. Eating better may also reduce the risk of being overweight or obese, a risk factor in colorectal cancer. Excess consumption of refined sugar and simple carbohydrates also increase colorectal cancer risk.[786] People who eat fiber-rich diets, particularly from vegetables, have a lower incidence of colorectal cancer.[787] Conversely, those who consume a diet high in animal fats with few vegetables have the greatest incidence of colorectal cancer.[788] Increased fiber intake, specifically from vegetables, combined with decreased red meat consumption, may reduce your colorectal cancer risk.

Regular bowel movements (at least once daily) limits the time waste stays in the colon and prevents damage to colon cells that may occur from contact with carcinogenic chemicals, bile salts, and animal-based foods. Infrequent bowel movement is associated with a greater risk of colorectal cancer.[789] Toilets commonly used in the United States can create problems with regular and complete bowel movements. Toilets that encourage the squatting position—commonly found in Asian and other countries—better support and properly align the bowel for complete elimination. The sitting position can promote constipation, hemorrhoids, other bowel disorders, and possibly even heart attacks from straining when the heart is already compromised. Toilets in the United States put the bowel in an unsupported, misaligned position, which can result in straining to eliminate. Interestingly, infants instinctively squat to eliminate waste, placing their intestinal organs and musculature in a much more optimal position to eliminate. To properly support the bowel and improve elimination when using a Western toilet, place your feet on a step stool directly in front of the toilet. This will move your knees closer to your abdomen, and simulate the squatting position to improve elimination and reduce the adverse effects of the sitting position.

PROBIOTICS

A proper proportion of healthy bacteria (probiotics) in the intestines may help prevent colorectal cancer. These living microorganisms exert health benefits far beyond aiding the digestive and elimination systems. They are beneficial to prevent and manage bowel disorders associated with colon cancer.[790-792] They may increase immune system function[793-795] and reduce skin disorders[796,797] as well as infections and illness.[798-802] Probiotics protect against colorectal cancer[803,804] through a variety of mechanisms, including inactivation of carcinogenic compounds, competition for intestinal space with pathogenic and putrefactive organisms, to enhancement of host immune response and encouragement of apoptosis of cancer cells.[805] The more probiotics that inhabit your gastrointestinal tract, the better the protection.

Colon Cancer Risk Reduction Role: Support bowel regularity to speed the elimination of potentially carcinogenic compounds, limit the amount of space available in the intestinal tract for harmful organisms, aid the immune response to harmful organisms, and encourage the destruction of cancer cells.

TURMERIC

Turmeric has demonstrated the ability to inhibit all stages of colon cancer.[806,807,808] Turmeric aids digestion and helps your body digest fats instead of accumulate them.[809] You can incorporate this powerful spice in your diet simply if you add a quarter teaspoon to appropriate meals. The current evidence strongly indicates that turmeric is a potent anti-cancer nutrient that directly effects cancer cells (it encourages their destruction).[810] In addition, it helps inhibit angiogenesis,[811,812] growth of new blood vessels, which cancerous tumors are dependent upon for progression. Last, studies with animals suggest that it may prevent the growth of intestinal polyps.[813] As was mentioned, turmeric may interact with anticoagulant and antiplatelet medications.

165

Colon Cancer Risk Reduction Role: Supports the digestive system, causes colorectal cancer cell death, blocks the formation of blood vessels intended to supply blood to cancerous tumors, aids the elimination of fats, and may prevent the formation of polyps.

Other nutrients that are considered beneficial in the prevention of polyps and colorectal cancer are calcium, folic acid, vitamin D, and the antioxidants vitamin E, vitamin C, carotenoids, and selenium. Antioxidants have shown the ability to enhance the action of chemotherapy agents in colorectal cancer.[814] If you take the recommended amounts of these nutrients in your daily multivitamin/mineral you should get the benefits these nutrients may provide.

STROKE

Stroke is a medical term used for a sudden interruption of blood flow and oxygen to any portion of the brain. It is caused by blockage or rupture of a blood vessel in the brain and may result in brain damage. There are two major types of stoke: ischemic and hemorrhagic. Ischemic stroke is caused when a blood vessel that supplies blood to the brain is blocked by a blood clot or other particles, such as cholesterol. Ischemic strokes are further divided into the subtypes: thrombotic stroke—a blood clot forms in an artery leading to the brain; and embolic stroke—a blood clot forms in a part of the body outside the brain and travels through the blood stream until it becomes lodged in the narrower arteries of the brain. A hemorrhagic stroke occurs when a blood vessel in the brain becomes weak, bursts open, and causes bleeding in the brain. Hemorrhagic strokes are also subdivided into intracerebral stroke—when a blood vessel in the brain bursts and spills in the actual brain tissue, damaging cells; and subarachnoid stroke—a blood vessel just outside the brain ruptures causing bleeding in between the brain and the thin tissues that cover the brain.

The number one risk factor for a stroke is high blood pressure. Another significant risk factor is atherosclerosis. Atherosclerosis causes the arteries to harden and narrow due to a buildup of fatty deposits in the arterial walls, which restricts blood flow. Other risk factors for stroke include: age, gender, smoking, diabetes, heart disease, brain aneurysms, race, ethnicity, family history, alcohol and illegal drug use, high cholesterol, physical inactivity, poor eating choices, obesity, stress, depression, and certain medical conditions (sickle cell anemia, vasculitis, vascular inflammation, and bleeding disorders).[815]

To reduce the risk of forming blood clots, you should eat a healthy diet full of high fiber foods, fruits, and vegetables. Include the right kind of fats, like omega-3 fatty acids, and avoid trans fats. Consume fish twice per week or take a fish oil supplement to increase DHA and EPA levels. Reduce salt and sugar intake. The so-called "cafeteria diet"—a diet consisting of high-calorie, high-sugar, and high-sodium has been linked to a greater risk of stroke, even among teens and young adults (age sixteen to twenty-two).[816] Foods high in anthocyanins (black or purple grapes, blueberries, cranberries, and red cabbage) should be consumed frequently. These foods reduce the risk of coronary disease and stroke through improved endothelial function and reduced inflammation.[817-819] Eating potassium rich foods (banana, dried prunes, lima beans, and potatoes) helps reduce blood pressure and stroke risk.[820,821] If you make better food choices you are more likely to reduce stroke risk.

Techniques to manage stress are beneficial in both stroke prevention and recovery. Atherosclerosis[822,823] and high blood pressure[824] are the two leading risk factors for strokes and are known to be exacerbated by stress. Regular physical activity reduces the risk of diabetes, heart disease, and stroke.[825] Aim for thirty minutes of moderate physical activity every day. Remember, this activity can be cumulative short bouts throughout the day. This may sound like a broken record, but regular physical activity combined with eating better will reduce obesity risk, another stroke risk factor.

Both hormone therapy and drug contraceptive use increase the risk of stroke, even when other risk factors are controlled for in studies. The use of drug contraceptives has been associated with up to a three-fold increase in stroke risk when compared to those who don't use drug contraceptives.[826-828] Hormone therapy is also associated with elevated stroke risk.[829-831] The good news is that once HRT is stopped the risk appears to reduce to normal. Consider your birth control options carefully and choose safer alternatives to hormone therapy.

As with virtually every disease smoking should be avoided. Heavy alcohol consumption is also associated with an increased risk. However, light to moderate alcohol consumption may be protective.[832] Given the addictive nature of alcohol, and its link to stroke risk factors like high blood pressure[833,834] and atherosclerosis,[835] it may be wise to avoid drinking altogether, or at the very least limit consumption of alcoholic beverages to light to moderate drinking. You could significantly improve your health if you stop one or both of these habits.

GARLIC

Garlic has the ability to reduce total cholesterol and increase HDL cholesterol.[673,674] The greater the total and LDL cholesterol levels the greater risk of atherosclerosis and high blood pressure. High blood pressure and atherosclerosis are the two leading causes of stroke. It is believed that garlic provides protection against atherosclerosis, and therefore stroke. Garlic improves endothelial function and protects lipids from oxidation.[836-840] Dysfunction of the inner lining of the blood vessels and lymphatic vessels, called the endothelium, involves an imbalance of vasodilating (blood vessel widening) and vasoconstricting (blood vessel constricting) substances, which shifts the blood vessels to a more constrictive state. This state is thought to be a key causal factor in atherosclerosis. Oxidized LDL is considered another causal factor in atherosclerosis. The restricted flow of blood to the brain and other parts of the body caused by atherosclerosis can increase the risk of stroke. Allicin, a chemical in garlic, makes blood platelets less sticky and therefore less likely to clot.[841] Typical dosages of garlic are 200 to 400 mg, three times daily. Those who take antimycobacterial drugs (drugs used for tuberculosis and other mycobacterium-caused diseases), drug contraceptives, HIV and hepatitis C drugs, anticoagulants, antiplatelet medications, and cyclosporine (a drug used to prevent transplant rejection and for the treatment of arthritis) should consult a physician or pharmacist before taking garlic due to potential interactions.

Stroke Risk Reduction Role: Helps reduce total cholesterol and prevent the oxidation of LDL cholesterol to reduce the risk of atherosclerosis, helps reduce blood pressure through reduced clumping of platelets, and improves blood vessel function.

CHRONIC LOWER RESPIRATORY DISEASE (CLRD)

CLRD is a term used for respiratory illnesses like chronic obstructive pulmonary disease, chronic bronchitis, and emphysema that affect millions of people of all ages. These lung diseases are largely caused by smoking, including secondhand smoke, accounting for approximately 80 to 90 percent of chronic lower respiratory deaths.[842] Indeed, according to the American Lung Association, men and women who smoke are up to thirteen times more likely to die from chronic obstructive pulmonary disease than those who do not. Other major risk factors include exposure to indoor or outdoor air pollutants, allergens, and occupational agents.[843] In addition, physical inactivity, poor nutritional choices, and post infectious chronic respiratory diseases are possible contributing factors to CLRD.

The most obvious action to take to avoid CLRD is to never smoke, quit smoking if you do smoke, and avoid exposure to environmental tobacco smoke. In addition, avoid heavily polluted environments and exposure to environmental irritants. Most irritant exposure occurs in the workplace or industrial areas, so wear proper safety and protective equipment at all times. Strive to breathe clean air even if it means going for a drive to find a cleaner air environment. Support your lung health through deep breathing exercises and physical activity, or think about taking up a wind musical instrument. Avoid foods that promote mucous congestion including dairy products, fried foods, and junk foods.

To prevent acute lower respiratory diseases from becoming chronic, proper treatment of these diseases is essential. Echinacea and goldenseal are excellent immune stimulating herbs, whereas mullein promotes the expulsion of mucous and is soothing for the respiratory tract. N-acetylcysteine and vitamin C are beneficial nutrient choices, which improve the ability to expectorate and enhance immune function. Potent antimicrobial essential oils like oregano, cinnamon, thyme, and clove are also good options to eliminate germs from the body that cause respiratory diseases. Of great importance with most respiratory diseases is to diffuse, or steam inhale, essential oils that support the respiratory system and/or encourage the expulsion of mucous, such as eucalyptus, peppermint, rosemary, pine, or cedarwood. Ensure you get adequate rest, plenty of clean fluids (to help thin and expel mucous), and avoid using cough suppressants, which thwart the body's ability to expel.

STOPPING DIABETES IN ITS TRACKS

Diabetes, also known as diabetes mellitus, is a chronic condition that affects the body's ability to use blood sugar (glucose) for energy. It is estimated that as many as one-third of Americans will suffer from diabetes by the year 2050 if current trends continue.[844] When carbohydrates are consumed they are absorbed from the intestines into the bloodstream. In response to the elevated blood sugar, the body signals the pancreas to produce insulin. Insulin interacts with and binds to cell receptor sites. Once attached to the cell receptor sites, the insulin stimulates the receptors to absorb glucose from the bloodstream. Glucose is then used by the cells to produce energy for bodily processes. If insufficient blood sugar is absorbed, hyperglycemia (high blood sugar) occurs. This excess blood sugar is diagnosed as diabetes. Diabetes occurs when the pancreas doesn't produce enough insulin in response to glucose or if cells of the body become resistant to insulin attachment.

Diabetes is divided into three types. Type 1 diabetes is a chronic condition where the body produces little or no insulin because the body's own immune system attacks and destroys the pancreas islet cells responsible for insulin production. This type requires insulin injections. Type 2 diabetes is by far the most common form, and is a condition in which the pancreas produces insufficient insulin or the body does not respond properly to insulin, called insulin resistance. The third type of diabetes called gestational diabetes develops during pregnancy in a woman who previously was not diagnosed with diabetes. It too affects blood glucose levels, which normally return to normal following delivery.

Diabetes is a significantly growing problem in the United States. In 2012, more than 9 percent of the population had diabetes, or roughly 29.1 million Americans.[845] The American Diabetes Association estimates that 86 million Americans have what is termed prediabetes, a condition in which blood sugar levels are higher than normal, but not high enough to be classified as diabetes yet. Astonishingly, they also estimate that more than half of Americans over age sixty-five have prediabetes.

The most common risk factors for type 1 diabetes include family history, genetics, age, and geography (risk increases the farther you travel from the equator). Other possible risk factors include exposure to certain viruses, early exposure to cow's milk, vitamin D deficiency, drinking water with nitrates, early or late introduction of cereal and gluten in an infant's diet, neonatal jaundice, and being born to a mother who had preeclampsia during pregnancy.[846] On the other hand, type 2 diabetes is largely preventable through eating better and regular physical activity. The risk factors for type 2 diabetes are age (forty-five or older), being overweight or obese, family history of diabetes, ethnicity (African Americans, Hispanics/Latinos, Native Americans, Asian Americans, and Pacific Islanders have greater risk), gestational diabetes, elevated blood pressure, physical inactivity, polycystic ovary syndrome (PCOS), vascular disorders, and pigmentation of the skin around the neck and armpits. The family history connection in type 2 diabetes may very well be an eating and lifestyle factor since many families eat the same meals and participate in similar amounts of physical activity.

Eating better is especially important in the management of type 2 diabetes since better food choices help balance and maintain normal blood sugar levels. In fact, wise food choices are the basis of managing diabetes. Some experts hypothesize that insulin receptor sites become clogged by fat or cholesterol and prevent insulin from attaching to these receptors. If insulin is unable to attach to cell receptors it creates insulin resistance. A well-balanced diet high in fiber, fruits, vegetables, lean meats, wholesome proteins, healthy fats, and appropriate amounts of whole grains (not refined) helps control blood sugar levels and reduces complications caused by diabetes. Foods with water-soluble fiber like apples, oranges, flaxseed, psyllium, oat bran, beans, nuts, and seeds, promote blood sugar balance. Consume foods high in nutritional value, or foods that provide significant nutrients in relation to their number of calories. Maintain a regular meal schedule (number of meals at regular times) with a relatively consistent amount of carbohydrates, fats, and proteins.[847] Consume smaller, more frequent meals (five or more per day, without increased total caloric intake) rather than three large meals, to help maintain more consistent insulin and blood sugar levels, particularly in obese populations.[848,849]

In general, wholesome carbohydrates (whole grains, fruits, and vegetables) are utilized more slowly by the body and therefore the change in blood sugar and insulin levels is more gradual. Often quoted is the fact that whole grain wheat bread has a similar glycemic index or greater than that of many candy bars. The glycemic index is a measurement of how quickly carbohydrate-containing foods affect blood sugar two hours after consumption. For example the average whole wheat bread has a glycemic index of 71, compared to a Snickers Bar with an index of 51 and Peanut M & Ms, which check in at 33. One major drawback to the glycemic index is that it doesn't simulate the way people typically consume foods. How often do people eat a single slice of whole wheat bread without anything else with it, like peanut butter or a slice of meat and cheese? It is rare that people will eat foods alone or one at a time. Instead, we eat a variety of carbohydrate foods (usually mixed with proteins and fats) in any single meal. Proteins and fats are metabolic regulators, which tend to decrease the glycemic effect of a meal. This is largely why the two candy bars mentioned score better than whole wheat bread, because both provide fat and protein (Peanut M&Ms—7.5 g fat and 2.9 g protein[850]; Snickers Bar—6.7 g fat and 2.5 g protein[851]) to regulate the rapid increase in blood sugar, whereas the bread contains no fat and 4 grams of protein.[852] Carbohydrates eaten alone will cause the most rapid increases in blood sugar levels. Conversely, a meal that includes a carbohydrate, fat, and protein will have a lesser effect on blood sugar levels.[853,854] Those with certain health conditions—high blood pressure, diabetes, high cholesterol, obesity, and autoimmune disorders should rigorously restrict grain and sugar intake until these conditions are under control.

Regular physical activity burns more calories and helps normalize metabolism. It also helps encourage cells to uptake glucose from the bloodstream.[855,856] This action may help significantly reduce the risk of diabetes. Individuals who are more active tend to have lower blood sugar levels. Research indicates that aerobic activities increase insulin sensitivity,[857,858] as does strength training.[859-861] Physical activity is also associated with decreased risk of diabetes complications like heart disease, stroke, and kidney failure.[862] Regular physical activity reduces one's diabetes risk.[863-865] In fact, scientists concluded that for every 2.2 pounds of weight lost by those who are overweight or obese, they can realize an additional 16 percent reduction in the risk of diabetes.[869]

CHROMIUM

Chromium may be beneficial in both the prevention and treatment of diabetes.[866-868] Chromium improves glucose tolerance and insulin sensitivity, helping to balances blood sugar levels. To reduce the risk of diabetes, 200 to 400 mcg of chromium may be a suitable preventative dose. Those with prediabetes or diabetes may need as much as 1,000 mcg. Chromium should not be taken concurrently with insulin because it may increase the risk of hypoglycemia. Chromium may also interact with the thyroid medication levothyroxine.[869]

Diabetes Risk Reduction Role: Improves insulin sensitivity and the body's response to glucose, which helps balance blood sugar levels.

ALPHA-LIPOIC ACID

Alpha-lipoic acid is an antioxidant that plays a critical role in the production of energy from glucose. It may reduce blood sugar levels[870] as well as decrease symptoms of diabetic neuropathy.[871] It is found in good quantities in flaxseed, walnuts, and grape-seed oil. The typical therapeutic dose of ALA is 600 to 1,200 mg daily. Alpha-lipoic acid may interact with chemotherapy and thyroid medications.

Diabetes Risk Reduction Role: Improves insulin sensitivity and the body's response to glucose, to help balance blood sugar levels.

STEVIA

Stevia is a zero-calorie, herbal sweetener and sugar substitute that is gaining popularity in the United States. It is derived from the *Stevia rebaudiana* plant native to South America. Stevia is much sweeter than regular table sugar, with standardized stevia extracts reported to be up to 250 times sweeter than sucrose. It is worth using as a sugar substitute and has a superb safety profile in Japan, where it has been used for decades as a food sweetener. One drawback to this sweetener is its bitter aftertaste. Some research even suggests stevia may be able to reduce plasma glucose levels and insulin levels without increasing the desire for more calories.[872] Theoretically, stevia may reduce the excretion of lithium, which could lead to excess lithium in the blood.[873]

Diabetes Risk Reduction Role: Provides a natural sugar substitute and balances blood sugar and insulin levels.

CINNAMON

Cinnamon extract or cinnamon essential oil has marked effects on blood glucose levels. It has been shown to lower fasting blood glucose levels,[874] and interestingly an animal study suggested that cinnamon oil may even improve the function of pancreatic islets beta-cells.[875] Beta-cells release the necessary amount of insulin to maintain normal blood sugar levels in response to increased sugar in the blood. It also protects the kidneys from damage associated with diabetes complications.[876] Those who take antidiabetic medications, anticoagulants, medications metabolized by the cytochrome P450 enzymes, and antiplatelet medications should not use cinnamon without first consulting with a physician or pharmacist.

Diabetes Risk Reduction Role: Supports normal function of the pancreatic islets beta-cells that produce insulin and helps decrease blood sugar levels

PRESERVING COGNITION TO PREVENT ALZHEIMER'S DISEASE

Alzheimer's disease (AD) is a progressive and irreversible brain disorder in which brain cells (neurons) deteriorate, resulting in cognitive dysfunction and possibly death. Memory loss, poor judgment, inability to reason, personality changes, and disorientation are the primary symptoms of AD. AD is the most common form of dementia—a term used to describe disorders that impair mental function to the extent it interferes with normal daily activities. Statistics from 2014 estimate that about 5.2 million people in the United States have AD,[877] with that number expected to rise significantly as more Baby Boomers reach their "golden years." The risk for AD doubles with every five years a person lives past age sixty-five. The common risk factors for AD include age (almost 50 percent of individuals older than eighty-five have AD), family history, genetics, and head trauma.[878] Additionally, because of higher levels of heavy metals (aluminum particularly) found in AD patients during autopsy, some scientists believe environmental toxins may contribute to AD. Although research has been inconsistent in establishing this fact,[879,880,881] aluminum is a neurotoxin and has been associated with neurological diseases, so the connection makes sense.[882]

Eat healthy and organic foods that nourish the body to help prevent AD. Research suggests that berries are some of the most nourishing and protective food for the brain. Their significant antioxidant capacity protect the brain from free-radical damage. Moreover, berries promote autophagy,[883] the brain's built-in housekeeping process that aids the clearance of damaging substances that accumulate in the brain during the aging process. Berries encourage the efficient function of neurons during the aging process. They also prevent neuronal damage, enhance neuronal communication, reduce inflammation, and help preserve memory, control, and reasoning abilities.[884-888] In addition, they support neuroplasticity, the ability of the brain to form new connections and learn new things throughout life,

Fish are a good source of DHA and EPA, which is critical to brain function for all ages from babies to seniors.[889-892] In fact, when combined with vitamin D, DHA helps optimize the immune system's ability to clear the brain of amyloid plaques.[893] Amyloid plaques are found in the spaces between brain neurons and greater amounts of plaque are associated with AD. The best way to get your DHA and EPA is to consume fish twice weekly. If you don't eat fish the next best thing is to take a fish oil supplement.

Eating ample amounts of fiber and super green foods combined with the consumption of plenty of clean water will improve detoxification. Accumulation of toxins and heavy metals in the brain has been linked to AD, so efficient detoxification is crucial. Avoid processed foods and food additives that increase your exposure to toxins. Choose non-aluminum cookware, avoid aluminum-based antiperspirants, stay away from soda in aluminum cans, and don't take antacids that contain aluminum. The healthier your food choices, the greater your nutritional support will be for proper brain function.

Research indicates the greater your education level, the lower your risk of AD.[894] Those with the least education had the most prevalence of AD, and AD progressed more quickly in these individuals.[895] This may be due to the increased brain activity involved in learning new skills, subjects, and information. Some scientists believe this benefit results from an increase in synapses (a junction between two nerve cells) due to increased cognitive requirements and brain usage, which establishes a denser reserve of synapses as people age. The mind should receive daily exercise just like the body to keep it sharp. Ways to challenge your brain and help maintain cognitive abilities as you age include:

- Read books daily that stimulate thought.
- Perform complicated tasks.
- Reduce TV watching to keep your mind sharp and prevent brain cell deterioration.
- Do puzzles.
- Learn a new language.
- Learn to play a musical instrument.
- Perform tasks with the non-dominant hand (i.e., eat and brush your teeth with your non-dominant hand).
- Memorize scriptural passages, poems, or historical documents.
- Stay active: physically, emotionally, mentally, spiritually, and socially.

The same risk factors (high cholesterol, high blood pressure, and diabetes) that contribute to heart disease can also increase the risk of AD. Regular physical activity combined with eating better may help mitigate these risks. Follow the same plan set forth to reduce the risk of heart disease and you just might save your mental abilities too.

SAGE

Sage is not only a spice; it is an effective medicinal herb and popular treatment for many health conditions in Europe, including upset stomach and inflammatory conditions. Sage is an effective mood enhancer and helps improve memory and cognitive function.[896-898] Studies using sixty drops of sage extract—not essential oil—daily have demonstrated effectiveness in managing

AD, significantly improving cognitive functions and possibly reducing agitation in AD patients.[899] Most trials have used the extract form, though some have used the dried sage leaf. Improved memory has also been observed in healthy young adults who were given sage essential oil.[900] As a cautionary warning, sage essential oil can contain significant quantities of thujone, which is known to be toxic—especially *Salvia officinalis*. It is not recommended to take *Salvia officinalis* internally because as little as twelve drops has reportedly caused seizures and a short coma in adults.[901] The study with healthy young adults used approximately one drop of Spanish sage (*Salvia lavandulifolia)* essential oil, which is devoid of thujone. Based on this fact, it is recommended to use one drop of Spanish sage essential oil orally per day, or small quantities of *Salvia officinalis* essential oil topically. In addition, sage may reduce the effectiveness of anticonvulsive drugs, which could counteract medications intended to prevent seizures.[902] It may also promote convulsions or interact with diabetic medications and central nervous system depressants.

AD Risk Reduction Role: Improves memory and cognitive abilities, suppresses the production of amyloid plaques, and balances mood.

ROSEMARY

Rosemary has been extensively studied for its effects on cognition and memory, and even William Shakespeare reportedly claimed that rosemary improved memory. A compound called carnosic acid, found in both rosemary and sage, suppresses the production of amyloid plaques in the brain.[903] When amyloid plaques form in the brain they may block the ability of brain cells to communicate with each other. Plaque formation is strongly associated with the risk of AD. A study that compared the effects of essential oil aromas observed that inhalation of rosemary significantly enhanced overall quality of long-term memory.[904] Applying rosemary with lemon in the morning and lavender and orange in the evening significantly improves personal orientation and cognitive function in elderly persons with dementia or AD.[905] Rosemary essential oil can increase the ability of healthy adults to remember things they needed to do in the future by up to 75 percent.[906] It may be beneficial to diffuse rosemary near those with dementia diseases or cognitive impairment. Rosemary could potentially interact with anticoagulant and antiplatelet medications, may inhibit cytochrome P450 enzymes responsible for multiple medications, and should be used with great caution around children under the age of six.

AD Risk Reduction Role:	Rosemary helps reduce the formation of amyloid plaques in the brain and may significantly enhance long-term memory, personal orientation, and short-term memory.

ANTIOXIDANTS

There is a growing body of evidence that suggests oxidative stress is associated with the initiation and progression of AD.[907-909] There is also sufficient evidence to recommend the use of antioxidants in the prevention of AD.[910-914] Optimum doses of antioxidants like vitamin C and E have shown promise in the prevention of AD.[915-917] They may also be beneficial to slow the progression of AD. The key is they need to be taken together.

AD Risk Reduction Role:	Improves long-term memory (even in healthy adults), enhances personal orientation and cognitive abilities of the elderly, and suppresses the production of amyloid plaques.

VITAMIN E

Vitamin E is associated with a decrease in functional decline among mild to moderate AD patients.[918] Foods rich in vitamin E (sunflower seeds, almonds, olives, and spinach) may help reduce AD risk. Studies with animals suggest that vitamin E stimulates autophagy.[919] It is a powerful antioxidant and known to protect brain lipids from oxidation.[920] Oxidation of brain lipoproteins (a combination of lipids and proteins) has been implicated as a cause of AD.[921] Vitamin E may also be taken as a supplement, but remember to take it with other antioxidants. The standard dosage used to reduce cognitive decline in people with AD is 2,000 IU daily. Vitamin E may interact with cyclosporine, statins, anticoagulants, and antiplatelet medications.

AD Risk Reduction Role:	Supports normal brain function and autophagy, and protects brain lipids from oxidative damage.

VITAMIN C

Scientists believe that a breakdown in the blood-brain barrier (BBB)—a filtering system set up to allow beneficial compounds in the brain and keep harmful substances out—may be a causal factor of AD. If the BBB dysfunctions, it is possible that more harmful substances can enter and stay in the brain tissue and disrupt cognitive function. Vitamin C reportedly strengthens the integrity of the BBB and reduces the formation of amyloid plaques, which could offer protection against AD.[922,923] German researchers discovered that a combination of vitamin C and vitamin E significantly decreases the oxidation of lipoproteins far better than vitamin E alone.[924] A comprehensive evaluation of antioxidants concluded that vitamin C, vitamin E, and beta-carotene reduced risk of AD, and considered them effective antioxidants for both its prevention and treatment.[925]

AD Risk Reduction Role: Strengthens the BBB to reduce the accumulation of harmful substances in the brain, reduces lipoprotein oxidation, supports normal cognitive function.

BOOSTING YOUR NATURAL DEFENSES AGAINST INFLUENZA AND PNEUMONIA

Influenza and pneumonia are both infections of the respiratory system. Influenza, commonly referred to as the flu, is a contagious respiratory disease caused by a virus. Pneumonia is an infection of one or both lungs caused by bacteria, virus, or fungi. Both are spread through close contact to someone already infected, usually by cough, sneeze, or other forms of germ transference. The US Centers for Disease Control and Prevention estimates 3 million people get pneumonia each year and as a result 1.1 million are hospitalized.[926] Approximately 5 to 20 percent of the US population get the flu each year, resulting in 200,000 hospitalizations.[927] Pneumonia results in over 52,000 deaths annually.[936] Flu causes just over 1,500 annual deaths.[928] The risk factors for influenza include: age (the very young and those over age sixty-five are most susceptible), occupation (it is logical that health care staff and child care workers are more likely to contract influenza given their close proximity to sick people and children), and living conditions (military barracks, nursing homes, or other facilities that house multiple residents). In addition, certain health conditions are also a factor such as a weak immune system (HIV/AIDS, chemotherapy, immunosuppressive medications), chronic lung disease, cardiovascular disease, and pregnancy.[929] As with the flu, pneumonia strikes the very young (under age two) and elderly (over age sixty-five) more frequently. A number of risk factors for pneumonia are controllable such as smoking, excess alcohol consumption, and exposure to chemical pollutants and toxic fumes. Other risk factors are not as controllable like lung diseases (cystic fibrosis, asthma, COPD, bronchiectasis), serious diseases (diabetes, heart disease, sickle cell anemia), being admitted to a hospital intensive care unit, having a weakened immune system, difficulty coughing, problems swallowing, a recent cold or flu, and malnourishment.[930]

The best preventive actions you can take for both conditions are to avoid contact with the organisms that cause these illnesses as well as maintain a strong immune system. Don't smoke. Smoking can damage your lungs' ability to prevent infection from foreign organisms. Get enough sleep so your immune system has the opportunity to perform its "cleanup" duties. Follow the recommendations to eat better, which will ensure you obtain adequate nutrients for optimal immune system function. Your multivitamin and mineral will also provide key nutrients necessary for efficient immune system function. If your job requires considerable social exposure to germs you may want to take extra vitamin C to boost immune system activity.

The following activities help prevent exposure:

1. Wash your hands frequently with soap and warm water. If soap and water are not available use an alcohol-based hand sanitizer.
2. Cover your nose and mouth with a tissue or handkerchief when you cough or sneeze; or cough and sneeze into your armpit or elbow.
3. Don't touch your eyes, nose, and mouth, particularly after you shake hands, or after you touch commonly shared items (i.e., doorknobs and shopping carts). Use sanitation wipes on shopping carts and public door handles before you touch them.
4. Avoid close contact with sick people when possible; and if you are sick avoid contact with others.

Supplements and homeopathic remedies are good choices for the prevention and treatment of respiratory illness. A few herbs that strengthen the immune system are andrographis, echinacea, elderberry, and goldenseal. These herbs are more often used to reduce severity and duration of respiratory infections, rather than to prevent them, but they may have a preventive effect also.

ANDROGRAPHIS

Commonly used in Ayurvedic medicine, andrographis supports immune system function and encourages healthy levels of immune cells. It enhances antibody activity and phagocytosis—the ingestion of pathogens by special immune cells.[931] Up to a 50 percent decrease in the occurrence of the common cold was noted when people took andrographis to prevent upper respiratory infections for two months.[932] Andrographis is often combined with Siberian ginseng to enhance its activity, which results in a significant reduction of the severity and duration of flu symptoms.[933] Therapeutic and preventive doses range from 178 to 300 mg three times daily. It is feasible that andrographis could interact with immunosuppressive medications, anticoagulants, antiplatelet medications, and antihypertensive drugs.

Flu and Pneumonia Risk Reduction Role: Supports normal immune system function and activity.

ECHINACEA

Echinacea has been used for centuries to shorten the duration and reduce symptoms of the flu. Scientific research has verified the effectiveness of echinacea for the relief of cold and flu symptoms and a reduction in the duration of illness when it is administered during early onset of illness.[934] It also combats bacterial upper respiratory infections by reducing inflammation and inactivating several common bacterium.[935] Echinacea comes in many varieties, so take the dosage recommended on the product label. Echinacea may increase blood levels of caffeine and interact with a variety of medications metabolized by the cytochrome P450 enzymes.[936] Theoretically, it could also counteract immunosuppressive medications.

Flu and Pneumonia Risk Reduction Role: Supports normal immune system function and kills bacteria that cause respiratory infections.

ELDERBERRY

Elderberry has a long history of use for the treatment of upper respiratory infections. A standardized extract, Sambucol, has been shown to inhibit several strains of the flu virus, including H1N1 (Swine flu), and reduces the duration of flu symptoms by about three days.[937,938] It helps prevent the infection of cells by the flu virus and is considered as effective as Tamiflu. The therapeutic dosage is usually 15 ml (1 tablespoon) two to four times daily. A preventive dose is likely 15 ml for adults and 5 ml for children. Like echinacea and andrographis, elderberry's stimulating effect on the immune system makes it possible to interfere with immunosuppressive medications.

Flu and Pneumonia Risk Reduction Role: Supports normal immune system function and reduces pathogenic infection of cells.

GOLDENSEAL

One of the most popular immune supportive herbs in America, goldenseal has earned a reputation as a harmful microorganism fighter. It is an effective natural antibiotic and immune system stimulator.[939-942] It has also demonstrated strong effectiveness against H1N1 Influenza A.[943] Goldenseal may possibly interact with cyclosporine, digoxin, and several medications metabolized through the cytochrome P450 pathways (NSAIDs, proton-pump inhibitors, aspirin, anti-seizure medications, immune modulators, blood sugar medications, blood pressure medications, antidepressants, antipsychotics, diabetic medications, antihistamines, antibiotics, and anesthetics).

Flu and Pneumonia Risk Reduction Role: Supports normal immune system function, kills bacteria, and prevents flu virus growth.

HOMEOPATHIC REMEDIES

Homeopathic remedies can be used effectively as both preventives and treatments for a number of respiratory infections. The two most commonly used flu preventives are Influenzinum 9C and Oscillococcinum. Influenzinum 9C is a flu preventive and treatment updated each year according to the most common strains of the flu being reported. Research suggests that it is as effective as the flu vaccine for flu prevention.[944] Oscillococcinum is a flu specific remedy, which reduces severity and length of flu symptoms at a rapid pace when taken during early onset. Many report that Oscillococcinum works quickly when administered during the early stages of the illness, and significantly reduces the number of sick days. It has also been investigated for its ability to prevent the flu, but the research has thus far been inconclusive.[945] For pneumonia, the homeopathic remedies aconite, ferrum phosphoricum, bryonia, kali muriaticum (often in conjunction with ferrum phosphoricum, alternating the two remedies), and phosphorus tri-iodatus (especially for chronic pneumonia) are frequently employed. These remedies are primarily used for the treatment of pneumonia once it occurs.

Flu and Pneumonia Risk Reduction Role: Homeopathic remedies can be used effectively to prevent the flu, and may also reduce its duration and severity of symptoms.

HOMEOPATHIC NOSODES

Homeoprophylaxis is a homeopathic method of disease prevention. It has proven approximately as effective as conventional vaccines for specific diseases.[946,947] Nosodes are homeopathic remedies prepared from a part of the disease itself. Similar in mechanism of action to vaccines, they are diluted infinitesimally so that no active microbes remain. Like vaccines, they are used as preventives for the disease they contain. Pneumococcinum is a pneumonia nosode. While homeopathic remedies and herbal immune enhancers do not guarantee disease avoidance, they are beneficial and frequently effective in both the treatment and prevention of acute and chronic contagious disease.

Flu and Pneumonia Risk Reduction Role: Nosodes can effectively be used to prevent pneumonia.

VITAMIN D

Another possibility is to increase your vitamin D intake during cold and flu season. Studies suggest that those who take higher doses of vitamin D (about 2,000 IU daily) can significantly reduce the incidence of seasonal flu.[948,949] A Japanese study that included 334 schoolchildren who received 1,200 IU of vitamin D or a placebo daily, observed that only 10.8 percent of the vitamin D group contracted the flu, versus 18.6 percent in the placebo control group. A meta-analysis of randomized controlled trials concluded that vitamin D provides protection against respiratory tract infections in general, suggesting it may help prevent pneumonia as well.[950] Considering the reasonable cost of vitamin D, this is a very affordable way to reduce the risk of upper respiratory infections.

Flu and Pneumonia Risk Reduction Role: Vitamin D may increase the ability of your immune system to ward off infections.

Conclusion

There is no one hundred percent foolproof way to avoid diseases or illness. It takes a synergistic effort of multiple facets of health and well-being. However, there are numerous ways in which we can support the body's effort to thwart disease risk, many, but not all of which, are reported in this book. It starts with what you eat. If you want your body to perform efficiently, you must provide it the nutrition it needs to do so. Fruits and vegetables are the cornerstone of this fuel for the body. Hydration is another key. Your body is predominantly water and must maintain hydration to perform optimally. Drink clean, filtered water daily. Meat can be on the menu, it just shouldn't be the staple of your diet. Instead, choose non-animal sources of protein, like nuts and beans. Fats are good. It may be hard to get this ingrained in your brain after decades of propaganda from organizations that promote all fats as bad, but there are good fats and your body needs them to function at its best. DHA and EPA are two of the most important fats when it comes to human health.

It is just as important to avoid or reduce harmful substances from entering your body. These substances can disrupt normal functions and make you perform less than you are capable of. Particularly harmful are high-fructose corn syrup, added sugar of any kind, artificial sweeteners, MSG, coffee, alcohol, some teas, pesticides, excess salt, sodium nitrite, and caffeine. As you are more mindful of what you let enter your body, you will realize better overall well-being, reduce your risk of disease, and increase the likelihood of a healthy life span.

Nutritional supplements are an inexpensive way to maintain health and reduce the risk of disease. These dietary companions are absolutely essential, given the vast amount of chemicals we are exposed to, surplus of stress, and reduced nutritional value of foods. Make use of the secrets of antioxidant supplementation and provide your body a variety of nutrients (balance) that are specific to organs, cells, or tissues (specificity). While not meant to be replacements for eating better, a daily infusion of optimum amounts of micronutrients through your supplement regimen aids all body systems.

Movement should be a way of life. You don't have to spend hours in the gym but you do need to make time for regular movement, whether all at once or in combined short bouts. Take advantage of MRT and HIIT that maximize your physical activity and your body's transformation. Regular physical activity will improve the efficiency of your cells, tissues, and organs, and therefore your overall well-being.

Your body is exposed to toxins on a daily basis. They are everywhere—in our food, water, air, medications, personal care products, household cleaners, and more. This superfluity of toxins is damaging to your health at the cellular level. Support your cells and body through regular detoxification. The liver, kidneys, bowel, lungs, skin, and lymph system could all use a break from the effects of toxins through a regular cleansing program. When you detoxify, you remove the heavy metals, chemicals, microbial compounds, and pathogens that impede homeostasis and help create an environment for peak vitality to occur.

You can't overlook that true health is only achieved with a focus on the whole person, and the whole person includes the body, mind, emotions, and spirit. What affects one aspect of your health will ultimately affect the others, whether positively or negatively. Reduce and manage stress. If you don't, you will allow your biochemistry to change dramatically and invite disease and illness to prosper. Find time every day to relax. Exude an optimistic attitude and look for the good in all situations. Maintain positive self-esteem and send positive communication to your cells. Don't let the negative talk bring your cells down. They need physical and psychological nourishment every day. Laugh and laugh often. Laughter truly is the best medicine and can profoundly influence your overall well-being. Build meaningful relationships with others. This doesn't have to be with a spouse or family member. You can have a meaningful relationship with an animal, the waitress at your favorite restaurant, or the grocery check-out clerk. Without meaningful relationships your well-being will stagnate. Get enough sleep. Your body needs it and so do your mind, emotions, and spirit. If you suffer from anxiety or depression, natural remedies may help. They work with the body to restore feelings of hope and joy, while simultaneously reducing anxious feelings.

Genes are not everything when it comes to disease risk. In fact, more often than not it takes an internal or external stimuli to trigger a gene that causes disease. You can reduce your risk of the top killers of Americans, including cancer, heart disease, Alzheimer's disease, and diabetes. It takes a joint effort of eating, regular movement, supplements, detoxification, stress management, and targeted remedies, but you can create a body environment that is less hospitable to disease.

It takes deliberate daily practice to make wellness a way of life. But if you do, even if it is one small step at a time, you will be on the way to realizing optimum health and a healthy life span. This type of health can't be achieved in a weekend or even through concerted efforts a few times a month. True optimum health will only be achieved if you make a determined effort to employ the most health-promoting dietary habits and lifestyle behaviors possible. You must incorporate a holistic approach that includes your mind, emotions, body, and spirit. As you do, you may just help to raise a healthier generation. It is never too late to reset your habits and improve your health.

References

1   Pathare YS, Wagh VD. "Herbal medicines and nutritional supplements used in the treatment of glaucoma: A review." *Res J Pharm Biol Chem Serv.* 2012 Jan–Mar;3(1):331–39.

2   Wang X, Ouyang Y, Liu J, et al. "Fruit and vegetable consumption and mortality from all causes, cardiovascular disease, and cancer:systematic review and dose-response meta-analysis of prospective cohort studies." *BMJ.* 2014 Jul 29;349:g4490.

3   Hung H-C, Joshipura KJ, Jiang R, et al. "Fruit and vegetable consumption and risk of major chronic disease." *J Natl Cancer Inst.* 2004 Nov 3;96(21): 1577–84.

4   Joshipura KJ, Hu FB, Manson JE, et al. "The effect of fruit and vegetable intake on risk for coronary heart disease." *Ann Interna Med.* 2001 Jun 19;134(12):116–14.

5   Mente A, de Koning L, Shannon HS, et al. "A systematic review of the evidence supporting a causal link between dietary factors and coronary heart disease." *Arch Intern Med.* 2009 Apr 13;169(7):659–69.

6   Joshipura KJ, Acherio A, Manson JE, et al. "Fruit and vegetable intake in relation to risk of ischemic stroke." *JAMA.* 1999 Oct 6;282(13):1233–9.

7   Boeing H, Bechthold A, Bub A, et al. "Critical review: vegetables and fruit in the prevention of chronic diseases." *Eur J Nutr.* 2012 Sep;51(6):637–63.

8   Mourouti N, Papavagelis C, Plytzanopoulou, et al. "Dietary patterns and breast cancer: a case-controlled study in women." *Eur J Nutr.* 2014 Jul 22. [Epub ahead of print]

9   Askari F, Parizi MK, Jessri M, et al. "Fruit and vegetable intake in relation to prostate cancer in Iranian men: a case controlled study." *Asian Pac J Cancer Prev.* 2014;15(13):5223–7.

10   Larsson SC, Hakansson N, Naslund I, et al. "Fruit and vegetable consumption in relation to pancreatic cancer risk: a prospective study." *Cancer Epidemiol Biomarkers Prev.* 2006 Feb;15(2):301–5.

11   Riboli E, Norat T. "Epidemiologic evidence of the protective effect of fruit and vegetables on cancer risk." *Am J Clin Nutr.* 2003 Sep;78 (3 Suppl):559S–69S.

12   Oyebode O, Gordon-Dseagu V, Walker A, et al. "Fruit and vegetable consumption and all-cause, cancer and CVD mortality: analysis of Health Survey for England data." *J Epidemiol Community Health.* 2014 Mar;68:856–62.

13   Rimm EB, Ascherino A, Giovannucci E, et al. "Vegetable, fruit, and cereal fiber intake and risk of coronary heart disease among men." *JAMA.* 1996 Feb 14;275(6):447–51.

14   Threapleton D, Greenwood D, Evans C, et al. "Dietary fiber intake and risk of first stroke. A systematic review and meta-analysis." *Stroke.* 2013 May;44(5):136–68.

15   Threapleton DE, Greenwood DC, Evans CE, et al. "Dietary fiber intake and risk of cardiovascular disease:systematic review and meta-analysis." *BMJ.* 2013 Dec 19;347:f6879.

16   Otles S, Ozgoz S. "Health effects of dietary fiber." *Acta Sci Pol Technol Ailment.* 2014 Apr–Jun;13(2):191–202.

17   Burns B. "Reactive arthritis in emergency medicine." Accessed October 29, 2014, from http://emedicine.medscape.com/article/331347-overview.

18   Spiller R, Aziz Q, Creed F. "Guidelines on the irritable bowel syndrome: mechanisms and practical management." *Gut.* 2007;56(12):1770–98.

19   Sartor RB, Mazmanian SK. "Intestinal microbes in inflammatory bowel diseases." *Am J Gastroenterol Suppl.* 2012;1:15–21.

20   Brown L, Rosner B, Willett W, et al. "Cholesterol-lowering effects of dietary fiber: a meta-analysis." *Am J Clin Nutr.* 1999 Jan;69(1):30–42.

21   Kwiterovich PO, Jr. "The role of fiber in the treatment of hypercholesterolemia in children and adolescents." *Pediatrics.* 1999 Nov;96(5 Pt 2):1005–9.

22   Keithley J, Swanson B. "Glucomannan and obesity: a critical review." *Altern Ther.* 2005 Nov–Dec;11(6):30–34.

23   Tang G. "Bioconversion of dietary provitamin A carotenoids to vitamin A in humans." *Am J Clin Nutr.* 2010 May;91(5):1468S–73S.

24   Davis C, Jing H, Rochford T, et al. "beta-Cryptoxanthin supplements or carotenoid-enhanced maize maintains liver vitamin A in Mongolian gerbils (Meriones unguicalatus) better than or equal to beta-carotene supplements." *Br J Nutr.* 2008 Oct;100(4):785–93.

25 The Harvard Medical School Family Health Guide. "Potassium lowers blood pressure." Accessed August 14, 2014, from http://www.health.harvard.edu/fhg/updates/update0705c.shtml.

26 Baines S, Powers J, Brown W. "How does the health and well-being of young Australian vegetarian and semi-vegetarian women compare with non-vegetarians." *Public Health Nutr.* 2007 May;10(5):436–42.

27 Greene-Finestone LS, Campbell MK, Evers SE, et al. "Attitudes and health behaviours of young adolescent omnivores and vegetarians: a chool-based study." *Appetite.* 2008 Jun;51(1):104–10.

28 Draper A, Lewis J, Malhotra N, et al. "The energy and nutrient intakes of different types of vegetarian: a case for supplements?" *Br J Nutr.* 1993 Jan;69(1):3–19.

29 Davey GK, Spencer EA, Appleby PN, et al. "EPIC-Oxford: lifestyle characteristics and nutrient intakes in a cohort of 33,883 meat-eaters and 31,546 non-meat-eaters in the UK." *Public Health Nutr.* 2003 May;6(3):259–69.

30 Key J, Appleby PN, Rosell MS. "Health effects of vegetarian and vegan diets." *Proc Nutr Soc.* 2006 Feb;65(1):35–41.

31 American Dietetic Association, Dietitians of Canada. Position of the American Dietetic Association and Dietitians of Canada: vegetarian diets. 2003 June;103(6):748–65.

32 United States Geological Survey. "The water in you." Accessed August 4, 2014, from http://water.usgs.gov/edu/propertyyou.html.

33 Boschmann M, Steiniger J, Hille U, et al. "Water-induced thermogenesis." *J Clin Endocrinol Metab.* 2003 Dec;88(12):6015–9.

34 Stookey JD. "The diuretic effects of alcohol and caffeine and total water intake misclassification." *Eur J Epidemiol.* 1999 Feb;15(2):181–8.

35 World Health Organization. "Pharmaceuticals in drinking-water." 2011. Accessed August 4, 2014, from http://www.who.int/water_sanitation_health/publications/2011/pharmaceuticals_20110601.pdf.

36 Radjenovic J, Petrovic M, Ventura F, Barcelo D. "Rejection of pharmaceuticals in nanofiltration and reverse osmosis membrane drinking water treatment." *J Membrane Sci.* 2008;42(14):361–10.

37 Eun HC, Lee AY, Lee YS. "Sodium hypochlorite dermatitis." *Contact Dermatitis.* 1984;11:45.

38 Watson SH, Kibler CS. "Drinking water as a cause of asthma." *J Allergies.* 1933;5:197–198.

39 Payment P, Siemiatycki J, Richardson L, et al. "A prospective epidemiological study of gastrointestinal health effects due to the consumption of drinking water." *Int J Enviro Health Res.* 1997;7(1):5–31.

40 Cantor KP, Lynch CF, Hildesheim ME, et al. "Drinking water source and chlorination byproducts. Risk of bladder cancer." *Epidemiology.* 1998 Jan;9(1):21–8.

41 Cantor KP. "Epidemiological evidence of carcinogenicity of chlorinated organics in drinking water." *Environ Health Perspect.* 1982 Dec;46:187–95.

42 Bain R, Cronk R, Hossain R, et al. "Global assessment of exposure to fecal contamination through drinking water based on systematic review." *Trop Med Int Health.* 2014 Aug;19(8):917–27.

43 No authors listed. "Higher red meat intake in young women increases breast cancer risk." *Nurs Stand.* 2014 Jul 2;28(44):16.

44 Kaluza J, Akesson A, Wolk, A. "Processed and unprocessed meat consumption and risk of heart failure: prospective study of men." *Circ Heart Fail.* 214 Jul;7(4):552–7.

45 Saneei P, Saadatnia M, Shaken F, et al. "A case-control study on red meat consumption and risk of stroke among a group of Iranian adults." *Public Health Nutr.* 2014 Jun 13:1–7.

46 Barnard N, Levin S, Trapp C. "Meat consumption as a risk factor for type 2 diabetes." *Nutrients.* 214 Feb 21;6(2):897–910.

47 Ronco AL, Mendilaharsu M, Boffetta P, et al. "Meat consumption, animal products, and the risk of bladder cancer: a case-control study in Uruguayan men." *Asian Pac J Cancer Prev.* 214;15(14):5805–9.

48 Ovesen LF. "Increased consumption of fruits and vegetables reduces the risk of ischemic heart disease." *Ugeskr Laeger.* 2005 Jun 20;167(25-31):3742–7.

49 Rogers AE, Zeisel SH, Groopman J. "Diet and carcinogenesis." *Carcinogenesis.* 1993 Nov;14(11):2205–17.

50 Ferdowsian HR, Barnard ND. "Effects of plant-based diets on plasma lipids." *Am J Cardiol.* 209 Oct 1;14(7):947–56.

51 Nagura J, Iso H, Watanabe Y, et al. "Fruit, vegetable and bean intake and mortality from cardiovascular disease among Japanese men and women: the JACC Study." *Br J Nutr.* 2009 Jul;102(2):285–92.

52 Berjia Fl, Poulsen M, Nauta M. "Burden of disease estimates associated to different red meat cooking practices." *Food Chem Toxicol.* 2014 Apr;66:237–44.

53 Bittman, M. "Rethinking the meat-guzzler." *New York Times* 2008.

54 World Cancer Research Fund. Animal foods. Accessed August 16, 2014, from http://www.dietandcancerreport.org/expert_report/recommendations/recommendation_animal_foods.php.

55 Taylor, E, Burley VJ, Greenwood DC, et al. "Meat consumption and risk of breast cancer in the UK women's cohort study." *British Journal of Cancer* 2007;96:1139–1146.

56 Genkinger, J, Koushik, A. "Meat consumption and cancer risk." *PLoS Med.* 2007 Dec;4(12):e345.

57 Benito-Garcia E, Feskanich D, Hu FB, et al. "Protein, iron, and meat consumption and risk for rheumatoid arthritis: a prospective cohort study." *Arthritis Res Ther.* 2007:9(1):R16.

58 Grant WB. "The role of meat in the expression of rheumatoid arthritis." *Br J Nutr.* 2000 Nov;84(5):589–95.

59 Lajous M, Bijon A, Fagherazzi G, et al. "Processed and unprocessed red meat consumption and hypertension in women." *Am J Clin Nutr.* 2014 Jul 30. [Epub ahead of print].

60 Chan DS, Lau R, Aune D, et al. "Red and processed meat and colorectal cancer incidence: meta-analysis of prospective studies." *PLoS One.* 2011;6(6):e20456.

61 Larsson S, Bergkvist L, Wolk A. "Processed meat consumption, dietary nitrosamines and stomach cancer risk in a cohort of Swedish women." *Int J Cancer.* 2006 Aug;119(6):915–19.

62 Micha R, Wallace S, Mozaffarin D. "Red and processed meat consumption and risk of incident coronary heart disease, stroke, and diabetes mellitus." *Epidemiol Prev.* 2010 May;121:2271–83.

63 Schulze MB, Manson JE, Willett WC, et al. "Processed meat intake and incidence of type 2 diabetes in younger and middle-aged women." *Diabetologia.* 2003 Nov;46(11):1465–1473.

64 Vang A, Singh PN, Lee JW, et al. "Meats, processed meats, obesity, weight gain and occurrence of diabetes among adults: findings from Adventist Health Studies." *Ann Nutr Metab.* 2008;52(2):96–104.

65 Akbaraly T, Sabia S, Hagger-Johnson G, et al. "Does overall diet in mid-life predict future aging phenotypes? A cohort study." *Am J Med.* 2013 May;126(5):411–19.

66 Perez L, Heim L, Sherzai A, et al. "Nutrition and vascular dementia." *J Nutr Health Again.* 2012 Apr;16(4):319–24.

67 Torfadottir JE, Valdimarsdottir UA, Mucci LA, et al. "Consumption of fish products across the lifespan and prostate cancer risk." *PLoS One.* 2013 Apr 17;8(4):e59799.

68 Campbell T, Campbell T II. *The China study.* Benbella Books: Dallas, Texas, 2004.

69 Lubin F, Wax Y, Modan B. "Role of fat, animal protein, and dietary fiber in breast cancer etiology: a case-control study." *J Natl Cancer Inst.* 1996;77(3):605–12.

70   Drasar BS, Irving D. "Environmental factors and cancer of the colon and breast." *Br J Cancer.* 1973 Feb;27(2):167–72.

71   Melnik BC. "Milk—the promoter of chronic Western diseases." *Med Hyptheses.* 2009 Jun;72(6):631–9.

72   Gerstein HC. "Cow's milk exposure and type I diabetes mellitus: a critical overview of the clinical literature." *Diabetes Care.* 1994 Jan;17(1):13–9.

73   Oski FA. "Is bovine milk a health hazard?" *Pediatrics.* 1985 Jan;75(1 Pt(2):182–6.

74   Ventura A, Canciani GP, Tamburlini G. "Congenital heart disease and cow's milk intolerance." *Helv Paediatr Acta.* 1984 Aug;39(3):269–74.

75   Melnik B. "Milk consumption: aggravating factor of acne and promoter of chronic diseases of Western societies." *J Dtsch Dermatol Ges.* 2009 Apr;7(4):364–70.

76   Malosse D, Perron H, Sasco A. "Correlation between milk and dairy product consumption and multiple sclerosis prevalence: a worldwide study." *Neuroepidemiology.*1992;11(4–6):304–12.

77   Ganmaa D, Sato A. "The possible role of female sex hormones in milk from pregnant cows in the development of breast, ovarian and corpus uteri cancers." *Med Hypotheses.* 2005;65(6):1028–37.

78   Ganmaa D, Li XM, Wang J, et al. "Incidence and mortality of testicular and prostatic cancers to world dietary practices." *Int J Cancer.* 2002 Mar 10:98(2):262–7.

79   Michaelsson K, Wolk A, Langenskiold, et al. "Milk intake and risk of mortality and fractures in women and men: cohort studies." *BMJ.* 2004;349:g6015. [Epub ahead of print]

80   Chan J, Giocannucci E. "Dairy products, calcium, and vitamin D and the risk of prostate cancer." *Epidemiology Revs.* 2001;23(1):87–92.

81   US National Library of Medicine, Genetics Home Reference. Lactose Intolerance. Accessed August 4, 2014, from http://ghr.nlm.nih.gov/condition/lactose-intolerance.

82   Lanou AJ, Berkow SE, Barnard ND. "Calcium, dairy products, and bone health in children and young adults: a reevaluation of the evidence." *Pediatrics.* 2005;115(3):736–43.

83   Recker R, Bammi A, Barger-Lux M, et al. "Calcium absorbability from milk products, an imitation milk, and calcium carbonate." *Am J Clin Nutr.* 1988;47:93–95.

84   Parra MF, Martinez de Morentino B, Cobo J, et al. "Acute calcium absorption from fresh or pasteurized yoghurt depending on the lactose digestibility status." *J Am Col Nutr.* 2007;26(3):288–94.

85 Liu S, Stampfer M, Hu F, et al. "Whole-grain consumption and risk of coronary heart disease: results from the Nurses' Health Study." *Am J Clin Nutr.* 1999 Sep;70(3):412–19.

86 McKeown N, Meigs J, Liu S, et al. "Whole-grain intake is favorably associated with metabolic risk factors for type 2 diabetes and cardiovascular disease in the Farmingham Offspring study." *Am J Clin Nutr.* 2002 Aug;76(2):390–98.

87 Steffen L, Jacobs D, Stevens J, et al. "Associations of whole-grain, refined-grain, and fruit and vegetable consumption with risks of all-cause mortality and incident coronary artery disease and ischemic stroke: the Atherosclerosis Risk in Communities (ARIC) study." *Am J Clin Nutr.* 2003 Sep;78(3):383–90.

88 Liu S, Willett W, Manson J, et al. "Relation between changes in intakes of dietary fiber and grain products and changes in weight and development of obesity among middle-aged women." *Am J Clin Nutr.* 2003 Nov;78(5):920–27.

89 Kristensen M, Toubro S, Jensen MG, et al. "Whole grain compared with refined grain wheat decreases the percentage of body fat following a 12-week energy-restricted dietary intervention in postmenopausal women." *J Nutr.* 2012 Apr;142(4):710–6.

90 McKeown MN, Trot LM, Jacques PF, et al. "Whole- and refined-grain intakes are differentially associated with abdominal visceral and subcutaneous adiposity in healthy adults: the Framingham Heart Study." *Am J Clin Nutr.* 2010 Nov;92(5):1165–71.

91 Drewnowski A. "The real contribution of added sugars and fats to obesity." *Epidemiological Rev.* 2007 June;29:160–71.

92 Yin J, Tezuka Y, Subehan, et al. "In vivo anti-osteoporotic activity of isotaxiresinol, a lignin from wood of Taxus yunnanensis." *Phytomedicine.* 2006 Jan;13(1–2):37–42.

93 George Mateljan Foundation. www.whfoods.com.

94 McCann M, et al. "Enterolactone restricts the proliferation of the LNCaP human prostate cancer cell line in vitro." *Mol Nutr Res.* 2008 May;52(5):567–80.

95 Karvonen M, Pitkanieni J, Tuomilehto. "The onset of type 1 diabetes in finnish children has become younger." *Diabetes Care.* 1999 Jul;22:1066–70.

96 McCann SE, Hootman KC, Weaver AM, et al. "Dietary intakes of total and specific lignans are associated with clinical breast tumor characteristics." *J Nutr.* 2012 Jan;142(1):91–98.

97   Peterson J, Johanna D, Adlercreutz H, et al. "Dietary lignans: physiology and potential for cardiovascular disease risk reduction." *Nutr Rev.* 2010 Oct;68(10):571–603.

98   Velasquez MT, Bhathena SJ. "Dietary phytoestrogens: a possible role in renal disease protection." *Am J Kidney Dis.* 2001 May;37(5):156–68.

99   Aune D, Chan D, Greenwood D, et al. "Dietary fiber and breast cancer risk: a systemic review and meta-analysis of prospective studies." *Ann Oncol.* 2012 Jun;23(6):1394–1402.

100 Durazzo A, Carcea M, Adlercreutz H, et al. "Effects of consumption of whole grain foods rich in lignans in healthy postmenopausal women with moderate serum cholesterol: a pilot study." *Int J Food Sci Nutr.* 2014 Aug;65(5):637–45.

101 Costa R, Summa M. "Soy protein in the management of hyperlipidemia." *Ann Pharmacother.* 2000 Jul–Aug;34(7):931–35.

102 Kgomotso T, Chiu F, Ng K. "Genistein- and aidzein 7-O-besta-D-glucuronic acid retain the ability to inhibit copper-mediated lipid oxidation of low density lipoprotein." *Mol Nutr Food Res.* 2008 Dec;52(12):1457–66.

103 Irace C, Marini H, Birro A, et al. "Genistein and endothelial function in postmenopausal women with metabolic syndrome." *Eur J Clin Invest.* 2013 Oct;43(10):1025–31.

104 Liese A, Roach A, Sparks K, et al. "Whole-grain intake and insulin sensitivity: the Insulin Resistance Atherosclerosis Study." *Am J Clin Nutr.* 2003 Nov;78(5):965–71.

105 Steffen L, Jacobs D, Jr., Murtaugh M, et al. "Whole grain intake is associated with lower body mass and greater insulin sensitivity among adolescents." *Am J Epidemiol.* 2003 Aug;158(3):243–50.

106 Liu S, Stampfer M, Hu F, et al. "Whole-grain consumption and risk of coronary heart disease: results from the Nurses' Health Study." *Am J Clin Nutr.* 1999 Sep;70(3):412–19.

107 Schartzkin A, Mouw T, Park Y, et al. "Dietary fiber and whole-grain consumption in relation to colorectal cancer in the NIH-AARP Diet and Health Study." *AM J Clin Nutr.* 2007 May;85(5):1353–60.

108 Kim DH, Sung B, Kang YJ, et al. "Anti-inflammatory effects of betaine on AOM/DSS-induced colon tumorigenesis in ICR male mice." *Int J Oncol.* 2014 Sep;45(3):1250–6.

109 Detopoulou P, Panagiotakos DB, Antonopoulou S, et al. "Dietary choline and betaine intakes in relation to concentrations of inflammatory markers in healthy adults: the ATTICA study." *Am J Clin Nutr.* 2008 Feb;87(2):424–30.

110 Likes R, Madl RL, Zeisel SH, et al. "The betaine and choline content of a whole wheat flour compared to other mill streams." *J Cereal Sci.* 2007;46(1):93–95.

111 Ferguson LR, Harris PJ. "Protection against cancer by wheat bran: role of dietary fibre and phytochemicals." *Eur J Cancer Prev.* 1999 Feb;8(1):17–25.

112 Qu H, Madl R, Takemoto D, et al. "Lignans are involved in the antitumor activity of wheat bran in colon cancer SW480 cells." *J Nutr.* 2005 Mar 1;135(3):598–602.

113 Pena-Rosas JP, Rickard S, Cho S. "Wheat bran and breast cancer: revisiting the estrogen hypothesis." *Arch Latinoam Nutr.* 1999 Dec;49(4):309–17.

114 Terry P, Lagergren J, Ye W, et al. "Inverse association between intake of cereal fiber and risk of gastric cardia cancer." *Gastroenterology.* 2001 Feb;120(2):387–91.

115 de Punder K, Pruimboom L. "The dietary intake of wheat and other cereal grains and their role in inflammation." *Nutrients.* 2013 Mar 12;5(3):771–87.

116 Vives MJ, Esteve M, Marine M, et al. "Prevalence and clinical relevance of enteropathy associated with systemic autoimmune diseases." *Dig Liver Dis.* 2012 Aug;44(8):636–42.

117 Visser J, Rozing J, Sapone A, et al. "Tight junctions, intestinal permeability, and autoimmunity celiac disease and type 1 diabetes paradigms." *Ann N Y Acad Sci.* 2009 May;1165:195–205.

118 Manukyan G, Ghazaryan K, Ktsoyan Z, et al. "Elevated systemic antibodies towards commensal gut microbiota in autoinflamamtory condition." *PLoS One.* 2008 Sep 9;3(9):e3172.

119 Sudha V, Spiegelman D, Hong BH, et al. "Consumer Acceptance and Preference Study (CAPS) on brown and undermilled Indian rice varieties in Chennai, India." *J Am Coll Nutr.* 2013;32(1):50–57.

120 Zhang G, Malik VS, Pan A, et al. "Substituting brown rice for white rice to lower diabetes risk: a focus-group study in Chinese adults." *J Am Diet Assoc.* 2010 Aug;110(8):1216–21.

121 Hu E, Malik V. "White rice consumption and risk of type 2 diabetes: meta-analysis and systematic review." *BMJ.* 2012;344:e1454.

122 Bahadoran Z, Mimiran P, Delshad H, et al. "White rice consumption is a risk factor for metabolic syndrome in Tehrani adults: a prospective approach in Tehran Lipid and Glucose Study." *Arch Iran Med.* 2014 Jun;17(6):435–40.

123 Yu D, Shu XO, Li H, et al. "Dietary carbohydrates, refined grains, glycemic load, and risk of coronary heart disease in Chinese adults." *Am J Epidemiol.* 2013 Nov 15;178(10):1542–49.

124 Palmer RMJ, Ashton DS, Moncada S. "Vascular endothelial cells synthesize nitric oxide from L-arginine." *Nature.* 1988 Jun 16;333:664–66.

125 Siani A, Pagano E, Lacone R, et al. "Blood pressure and metabolic changes during dietary L-arginine supplementation in humans." *A, J Hyperten.* 2000;13:547–51.

126 Beal DT, Wood W, Wu M, et al. "When do habits persist despite conflict with motives?" *Pers Soc Psychol Bull.* 2011 Nov;37(11):1428–37.

127 Kritchevsky S. "B-carotene, carotenoids and the prevention of coronary heart disease." *J Nutr.* 1999 Jan 1;129(1):5–8.

128 Weigert G, Kava S, Pemp B, et al. "Effects of lutein supplementation on macular pigment optical density and visual acuity in patients with age-related macular degeneration." *Invest Opthamol Vis Sci.* 2011 Oct 17;52(11):8174–8.

129 Adam K, Liu R. "Antioxidant activity of grains." *J of Agric Food Chem.* 2002;50(21):6182–87.

130 Tosh SM. "Review of human studies investigating the post-prandial blood-glucose lowering ability of oat and barley food products." *Eur J Clin Nutr.* 2013 Apr;67(4):31–7.

131 Lammert A, Kratzsch J, Sellhorst J, et al. "Clinical benefit of a short-term dietary oatmeal intervention in patients with type 2 diabetes ad sever insulin resistance:A pilot study." *Exp Clin Endocrinol Diabetes.* 2008 Feb;116(2):132–34.

132 Ostadrahimi A, Ziaei JE, Esfahani A, et al. "Effect of beta glucan on white blood cell counts and serum levels of IL-4 and IL-12 in women with breast cancer undergoing chemotherapy: a randomized double-blind placebo-controlled clinical trial." *Asian Pac J Cancer Prev.*2014;15(14):5733–9.

133 Beck EJ, Tapsell LC, Batterham MJ, et al. "Increase in peptide Y-Y levels following oat beta-glucan ingestion are dose-dependent in overwight adults." *Nutr Res.* 2009 Oct;29(10):705–09.

134 Beck EJ, Tosh SM, Batterham MJ, et al. "Oat beta-glucan increases post-prandial cholecystokinin levels, decreases insulin response and extends subjective satiety in overweight subjects." *Mol Nutr Food Res.* 2009 Oct;53(10):1343–51.

135 Braaten JT, Wood PJ, Scott FW, et al. "Oat beta-glucan reduces blood cholesterol concentration in hypercholesterolemic subjects." *Eur J Clin Nutr.* 1994 Jul;48(7):465–74.

136 Sadig Butt M, Tahir-Nadeem M, Khan MK, et al. "Oat: unique among the cereals." *Eur J Nutr.* 2008 Mar;47(2):68–79.

137 Thongooun P, Pavadhgul P, Bumrungpert A, et al. "Effect of oat consumption on lipid profiles in hypercholesterolemic adults." *J Med Assoc Thai.* 2013 Dec;96 Suppl 5:S25–32.

138 Othman RA, Moghadasian MH, Jones PJ. "Cholesterol-lowering effects of oat N-glucan." *Nutr Rev.* 2011 Jun;69(6):299–309.

139 Andon M, Anderson J. "State of the art reviews: the oatmeal-cholesterol connection: 10 years later." *Am J of Lifestyle Med.* 2008 Jan/Feb;2(1):51–57.

140 Davidson M, Dugan L, Burns J, et al. "The hypercholesterolemic effects of B-glucan in oatmeal and oat bran." *JAMA.* 1991 Apr 10;265(14):1833–9.

141 Virtranen SM, Kaila M, Pekkanen J, et al. "Early introduction of oats associated with decreased risk of persistent asthma and early introduction of fish with decreased risk of allergic rhinitis." *Br J Nutr.* 2010 Jan;103(2):266–73.

142 Otsuka H, Inaba M, Fujikura T, et al. "Histochemical and functional characteristics of metachromatic cells in the nasal epithelium in allergic rhinitis: studies of nasal scrapings and their dispersed cells." *J Allergy Clin Immunol.* 1995 Oct;96(4):528–36.

143 Joskiva M, Franova S, Sadlonova V. "Acute bronchodilator effect of quercetin in experimental allergic asthma." *Bratisl Lek Listy.* 2011;112(1):9–12.

144 Malishevskaia IV, Ilashchuk TA, Okipniak IV. "Therapeutic efficacy of quercetin in patients with ischemic heart disease with underlying metabolic syndrome." *Georgian Med News.* 2013 Dec;(225):67–71.

145 Lee KH, Park E, Lee HJ, et al. "Effects of daily quercetin-rich supplementation on cardiometabolic risks in male smokers." *Nutr Res Pract.* 2011 Feb;5(1):28–33.

146 Ji JJ, Lin Y, Huang SS, et al. "Quercetin: a potential natural drug for adjuvant treatment of rheumatoid arthritis." *Afr J Tradit Complement Altern Med.* 2013 Apr 12;10(3):418–21.

147 Maso V, Calgarotto AK, Franchi Junior GC, et al. "Multi-target effects of quercetin in leukemia." *Cancer Prev Res (Phila).* 2014 Oct 7. [Epub ahead of print]

148 Zevallos VF, Herencia LI, Chang F, et al. "Gastrointestinal effects of eating quinoa (Chenopodium quinoa Willd.) in celiac patients." *Am J Gastroenterol.* 2014 Feb;109(2):270–78.

149 Mendonca S, Saldiva P, Cruz R, et al. "Amaranth protein presents cholesterol-lowering effect." *Food Chem.* 2009 Oct;116(3):738–42.

150 Berger A, Gremaud G, Baumgartner M, et al. "Cholesterol-lowering properties of amaranth grain and oil in hamsters." *Vit Nutr Res.* 2003 Jan;73(1):39–47.

151 Plate A, Areas J. "Cholesterol-lowering effect of extruded amaranth (Amaranthus caudatus L) in hypercholesterolemic rabbits." *Food Chem.* 2002 Jan;76(1):1–6.

152 Behall K, Scholfield D, Hallfrisch J. "Diets containing barley significantly reduce lipids in mildly hypercholesterolemic men and women." *Am J Clin Nutr.* 2004 Nov;80(5):1185–93.

153 Behall K, Scholfield D, Hallfrisch J. "Barley β–glucan reduces plasma glucose and insulin responses compared with resistant starch in men." *Nutr Res.* 2006 Dec;26(12):644–50.

154 Akramiene D, Kondrotas A, Didziapetriene J, et al. "Effects of beta-glucans on the immune system." *Medicina (Kaunas, Lithuania).* 2007;43(8):597–606.

155 Fullerton SA, Samadi AA, Tortorelis DG, et al. "Induction of apoptosis in human prostatic cancer cells with beta-glucan (Maitake mushroom polysaccharide)." *Mol Urol.* 2000;4(1):7–13.

156 Samaha F, Iqbal N, Seshadri P, et al. "A low-carbohydrate as compared with a low-fat diet in sever obesity." *N Engl J Med.* 2003 May 22;348:2074–81.

157 McManus K, Antinoro L, Sacks F. "A randomized controlled trial of a moderate-fat, low-energy diet compared with a low fat, low-energy diet for weight loss in overweight adults." *Int J Obes Relat Metab Disord.* 2001 Oct;25(10):1503–11.

158 Summerbell CD, Cameron C, Glasziou PP. "Advice on low-fat diets for obesity." *Cochrane Database Syst Rev.* 2008 Jul 16:(3):CD003640.

159 Howard B, Van Horn L, Hsia J, et al. "Low-fat dietary pattern and risk of cardiovascular disease." *JAMA.* 2006;295(6):655–66.

160 Howard BV, Van Horn L, Hsia J, et al. "Low-fat dietary pattern and risk of cardiovascular disease: the Women's Health Initiative Randomized Controlled Dietary Modification Trial." *JAMA.* 2006 Feb 8;295(6):655–66.

161 Hu F, Stampfer M, Manson J, et al. "Dietary fat intake and the risk of coronary heart disease in women." *N Eng J Med.* 1997 Nov 20;337(21): 1491–99.

162 Tanasescu M, Cho E, Manson JE, et al. "Dietary fat and cholesterol and the risk of cardiovascular disease among women with type 2 diabetes." *Am J Clin Nutr.* 2004 Jun;79(6):999–1004.

163 Siri-Tarino PW, Sun Q, Hu FB, et al. "Saturated fat, carbohydrate, and cardiovascular disease." *Am J Clin Nutr.* 2010 Mar;91(3):502–9.

164 Sartika RA. "Dietary trans fatty acids intake and its relation to dyslipidemia in a sample of adults in Depok city, West Javva, Indonesia." *Malays J Nutr.* 2011 Dec;17(3):337–46.

165 Kavanagh K, Jones K, Sawyer J, et al. "Trans fat diet induces abdominal obesity and changes in insulin sensitivity in monkeys." *Obesity*. 2007 July;15(7):1675–84.

166 Salmerion J, Hu F, Manson J. "Dietary fat intake and risk of type 2 diabetes in women." *Am J Clin Nut.* 2001 Jun;73(6):1019–26.

167 Vessby B, Uusitupa M, Hermansen K, et al. "Substituting dietary saturated for monounsaturated fat impairs insulin sensitivity in healthy men and women: the KANWU study." *Diabetologia*. 2001;44(3):312–9.

168 Brouwer IA, Wanders AJ, Katan MB. "Effect of animal and industrial trans fatty acids on HDL and LDL cholesterol levels in humans—a quantitative review." *PLoS One*. 2010 Mar 2;5(3):e9434.

169 Willett WC, Stampfer MJ, Manson JE, et al. "Intake of trans fatty acids and risk of coronary heart disease among women." *Lancet*. 1993 March;341(8845):581–85.

170 No authors listed. "FDA deems trans fats unsafe. These artery-clogging fats may linger in the food supply for a while. Learn how to avoid them." *Harv Health Lett*. 2014 Feb;24(6):6–7.

171 Willet W. "The case for banning trans fats. The FDA's new policy on these deadly artificial fatty acids is long overdue." *Sci Am*. 2010 Mar;310(3):13.

172 Kiage JN, Merrill PD, Judd SE, et al. "Intake of trans fat and incidence of stroke in the Reasons for Geographic and Racial Differences in Stroke (REGARDS) cohort." *Am J Clin Nutr*. 2014 May;99(5):1071–76.

173 Kiage JN, Merrill PD, Robinson CJ, et al. "Intake of trans fat and all-cause mortality in the Reasons for Geographical and Racial Difference in Stroke (REGARDS) cohort." *Am J Clin Nutr*. 2013 May;97(5):1121–18.

174 Igbal MP. "Trans fatty acids—A risk factor for cardiovascular disease." *Pak J Med Sci*. 2014 Jan;30(1):194–97.

175 American Heart Association Nutrition Committee, Lichtenstein AH, Appel LJ, et al. "Diet and lifestyle recommendations revision 2006: scientific statement from the American Heart Association Nutrition Committee." *Circulation*. 2006 Jul 4;114(1):82–96.

176 Chowdhury E, Warnakula S, Kunutsor S, et al. "Assocation of dietary, circulating, and supplement fatty acids with coronary risk: A systematic review." *Ann Intern Med*. 2014;160(6):398–406.

177 US Centers for Disease Control and Prevention. "Saturated fat." Accessed August 18, 2014, from http://www.cdc.gov/nutrition/everyone/basics/fat/saturatedfat.html.

178 US Centers for Disease Control and Prevention. "Trans fat." Accessed August 18, 2014, from http://www.cdc.gov/nutrition/everyone/basics/fat/transfat.html.

179 The Cheesecake Factory. Nutrition chart. Accessed August 18, 2014, from http://www.cheesecakefactorynutrition.com/restaurant-nutrition-chart. php?.

180 Red Robin. "Customizer hub." Accessed August 18, 2014, from http://www.redrobin.com/customizer_hub_mobile#.

181 Outback Steakhouse. Accessed August 18, 2014, from http://www.outback.com/nutrition.

182 IHOP. "Nutrition information." Accessed August 18, 2014, from http://www.ihop.com/-/media/ihop/pdFs/nutritionalinformation.ashx.

183 Applebee's. "Nutritional information." Accessed August 18, 2014, from https://www.applebees.com/-/media/docs/Applebees_Nutritional_Info. pdf.

184 Burdge GC, Jones AE, Wooton SA. "Eicosapentaenoic acids are the principal products of alpha-linolenic acid metabolism in young men." *Br J Nutr.* 2002;88(4):355–64.

185 Burdge GC, Wooton SA. "Conversion of alpha-linolenic acid to eicosapentaenoic, docosapentaenoic and docosahexaenoic in young women." *Br J Nutr.* 2002;88(4):411–20.

186 Zheng JS, Hu XJ, Zhao YM, et al. "Intake of fish and marine n-3 polyunsaturated fatty acids and risk of breast cancer: meta-analysis of data from 21 independent prospective cohort studies." *BMJ.* 2013 June;346:f3706.

187 Mizwixki MT, Liu G, fiala M, et al. "1α,25-dihydroxyvitamin D3 and resolving D1 retune the balance between amyloid-β phagocytosis and inflammation in Alzheimer's disease patients." *J Alzheimers Dis.* 2013;34(1):155–70.

188 Simopoulos AP. "Omega-3 fatty acids in inflammation and autoimmune diseases." *J Am Coll Nutr.* 2002 Dec;21(6):495–505.

189 Calder PC. "N-3 polyunsaturated fatty acids and cytokine production in health and disease." *Ann Nutr Metab.* 1997;41(4):203–34.

190 Mori T, Beilin L. "Omega-3 fatty acids and inflammation." *Cur Atheroscler Rep.* 2004;6(6):461–67.

191 Breslow J. "n-3 fatty acids and cardiovascular disease." *Am J Clin Nutr.* 2006 Jun;83(6):s1477–82.

192 Calder PC. "N-3 fatty acids and cardiovascular disease: evidence explained and mechanisms explored." *Clin Sci (Lond).* 2004 Jul;107(1):1–11.

193 Kremer J. "n-3 fatty acid supplements in rheumatoid arthritis." *Am J Clin Nutr.* 2000 Jan;71(1):349s–51s.

194 Thorsdottir I, Tomasson H, Gunnarsdottir, et al. "Randomized trial of weight-loss-diets for young adults varying in fish and fish oil content." *Int J Obesity.* 2007;31:1560–66.

195 Horrocks L, Yeo Y. "Health benefits of docosahexaenoic acid (DHA)." *Pharm Res.* 1999 Sep;40(3):211–25.

196 Conner W. "Importance of n-3 fatty acids in health and disease." *Am J Clin Nutr.* 2000 Jan;71(1):1715–55.

197 Harris W, Pottala J, Sands S, et al. "Comparison of the effects of fish and fish-oil capsules on the n-3 fatty acid content of blood cells and plasma phospholipids." *Am J Clin Nutr.* 2007 Dec;86(6):1621–1625.

198 Kris-Etherton P, Grieger J, Etherton T. "Dietary reference intakes of DHA and EPA." *Prostaglandins Leukot Essent Fatty Acids.* 2009 Aug–Sep;81(2–3):99–104.

199 Harris WS, Mozaffarian D, Lefevre M, et al. "Towards establishing dietary reference intakes for eicosapentaenoic and docosahexaenoic acids." *J Nutr.* 2009 Apr;139(4):804S–19S.

200 Hu FB, Bronner L, Willett WC, et al. "Fish and omega-3 fatty acid intake and risk of coronary heart disease in women." *JAMA.* 2002 Apr 10;287(14):1815–21.

201 Skerrett PJ, Hennekens CH. "Consumption of fish and fish oils and decreased risk of stroke." *Prev Cardiol.* 2003 Winter;6(1):38–41.

202 Laidlaw M, Cokerline CA, Rowe WJ. "A randomized clinical trial to determine the efficacy of manufacturers' recommended doses of omega-3 fatty acids from different sources in facilitating cardiovascular disease risk reduction." *Lipids Health Dis.* 2014 Jun 21;13:99.

203 Ilich JZ, Kelly OJ, Kim Y, et al. "Low-grade chronic inflammation perpetuated by modern diet as a promoter of obesity and osteoporosis." *Arh Hig Rada Toksikol.* 2014 Jun;65(2):139–48.

204 Simopoulos AP. "The importance of the ratio of omega-6/omega-3 essential fatty acids." *Biomed Pharmacother.* 2002 Oct;56(8):365–79.

205 US Department of Health and Human Services. "How much sugar do you eat? You may be surprised." Accessed August 4, 2014, from http://www.dhhs.state.nh.us/dphs/nhp/adults/documents/sugar.pdf.

206 Pepsi Bottling Company. Accessed August 18, 2014, from http://www.pepsiproductfacts.com.

207 Calorie Count. "Calories in Cherry Limeade." Accessed August 18, 2014, from http://caloriecount.about.com/calories-sonic-cherry-limeade-i56941.

208 Turina M, Fry DE, Polk HC Jr. "Acute hyperglycemia and the innate immune system: clinical, cellular, and molecular aspects." *Crit Care Med.* 2005 Jul;33(7):1624–33.

209 Yabao RN, Duante CA, Velandria FV, et al. "Prevalence of dental caries and sugar consumption among 6–12 year old schoolchildren in La Trinadad, Benguet, Philippines." *Eur J Nutr.* 2005 Dec;59(12):1429–38.

210 Johnson R, Segal M, Saution M, et al. "Potential role of sugar (fructose) in the epidemic of hypertension, obesity and the metabolic syndrome, diabetes, kidney disease, and cardiovascular disease." *Am J Clin Nutr.* 2007 Oct;86(4):899–906.

211 Thornley S, Stewart A, Marshall R, et al. "Per capita sugar consumption is associated with sever childhood asthma: an ecological study of 53 countries." *Prim Care Respir J.* 2011 Mar;20(1):75–8.

212 Westover AN, Marangell LB. "A cross-national relationship between sugar consumption and major depression?" *Depress Anxiety.* 2002;16(3):118–20.

213 Lewis J. "Health briefings." *Fort Worth Star Telegram.* Reported to the Society for Pediatric Research in Anaheim, CA, on May 9, 1990, by Yale medical researchers.

214 Venkateswaran V, Haddad A, Fleshner N, et al. "Association of diet-induced hyperinulinemia with accelerated growth of prostate cancer (LNCaP) xenografts." *JNCI J Natl Cancer Inst.* 2007;99(23):1793–1800.

215 Goran MI, Ulijaszek SJ, Ventura EE, et al. "High fructose corn syrup and diabetes prevalence:a global perspective." *Glob Public Health.* 213;8(1):55–64.

216 Miller A, Adeli K. "Dietary fructose and the metabolic syndrome." *Curr Opin Gastroenterol.* 2008 Mar;24(2):204–9.

217 Ferder L, Ferder M, Inserra F. "The role of high-fructose corn syrup in metabolic syndrome and hypertension." *Curr Hypertension Reports.* 2010 Apr;12(2):105–12.

218 Gaby AR. "Adverse effects of dietary fructose." *Altern Med Rev.* 2005 Dec;10(4):294–306.

219 Stanhope K, Havel P. "Endocrine and metabolic effects of consuming beverages sweetened with fructose, glucose, sucrose, or high-fructose corn syrup." *Am J Clin Nutr.* 2008 Dec;88(6):1733S–1737S.

220 Stanhope KL, Bremer AA, Medici V, et al. "Consumption of fructose and high fructose corn syrup increase postprandial triglycerides, LDL-cholesterol, and apolipoprotein-B in young men and women." *J Clin Endocrinol Metab.* 2011 Oct;96(10):E1596–605.

221 Dufault R, LeBlanc B, Schnoll R, et al. "Mercury from chlor-alkali plants: measured concentrations in food product sugar." *Environmental Health.* 2009;8:2.

222 Larson N, DeWolfe J, Story M, et al. Adolescent consumption of sports and energy drinks: linkages to higher physical activity, unhealthy beverage patterns, cigarette smoking, and screen media use. *J Nutr Ed Behavior.* 2014;46(3):181.

223 Reissig C, Strain EC, Griffiths RR, "Caffeinated energy drinks—A growing problem." *Drug Alcohol Dep.* 2009;99(1–3):1–10.

224 Center for Behavioral Health Statistics and Quality. "The DAWN Report: update on emergency department visits involving energy drinks: a continuing public health concern, 2013." Accessed August 18, 2014, from http://www.samhsa.gov/data/spotlight/spot124-energy-drinks-2014.pdf.

225 Reissig C, Strain E, Griffiths R. "Caffeinated energy drinks—A growing problem." *Drug Alcohol Dependency.* 2009 Jan 1;99(1–3):1–10.

226 Worthley MI, Prabhu A, De Sciscio P, et al. "Detrimental effects of energy drink consumption on platelet and endothelial function." *Am J Med.* 2012 Feb;123(2):184–7.

227 Eteng MU, Eyong EU, Akpanyung EO, et al. "Recent advances in caffeine and theobromine toxicities: a review." *Plant Foods Hum Nutr.* 1997 Oct;51(3):231–43.

228 Wang Y, Waller DP, Hikim AP, et al. "Reproductive toxicity of theobromine and cocoa in male rats." *Reprod Toxicol.* 1992;6(4):347–53.

229 Slattery ML, West DW. "Smoking, alcohol, coffee, tea, caffeine, and theobromine: risk of prostate cancer in Utah (United States)." *Cancer Causes Control.* 1993 Nov;4(6):559–63.

230 Olthof M, Hollman P, Zock P, and Katan M. "Consumption of high doses of chlorogenic acid, present in coffee, or of black tea increases plasma total homocysteine concentrations in humans." *J Clin Nutr.* 2001 Mar;73(3):532–8.

231 Rossignol AM, Bonnlander H. "Prevalence and severity of the premenstrual syndrome. Effects of foods and beverages that are sweet or high in sugar content." *J Reprod Med.* 1991 Feb;36(2):131–36.

232 Environmental Protection Agency. "Review of fluoride drinking water standard." Accessed August 14, 2014, from http://water.epa.gov/drink/contaminants/basicinformation/fluoride.cfm.

233 Du GJ, Zhang Z, Wen XD, et al. "Epigallocatechin Gallate (EGCG) is the most effective cancer chemopreventive polyphenol in green tea." *Nutrients.* 2012 Nov 8;4(11):1679–91.

234 Rhode J, Jacobsen C, Kromann-Andersen H. "Toxic hepatitis triggered by green tea." *Ugeskr Laeger.* 2011 Jan 17;173(3):205–6.

235 Bonkovsky HL. "Hepatotoxicity associated with supplements containing Chinese green tea (Camellia sinensis)." *Ann Intern Med.* 2006 Jan 3;144(1):68–71.

236 Verhelst X, Burvenich P, Van Sassenbroeck D, et al. "Acute hepatitis after treatment for hair loss with oral green tea extracts (Camellia sinensis)." *Acta Gastroenterol Belg.* 2009 Apr–Jun;72(2):262–4.

237 Molinar M, Watt KD, Kruszyna T, Nelson R, et al. "Acute liver failure induced by green tea extracts: case report and review of the literature." *Liver Transpl.* 2006 Dec;12(12):1892–95.

238 Yellapu RK, Mittal V, Grewal P, et al. "Acute liver failure caused by 'fat burners' and dietary supplements: a case report and literature review." *Can J Gastroenterol.* 2011 Mar;25(3):157–60.

239 Mayo Clinic. "Caffeine content for coffee, tea, soda and more." Accessed August 5, 2014, from http://www.mayoclinic.org/healthy-living/nutrition-and-healthy-eating/in-depth/caffeine/art-20049372.

240 Liu J, Sui X, Lavie CJ, et al. "Association of coffee consumption with all-cause and cardiovascular disease mortality." *Mayo Clin Proc.* 2013 Oct;88(10):1066–74.

241 Happonen P, Voutilainen S, Salonen J. "Coffee drinking is dose-dependently related to the risk of acute coronary events in middle-aged men." *J Nutr.* 2004 Sep 1;134(9):2381–86.

242 Bak A, Grobbee D, "The effect on serum cholesterol levels of coffee brewed by filtering or boiling." *N Eng J Med.* 1989;321:1432–37.

243 Mikuls TR, Cerhan JR, Criswell LA, et al. "Coffee, tea, and caffeine consumption and risk of rheumatoid arthritis: results from the Iowa Women's Health Study." *Arthritis Rhematism.* 2002 Jan;46(1):83–91.

244 Morck TA, Lynch SR, Cook JD. "Inhibition of food iron absorption by coffee" *Am J Clin Nutr.* 1983 Mar;37(3):416–20.

245 Sugiyama K, Kuriyama S, Akhter M, et al. "Coffee consumption and mortality due to all causes, cardiovascular disease, and cancer in Japanese women." *J Nutr.* 2010 May;140(5):1007–13.

246 van Dam R, Freskens E. "Coffee consumption and risk of type 2 diabetes mellitus." *Lancet.* 2002 Nov 9;360(9344):1477–78.

247 Lopez-Garcia E, van Dam R, Qi L, et al. "Coffee consumption and markers of inflammation and endothelial dysfunction in healthy and diabetic women." *Am J Clin Nutr.* 2006 Oct;84(4):888–93.

248 Lopez-Garcia E, Rodriquez-Artaleo F, Rexrode K, et al. "Coffee consumption and risk of stroke in women." *Circulation.* 2009;119:1116–23.

249 Diehl A. "Liver disease in alcohol abusers: clinical perspective." *Alcohol.* 2002 May;27(1):7–11.

250 Thomas V, Rockwood K. "Alcohol abuse, cognitive impairment, and mortality among older people." *J Am Geriatrics Soc.* 2001 Apr;49(4):415–20.

251 Gonzales K, Roeber J, Kanny D, et al. "Alcohol-attributable deaths and years of potential life lost—11 States, 2006–2010." 2014 Mar;63(10):213–16.

252 Center for Addiction and Substance Abuse, Columbia University. "The cost of substance abuse to America's health system, Report 1." *Medicaid Hospital Costs.* 1994.

253 Hunkeler EM, Hung YY, Rice DP, et al. "Alcohol consumption patterns and health care costs in an HMO." *Drug Alcohol Depend.* 2001 Oct 1;64(2):181–90.

254 Salome HJ, French MT, Matzger H, et al. "Alcohol consumption, risk of injury, and high-cost medical care." *J Behav Health Serv Res.* 2005 Oct–Dec;32(4):368–80.

255 Harwood, H. "Updating estimates of the economic costs of alcohol abuse in the United States: estimates, update methods, and data." Report prepared by The Lewin Group for the National Institute on Alcohol Abuse and Alcoholism. 2000. Based on estimates, analyses, and data reported in Harwood, H,. Fountain, D, Livermore. *The Economic Costs of Alcohol and Drug Abuse in the United States 1992.* Report prepared for the National Institute on Drug Abuse and the National Institute on Alcohol Abuse and Alcoholism, National Institutes of Health, Department of Health and Human Services. NIH Publication No. 98–4327. Rockville, MD: National Institutes of Health, 1998.

256 Thomson AD. "Mechanisms of vitamin deficiency in chronic alcohol misusers and the development of the Wernicke-Korsakoff Syndrome." *Alcohol and Alcoholism.* 2000 May–Jun;35(1):2.7.

257 Fullwood D. "Alcohol-related liver disease." *Nurs Stand.* 2014 Jul 16;28(46):42–7.

258 Bofetta P, Hashibe M. "Alcohol and cancer." *The Lancet Oncology.* 2006 Feb;7(2):149–56.

259 Bode C, Bode JC. "Alcohol's role in gastrointestinal tract disorders." *Alcohol Health Red World.* 1997;21(1):76–83.

260 Environmental Protection Agency. www.epa.gov.

261 Parron T, Requena M, Hernandez AF, et al. "Environmental exposure to pesticides and cancer risk in multiple human organ systems." *Toxicol Lett.* 2013 Nov 20:S0378–4274.

262 Parron T, Requena M, Hernandez AF, et al. "Association between environmental exposure to pesticides and neurodegenerative diseases." *Toxicol Appl Pharmacol.* 2011 Nov 1;256(3):379–85.

263 Olney J. "Excitatory amino acids and neuropsychiatric disorders." *Biol Psychiatry* 26:505–525, 1989.

264 Bunyan J, Murrell A, Shah P. "The induction of obesity in rodents by means of monosodium glutamate." *Br J Nutr.* 1976 Jan;35(1):25–39.

265 US Food and Drug Administration. Accessed August 5, 2014, from http://www.fda.gov/ohrms/dockets/dailys/03/Jan03/012203/02P-0317_emc-000196.txt.

266 Graudal N, Jurgens G, Baslund B, et al. "Compared with usual sodium intake, low- and excessive-sodium diets are associated with increased mortality: A meta-analysis." *Am J Hypertension.* 2014 Apr 26. [Epub ahead of print]

267 Xie TP, Zhao YF, Chen LQ, et al. "Long-term exposure to sodium nitrite and risk of esophageal carcinoma: a cohort study for 30 years." *Dis Esophagus.* 2011 Jan;24(1):30–2.

268 US Centers for Disease Control and Prevention. "Healthy weight—it's not a diet, it's a lifestyle." Accessed August 19, 2014, from http://www.cdc.gov/healthyweight/losing_weight/keepingitoff.html.

269 National Institutes of Health, US Department of Health and Human Services. *Opportunities and challenges in digestive disease research: Recommendations of the National Commission on Digestive Diseases.* 2009. NIH Publication 08-6514.

270 Everhart JE. "The burden of digestive diseases in the United States." National Institue of Diabetes and Digestive and Kidney Disorders, US. Department of Health and Human Services. 2008. NIH Publicatoin 09-6433.

271 Muller S, Marz R, Schmolz M, et al. "Placebo-controlled randomized clinical trial on the immunomodulating activities of low- and high-dose bromelain after oral administration—new evidence on the antiinflammatory mode of action of bromelain." *Phytother Res.* 2013 Feb;27(2):199–204.

272 Secor ER Jr, Shah SJ, Guernsey LA, et al. "Bromelain limits airway inflammation in an ovalbumin-induced murine model of established asthma." *Altern Ther Health Med.* 2012 Sep–Oct;18(5):9–17.

273 Onken JE, Greer PK, Calingaert B, et al. "Bromelain treatment decreases secretion of pro-inflammatory cytokines and chemokines by colon biopsies in vitro." *Clin Immunol.* 2008 Mar;126(3):345–52.

274 Kerkhoffs GM, Struijs PA, de Wit C, et al. "A double blind, randomized, parallel group study on the efficacy and safety of treating acute lateral ankle sprain with oral hydrolytic enzymes." *Br J Sports Med.* 2004 Aug;38(4):431–5.

275 Kamenícek V, Holán P, Franěk P. "Systemic enzyme therapy in the treatment and prevention of post-traumatic and postoperative swelling." *Acta Chir Orthop Traumatol Cech.* 2001;68(1):45–9.

276 Klein G, Kullich W, Schnitker J, Schwann H. "Efficacy and tolerance of an oral enzyme combination in painful osteoarthritis of the hip. A double-blind, randomised study comparing oral enzymes with non-steroidal anti-inflammatory drugs." *Clin Exp Rheumatol.* 2006 Jan–Feb;24(1):25–30.

277 US Food and Drug Administration. "FDA drug safety communication: Possible increased risk of fractures of the hip, wrist, and spine with the use of proton pump inhibitors." 2011. Accessed November 4, 2014, from http://www.fda.gov/Drugs/DrugSafety/PostmarketDrugSafety InformationforPatientsandProviders/ucm213206.htm.

278 Marks IN, Boyd E. "Mucosal protective agents in the long-term management of gastric ulcer." *Med J Aust.* 1985 Feb 4;142(3):S23–25.

279 Rees WD, Rhodes J, Wright JE, et al. "Effect of deglycyrrhizinated liquorice on gastric mucosal damage by aspirin." *Scand J Gastroenterol.* 1979;14(5):605–07.

280 Bennett A. "Gastric mucosal formation of prostanoids and the effects of drugs." *Acta Physiol Hung.* 1984;64(3–4):215–17.

281 World Health Organization. "Micronutrient deficiencies." Accessed August 20, 2014, from http://www.who.int/nutrition/topics/vad/en/.

282 World Health Organization. "Micronutrient deficiencies. Iron deficiency anaemia." Accessed August 20, 2014, from http://www.who.int/nutrition/topics/vad/en/.

283 Ames B. "Increasing longevity by tuning up metabolism." *EMBO Reports.* 2005 Jul;6(S1):S20–24.

284 Fairfield KM, Fletcher RH. "Vitamins for chronic disease prevention in adults: scientific review." *JAMA.* 2002 Jun 19;287(23):3116–26.

285 Council for Responsible Nutrition. 2008 HCP Impact Study. "Life… supplemented" HCP Impact Study Results. Accessed August 5, 2009, from http://newhope360.com/health-conditions/2008-life-supplement-ed-hcp-impact-study-results-released.

286 Kristi AR, Darke AK, Morris DJ, et al. "Baseline selenium status and effects of selenium and vitamin E supplementation on prostate cancer risk." *J Nat Cancer Inst.* 2014 Feb. [Epub ahead of print]

287 Klein EA, Thompson IM, Tangen CM, et al. "Vitamin E and the risk of prostate cancer risk." *JAMA*. 2011;306(14):1549–56.

288 Gavaghan J. "Hooked on chicken nuggets: Girl, 17, who has eaten nothing else since age TWO rushed to hospital after collapsing." Accessed August 21, 2014, from http://www.dailymail.co.uk/health/article-2092071/Stacey-Irvine-17-collapses-eating-McDonalds-chicken-nuggets-age-2.html.

289 Internet FAQ Archives. "Dietary trends, American." Accessed April 11, 2009, from http://www.faqs.org/nutrition/Diab-Em/Dietary-Trends-American.html.

290 Centers for Disease Control and Prevention. "Micronutrient facts." Accessed August 5, 2014, from http://www.cdc.gov/immpact/micronutrients/index.html.

291 Neff R, Hartle J, Laestadius L, et al. "A comparative study of allowable pesticide residue levels on produce in the United States." *Global and Health*. 2012;8:2.

292 Davis, D. "Tradeoffs in agriculture and nutrition." *Food Technology*. 2005 Mar;59(3):120.

293 Jack, A. "The disappearing nutrients in America's fruit orchards." Accessed August 6, 2014, from http://www.thenhf.com/the-disappearing-nutrients-in-americas-orchards/.

294 Leopold Center for Sustainable Agriculture. "Checking the food odometer: comparing food miles for local versus conventional produce sales to Iowa institutions." Accessed August 8, 2014, from http://www.leopold.iastate.edu/sites/default/files/pubs-and-papers/2003-07-checking-food-odometer-comparing-food-miles-local-versus-conventional-produce-sales-iowa-institution.pdf.

295 Huang S, Huang K. "Increased US imports of fresh fruit and vegetables." 2007 Sep. Accessed August 14, 2014, from http://www.unitedfresh.org/assets/files/Increased%20U. S.%20FFV%20Imports.pdf.

296 Chen, A, Katz, D. "Aging and neuroepidemiology group." *Am J Epidemiol*. 2009 Jun.

297 Grune T, Lietz G, Palou A, et al. "Beta-carotene is an important vitamin A source for humans." *J Nutr*. 2010;140:2268S–85S.

298 Garland CF, Garland FC, Gorham ED. "The role of vitamin D in cancer prevention." *AM J Public Health*. 2006 Feb;96(2):252–61.

299 Withim MD, Nadir MA, Struthers AD. "Effect of vitamin D on blood pressure: a systematic review and meta-analysis." *J Hypertesion*. 2009;27(10):1948–54.

300 Agmon-Levin N, Theodor E, Segal RM, et al. "Vitamin D in systemic and organ-specific autoimmune diseases." *Clin Rev Allergy Immunol.* 2013 Oct;45(2):256–66.

301 Grober U, Spitz J, Reichrath J, et al. "Vitamin D: update 2013: from rickets prophylaxis to general preventive healthcare." *Dermatoendocrinol.* 2013 Jun 1;5(3):331–47.

302 Hossein-nezhad A, Spira A, Holick MF. "Influence of vitamin D status and vitamin D3 supplementation on genome wide expression of white blood cells: a randomized double-blind clinical trial." *PLoS One.* 2013;8(3):e58725.

303 Hossein-nezhad A, Spira A, Holick MF. "Influence of vitamin D status and vitamin D3 supplementation on genome wide expression of white blood cells: a randomized double-blind clinical trial." *PLoS One.* 2013;8(3):e58725.

304 Garland, CF, Kim JJ, Mohr SB, et al. "Meta-analysis of all-cause mortality according to serum 25-hydroxyvitamin D." *Am J Public Health.* 2014 Aug;14(8):e43–50.

305 Itty S, Day S, Lyles KW, et al. "Vitamin D deficiency in neovascular versus nonneovascular age-related macular degeneration." *Retina.* 2014 Jun 18. [Epub ahead of print]

306 Spedding S. "Vitamin D and depression:a systematic review and meta-analysis comparing studies with and without biological flaws." *Nutrients.* 2014 Apr 11;6(4):151–18.

307 Wilson VK, Houston DK, Kilpatrick L, et al. "Relationship between 25-hydroxyvitamin D and cognitive function in older adults: the Health, Aging and Body Composition Study." *J Am Geriatr Soc.* 2014 Apr;62(4):636–41.

308 Goksugar SB, Tufan AE, Semiz M, et al. "Vitamin D status in children with attention-deficit-hyperactivity disorder." *Pediatr Int.* 2014 Jan 13. [Epub ahead of print]

309 Kamal M, Bener A, Ehlayel MS. "Is high prevalence of vitamin D deficiency a correlate for attention deficit hyperactivity disorder?" *Atten Defic Hyperact Disord.* 2014 Jun;6(2):73–8.

310 Vieth R. "Vitamin D supplementation, 25-hydroxyvitamin D concentrations, and safety." *Am J Clin Nutr.* 1999 May;69(5):842–56.

311 Meydani SM, Meydani M, Blumberg JB, et al. "Vitamin E supplementation and in vivo immune response in healthy elderly subjects. A randomized controlled trial." *JAMA.* 1997 May7;277(17):1380–6.

312 Lanham-New S. "Importance of calcium, vitamin D and vitamin K for osteoporosis prevention and treatment." *Proceedings of the Nutrition Society.* 2008;67:163–76.

313 Binkley NC, Krueger DC, Engelke JA, et al. "Vitamin K supplementation reduces serum concentrations of under-y-carboxylated osteocalcin in healthy young and elderly adults." *Am J Clin Nutr.* 2000 Dec;72(6):1523–28.

314 Iwamoto J, Sato Y, Takeda T, et al. "High-dose vitamin K supplementation reduces fracture incidence in postmenopausal women: a review of the literature." *Nutr Res.* 2009 Apr;29(4):221–28.

315 Sconce E, Avery P, Wynne H, et al. "Vitamin K supplementation can improve stability of anticoagulation for patients with unexplained variability in response to Warfarin." *Blood.* 2007 Mar 15;109(6):2419–23.

316 American Academy of Pediatrics. "Controversies concerning vitamin K and the newborn." *Pediatrics.* 2003 Jul;112:191.

317 Mimori Y, Katsuoka H, Nakamura S. "Thiamine therapy for Alzheimer's disease." *Met Brain Disease.* 1996 March;11(1)89–94.

318 Baker H, Frank O. "Absorption, utilization and clinical effectiveness of allithiamines to water-soluble thiamines." *J Nutr Sci Vitaminol (Tokyo).* 1976 Aug;22(SUPPL):63–68.

319 Haupt E, Ledermann H, Kopcke W. "Benfotiamine in the treatment of diabetic polyneuropathy—a three week randomized, controlled pilot study (BEDIP study)." *Int J Clin Pharmacol Ther.* 2005 Feb;43(2):71–7.

320 Hammes HP, Du X, Edelstein D, et al. "Benfotiamine blocks three major pathways of hyperglycemic damage and prevents experimental diabetic retinopathy." *Nat Med.* 2003 Mar;9(3):294–99.

321 Pataki L, Matkovics B, Novak Z, et al. "Riboflavin (vitamin B2) treatment of nonatal pathological jaundice." *Acta Paedatr Hung.* 1985;26(4):341–45.

322 Tisdall FF, McCreary JF, Pearce H. "The effect of riboflavin on corneal vascularization and symptoms of eye fatigue in RCAF personnel." *Can Med Assoc J.* 1943 Jul;49(1):5–13.

323 Mares-Perlman JA, Brady WE, Klein BE, et al. "Diet and nuclear lens opacities." *Am J Epidemiol.* 1995 Feb 15;141(4):322–34.

324 Schoenen J, Lenaerts M, Bastings E. "High-dose riboflavin as a prophylactic treatment of migraine: results of an open pilot study." *Cephalalgia.* 1994 Oct;14(5):328–29.

325 Powers H. "Riboflavin (vitamin B-2) and health." *Am J Clin Nutr.* 2003 Jun;77(6):1352–60.

326 Carlson LA. "Nicotinic acid:the broad-spectrum lipid drug. A 50th anniversary review." *J Int Med.* 2005 Aug;258(2):94–114.

327 Carlson LA, Hamsten A, Asplund A. "Pronounced lowering of serum levels of lipoprotein LP(a) in hyperlipidaemic subjects treated with nicotinic acid." 1989 Oct;226(4):271–76.

328 Hutt V, Wechsler JG, Klor HU, et al. "Effect of clofibrate-inositol nicotinate combination on lipids and lipoproteins in primary hyperlipoproteinemia of types IIa, IV and V." *Arzneimittelforschung.* 1983;33(5):776–79.

329 Elam M, Hunninghake DB, Davis KB, et al. "Effects of niacin on lipid and lipoprotein levels and glycemic control in patients with diabetes and peripheral arterial disease: the ADMIT study: a randomized trial. Arterial Disease Multiple Intervention Trial." *JAMA.* 2000 Sep13;284(10):1263–70.

330 Guyton JR, Bays HE. "Safety considerations with niacin therapy." *Am J Cardiology.* 2007 Mar 19;99(6):S22–S31.

331 Kashanian M, Mazinani R, Jalalmanesh S. "Pyridoxine (vitamin B6) therapy for premenstrual syndrome." *Int J Gynaecol Obstet.* 2007 Jan;96(1):43–4.

332 Matok I, Clark S, Miodovnik M, et al. "Studying the antiemetic effect of vitamin B6 for morning sickness; pyridoxine and pyridoxal are prodrugs." *J Clin Pharmacol.* 2014 Jul 22. [Epub ahead of print]

333 Rossignol DA. "Novel and emerging treatments for autism spectrum disorders: a systematic review." *Ann Clin Psychology.* 2009 Oct–Dec;21(4):213–36.

334 Pearl PL, Gospe SM Jr. "Pyridoxine or opyridoxyl-5-phosphate for neonatal epilepsy: the distinction just got murkier." *Neurology.* 2014 Apr 22;82(16):1392–4.

335 Albin RL, Albers JW, Greenberg HS, et al. "Acute sensory neuropathy-neuronopathy from pyridoxine overdose." *Neurology.* 1987 Nov;37(11):1729–32.

336 Larrieta E, Vega-Monroy ML, Vital P, et al. "Effects of biotin deficiency on pancreatic islet morphology, insulin sensitivity and glucose homeostasis." *J Nutr Biochem.* 2012 Apr;23(4):392–9.

337 Study of the Effectiveness of Additional Reductions in Cholesterol and Homocysteine (SEARCH) Collaborative Group. "Effects of homocysteine-lowering with folic acid plus vitamin B12 vs placebo on mortality and major morbidity in myocardial infarction survivors: a randomized trial." *JAMA.* 2010 June;303(24):2486–94.

338 Harten P. "Reducing toxicity of methotrexate with folic acid." *Z Rheumatol.* 2005 Jun;64(5):353–8.

339 Shea B, Swinden MV, Tanjong Ghogomu E, et al. "Folic acid and collinic acid for reducing side effects in patients receiving methotrexate for rheumatoid arthritis." *Cochrane Database Syst Rev.* 2013 May 31;5:CD000951.

340 Health Quality Ontario. "Vitamin B12 and cognitive function: an evidence-based analysis." *Ont Health Technol Assess Ser.* 2013 Nov1;13(23):1–45.

341 Fenech M, Aitken A, Rinaldi J. "Folate, vitamin B12, homocysteine status and DNA damage in young Australian adults." *Carcinogenesis.* 1998;19(7):1163–71.

342 Lederle, F. "Oral cobalamin for pernicious anemia medicine's best kept secret." *JAMA* 1991 Jan 2;265(1):96–7.

343 Lin J, Kelsberg G, Safranek S. "Clinical inquiry: is high-dose oral B12 a safe and effective alternative to a B12 injection." *J Farm Pract.* 2012 Mar;61(3):162–3.

344 Freeman AG. "Sublingual cobalamin for pernicious anaemia." *Lancet.* 1999 Dec 11;354(9195):2080.

345 No authors listed. "Oral or intramuscular vitamin B12?" *Drug Ther Bull.* 2009 Feb;47(2):19–21.

346 Metha AK, Singh BP, Arora N, et al. "Choline attenuates immune inflammation and suppresses oxidative stress in patients with asthma." *Immunobiology.* 201 Jul;215(7):527–34.

347 Mehta AK, Arora N, Gaur SN, et al. "Choline supplementation reduces oxidative stress in mouse model of allergic airway disease." *Eur J Clin Invest.* 2009 Oct;39(10):934–41.

348 Buckman A, Dubin M, Moukarzel A, et al. "Choline deficiency: a cause of hepatic steatosis during parenteral nutrition that can be reversed with intravenous choline supplementation." *Hepatology.* 1995 Nov;22(5):1399–1403.

349 Ambali S, Orieji C, Abubakar W, et al. "Ameliorative effect of vitamin C on alterations in thyroid hormones concentrations induced by subchronic coadminsitrations of chlorpyrifos and lead in Wistar rats." *J Thyroid Res.* 2011;2011:214924.

350 McRae MP. "Vitamin C supplementation lowers serum low-density lipoprotein cholesterol and triglycerides: a meta-analysis of 13 randomized controlled trials." *J Chiropr Med.* 2008 Jun;7(2):48–58.

351 Vinson JA, Bose P. "Comparative bioavailability to humans of ascorbic acid alone or in a citrus extract." *Am J Clin Nutr.* 1988;48(3):601–04

352 Nielsen FH, Hunt CD, Mullen LM, et al. "Effect of dietary boron on mineral, estrogen, and testosterone metabolism in postmenopausal women." *FASEB J.* 1987 Nov;1(5):394–97.

353 Naghii MR, Mofid M, Asgari AR, et al. "Comparative effects of daily and weekly boron supplementation on plasma steroid hormones and proinflammatory cytokines." *J Trace Elem Med Biol.* 2011 Jan;25(1):54–58.

354 Hunt CD, Herbel JL, Idso JP. "Dietary boron modifies the effects of vitamin D3 on indices of energy substrate utilization and mineral metabolism in the chick." *J Bone Miner Res.* 1994 Feb;9(2):171–82.

355 Hunt CD. "The biochemical effects of physiologic amounts of dietary boron in animal nutrition models." *Environ Health Perspect.* 1994 Nov;102 Suppl 7:35–42.

356 Hunt CD, Idso JP. "Dietary boron as a physiological regulator of the normal inflammatory response: a review and current research progress." *J Trace Elem Exp Med.* 1999;12:221–33.

357 Zhang ZF, Winton MI, Rainey C, et al. "Boron is associated with decreased risk of human prostate cancer." Presented at Experimental Biology 2001 March 31–April 4;Orlando, FL.

358 Barranco WT, Eckhert CD. "Boric acid inhibits human cancer cell proliferation." *Cancer Lett.* 2004 Dec 8;216(1):21–29.

359 Bonjour JP, "Calcium and phosphate: a duet of ions playing for bone health." *J AM Coll Nutr.* 2011 Oct;30(5 Suppl 1):438S–48S.

360 Thys-Jacobs S, Starkey P, Bernstein D, et al. "Calcium carbonate and the premenstrual syndrome: effects on premenstrual and menstrual symptoms. Premenstrual Syndrome Study Group." *Am J Obstet Gynecol.* 1998 Aug;179(2):444–452.

361 Cichosz G, Czeczot H. "Calcium—essential for everybody." *Pol Merkur Lekarski.* 2014 Jun;36(216):407–11.

362 Margolis K, Ray R, Horn L, et al. "Effect of calcium and vitamin D supplementation on blood pressure." *Hypertension.* 2008;52:847–55.

363 Gulson BL, Mizon KJ, Palmer JM, et al. "Contribution of lead from calcium supplements to blood lead." *Environ Health Perspec.* 2001 Mar;109(3):283–88.

364 Xiao Q, Murphy RA, Houston DK, et al. "Dietary and supplemental calcium intake and cardiovascular disease mortality: the National Institutes of Health–AARP diet and health study." *JAMA Intern Med.* 2013 Apr 22;173(8):639–46.

365 Michaelsson K, Mellhus H, Warensjo lemming E, et al. "Long term calcium intake and rates of all cause and cardiovascular mortality: community based prospective longitudinal cohort study." *BMJ.* 2013 Feb 12;346:f228.

366 Hoffman NJ, Penque BA, Habegger KM, et al. "Chromium enhances insulin responsiveness via AMPK." *J Nutr Biochem.* 2014 May;25(5):565–72.

367 Press R, Geller J, Evens G. "The effect of chromium picolinate on serum cholesterol and apolipoprotein fractions in human subjects." *West J Med.* 1990 Jan;152(1):41–45.

368 Anderson RA. "Effects of chromium on body composition and weight loss." *Nutr Rev.* 1998 Sep;56(9):266–70.

369 Balk E, Tatsioni A, Lichtenstein A, et al. "Effect of chromium supplementation on glucose metabolism and lipds: a systematic review of randomized controlled trials." *Diabetes Care.* 2007 Aug;30(8):2154–63.

370 Laurberg P, Cerqueira C, Ovesen L, et al. "Iodine intake as a determinant of thyroid disorders in populations." *Best Pract Res Clin Endocrinol Metab.* 2010 Feb;24(1):13–27.

371 World Health Organization. "Micronutrient deficiencies. Iodine deficiency disorders." Accessed August 21, 2014, from http://www.who.int/nutrition/topics/idd/en/.

372 Delange F. "Iodine deficiency as a cause of brain damage." *Postgrad Med J.* 2001 Apr;77(906):217–20.

373 Hunnicutt K, He K, Xun P. "Dietary iron intake and body iron stores are associated with risk of coronary heart disease in a meta-analysis of prospective cohort studies." *J Nutr.* 2014;144(3):359.

374 Tohno S, Tohno Y, Masuda M, et al. "A possible balance of magnesium accumulations among bone, cartilage, artery, and vein in single human individuals." *Biol Trace Elem Res.* 1999 Dec;70(3):233–41.

375 Dimai HP, Porta S, Wirnsberger, et al. "Daily oral magnesium supplementation suppresses bone turnover in young adult males." *J Clin Endocrinol Metab.* 1998 Aug;83(8):2742–48.

376 Aydin H, Deyneli O, Yavuz D, et al. "Short-term oral magnesium supplementation suppresses bone turnover in postmenopausal osteoporotic women." *Biol Trace Elem Res.* 2010 Feb;133(2):136–43.

377 Antman E. "Magnesium in acute MI." *Circulation.* 1995;92:2367–2372.

378 Li J, Zhang Q, Zhang M, et al. "Intravenous magnesium for acute myocardial infarction." *Cochrane Database Syst Rev.* 2007 Apr 18;(2):CD02755.

379 Stuglinger HG, Kiss K, Smetana R. "Significance of magnesium in cardiac arrhythmias." *Wien Med Wochenschr.* 2000;150(15–16):330–34.

380 Ho KM. "Intravenous magnesium for cardiac arrhythmias: jack of all trades." *Magnese Res.* 2008 Mar;21(10):65–8.

381 Belfort M, Moise K. "Effect of magnesium sulfate on maternal brain blood flow in preeclampsia: a randomized, placebo-controlled study." *Am J Obstet Gynecol.* 1992 Sep;167(3):661–6.

382 Duley L, Henderson-Smart DJ, Walker GJ, et al. "Magnesium sulphate versus diazepam for eclampsia." *Cochrane Database Syst Rev.* 2010 Dec 8;(12):CD000127.

383 Attlas J, Weisz G, Almog S, et al. "Oral magnesium intake reduces permanent hearing loss induced by noise exposure." *Am J Otolaryngology.* 1994 Jan–Feb;15(1):26–32.

384 Mauskop A, Altura BM. "Role of magnesium in the pathogenesis and treatment of migraines." *Clin Neurosci.* 1998;5(1):24–7.

385 Mauskop A, Varughese J. "Why all migraine patients should be treated with magnesium." *J Neural Transm.* 2012 May;119(5):575–9.

386 Ray SS, Das D, Ghosh T, et al. "The levels of zinc and molybdenum in hair and food grain in areas of high and low incidence of esophageal cancer: a comparative study." *Glob J Health Sci.* 2012 Jun 25;4(4):168–75.

387 Davies BE, Anderson RJ. "The epidemiology of dental caries in relation to environmental trace elements." *Experientia.* 1987 Jan 15;43(1):87–92.

388 Vyskocil A, Viau C. "Assessment of molybdenum toxicity in humans." *J Appl Toxicol.* 1999 May–Jun;19(3):185–192.

389 Stenvinkel P, Irving GF, Wegener S, et al. "Phosphate additives in food a potential public health risk. High phosphate levels can lead to cardiovascular disease." *Lakartidningen.* 2014 Jul;111(27–28):1176–79.

390 Ritz E, Hahn K, Ketteler M, et al. "Phosphate additives in food—a health risk." *Dtsch Arztebl Int.* 2012 Jan;109(4):49–55.

391 Toussaint ND, Pedagogos E, Tan Sj, et al. "Phosphate in early chronic kidney disease: associations with clinical outcomes and a target to reduce cardiovascular risk." *Nephrology (Carlton).* 2012 Jul;17(5):433–44.

392 Tonelli M, Sacks F, Pfeffer M, et al. "Relation between serum phosphate level and cardiovascular devent rate in people with coronary disease." *Circulation.* 2005;112:2627–33.

393 Draper HH, Scythes CA. "Calcium, phosphorus, and osteoporosis." *Fed Proc.* 1981 Jul;40(9):2434–38.

394 Pinheiro M, Schuch N, Genaro P, et al. "Nutrient intakes related to osteoporotic fractures in men and women—the Brazillian Osteoporosis Study (BRAZOS)." *Nutr J.* 2009 Jan 29;8:6.

395 Leehey DJ, Ing TS. "Correction of hypercalcemia and hypophosphatemia by hemodialysis using a conventional, calcium-containing dialysis solution enriched with phosphorus." *Am J Kidney Dis.* 1997 Feb;29(2):288–90.

396 Whelton P, He J, Cutler J, et al. "Effects of oral potassium on blood pressure: meta-analysis of randomized controlled trials." *JAMA.* 1997;277(20):1624–32.

397 Schrauzer GN. "Anticarcinogenic effects of selenium." *Cell Mol Life Sci.* 2000 Dec;57(13–14):1864–73.

398 Ip C. "Lessons from basic research in selenium and cancer prevention." *J Nutr.* 1998 Nov 1;128(11):1845–54.

399 Clark L, Combs G, Turnbull B, et al. "Effects of selenium supplementation for cancer prevention in patients with carcinoma of the skin: a randomized controlled trial." *JAMA.* 1996 Dec 25;276(24):1957–63.

400 Li Z, Meng J, Xu TJ, et al. "Sodium selenite induces apoptosis in colon cancer cells via Bax-dependent mitochondrial pathway." *Eur Rev Med Pharmacol Sci.* 2013 Aug;17(16):2166–71.

401 Epplein M, Burk RF, Cai Q, et al. "A prospective study of plasma seleno-protein P and lung cancer risk among low-income adults." *Cancer Epidemiol Biomarkers Prev.* 2014 Jul;23(7):1238–44.

402 Lou H, Wu R, Fu Y. "Relation between selenium and cancer of the cervix." *Zhonghua Zhong Liu Za Zhi.* 1995 Mar;17(2):112–14.

403 Wei WQ, Abnet CC, Qiao YL, et al. "Prospective study of serum selenium concentrations and esophageal and gastric cardia cancer, heart disease, stroke, and total death." *Am J Clin Nutr.* 2004 Jan;79(1):80–85.

404 Scott R, MacPherson A, Yates RW, et al. "The effect of oral selenium sup-plementation on human sperm motility." *Br J Urol.* 1998 Jul;82(1):76–80.

405 Kucharzewski M, Braziewicz J, Majewaska U, et al. "Concentration of selenium in the whole blood and the thyroid tissue of patients with various thyroid diseases." *Biol Trace Elem Res.* 2002 Jul;88(1):25–30.

406 Kohrle J. "The trace element selenium and the thyroid gland." *Biochimie.* 1999 May;81(5):527–33.

407 Rayman MP. "The importance of selenium to human health." *Lancet.* 2000 Jul 15;356(9225):233–41.

408 Kohrle J. "Selenium and the control of thyroid metabolism." *Thyroid.* 2005 Aug;15(8):841–53.

409 Hawkes WC, Keim NL. "Dietary selenium intake modulates thyroid hormone and energy metabolism in men." *J Nutr.* 2003 Nov 1;133(11):3443–48.

410 Broome CS, McArdle F, Kyle J, et al. "An increase in selenium intake improves immune function and poliovirus handling in adults with marginal selenium status." *Am J Clin Nutr.* 2004 Jul;80(1):154–62.

411 Yazdi MH. "Effect of supplementation of biogenic selenium nanoparticles on white blood cell profile of BALB/c mice and mice exposed to X-ray radiation." *Avicenna J Med Biotechnol.* 2013 Jul;5(3):158–67

412 Flores-Mateo G, Navas-Acien A, Pastor-Barriuso R, et al. "Selenium and coronary heart disease: a meta-analysis." *Am J Clin Nutr.* 2006 Oct;84(4):762–73.

413 Virtamo J, Valkeila E, Alfthan, et al. "Serum selenium and the risk of coro-nary heart disease and stroke." *Am J Epidemiol.* 1985 Aug;122(2):276–82.

414 Rayman MP, Stranges S, Griffin BA, et al. "Effect of supplementation with high-selenium yeast on plasma lipids, A randomized trial." *An Int Med.* 2011 May 17;154:656–65.

415 American Heart Association. "Eating too much salt led to nearly 2.3 million heart-related deaths worldwide in 2010." American Heart Association Meeting Report. 2013. Accessed August 22, 2014, from http://news-room. heart.org/news/eating-too-much-salt-led-to-nearly-2-3-million-heart-related-deaths-worldwide-in-2010.

416 Mozaffarian D, Fahimi S, Singh G, et al. "Abstract 028: The global impact of sodium consumption on cardiovascular mortality: a global, regional, and national comparative risk assessment." *Circulation.* 2013;127:A028.

417 Graudal N, Jurgens G, Baslund B, et al. "Compared with usual sodium intake, low- and excessive-sodium diets are associated with increased mortality: a meta-analysis." *Am J Hypertension.* 2014 Apr 26. [Epub ahead of print]

418 US Centers for Disease Control and Prevention. "Most Americans should consume less sodium." Accessed August 22, 2014, from http://www.cdc.gov/salt/.

419 Prasad A. "Zinc in human health: effect of zinc on immune cells." *Mol Med.* 2008 May–Jun;14(5–6):353–57.

420 Liu MJ, Bao S, Galvez-Peralta M, et al. "ZIP8 regulates host defense through zinc-mediated inhibition of NF-kB." *Cell Reports.* 2013 Feb;3(2):386–400.

421 Arslan K, Karahan O, Okus A, et al. "Comparison of topical zinc oxide and silver sulfadiazine in burn wounds: an experimental study." *Ulus Travma Acil Cerrahi Derg.* 2012 Sep;18(5):376–83.

422 Maxwell C, Volpe SL. "Effect of zinc supplementation on thyroid hormone function. A case study of two college females." *Ann Nutr Metab.* 2007;51(2):188–94.

423 Ertek S, Cicero AF, Caglar O, et al. "Relationship between serum zinc levels, thyroid hormones and thyroid volume following successful iodine supplementation." *Hormones (Athens).* 2010 Jul–Sep;9(3):263–68.

424 Johnson AR, Munoz A, Gottlieb JL, et al. "High dose zinc increases hospital admissions due to genitourinary complications." *J Urol.* 2007 Feb;177(2):639–43.

425 Yan M, Hardin K, Ho E. "Differential response to zinc-induced apoptosis in benign prostate hyperplasia and prostate cancer cells." *J Nutr Biochem.* 2010 Aug 21(8):687–94.

426 Escolar G, Bulbena O. "Zinc compounds, a new treatment for peptic ulcer." *Drugs Exp Clin Res.* 1989;15(2):83–9.

427 Jimenez E, Bosch F, Galmes JL, et al. "Meta-analysis of efficacy of zinc acexamate in peptic ulcer." *Digestion.* 1992;51(1):18–26.

428 Dodig-Curkovic K, Dovhanj J, Curkovic M, et al. "The role of zinc in the treatment of hyperactivity disorder in children." *Acta Med Croatica.* 2009 Oct;63(4):307–43.

429 Mahajan BB, Dhawan M, Singh R. "Herpes genitalis—topical zinc sulfate: an alternative therapeutic and modality." *Indian J Sex Trans Dis.* 2013 Jan;34(1):32–4.

430 Qiu M, Chen Y, Chu Y, et al. "Zinc ionophores pyrithione inhibits herpes simplex virus replication through interfering with proteasome function and NF-kB activation." *Antiviral Res.* 2013 Oct;100(1):44–53.

431 Atasoy HB, Ulusoy ZI. The relationship between zinc deficiency and children's oral health. *Pediatr Dent.* 2012 Sep–Oct;34(5):383–6.

432 Arterburn LM, Hall EB, Oken H. "Distribution, interconversion, and dose response of n-3 fatty acids in humans." *Am J Clin Nutr.* 2006 Jun;83(6):S1467–76.

433 Bunea R, El Farrah K, Deutsch L. "Evaluation of the effects of Neptune Krill Oil on the clinical course of hyperlipidemia." *Altern Med Rev.* 2004 Dec;9(4):420–8.

434 ConsumerLab.com. "Product review: fish oil and omega-3 fatty acid supplements review (including krill, algae, calamari, green-lipped mussel oil)." Accessed August 7, 2014, from https://www.consumerlab.com/reviews/fish_oil_supplements_review/omega3/.

435 Albert B, Cameron-Smith D, Hofman P, et al. "Oxidation of marine omega-3 supplements and human health." *Biomed Res Int.* 2013;2013:464921.

436 Garcia-Hernandez VM, Gallar M, Sanchez-Soriano J, et al. "Effect of omega-3 dietary supplements with different oxidation levels in the lipid profile of women: a randomized controlled trial." *Int J Food Sci Nutr.* 2013 Dec;64(8):993–1000.

437 Saini R. "Coenzyme A10: the essential nutrient." *J Pharm Bioallied Sci.* 2011 Jul;3(3):466–67.

438 Singh RB, Wander GS, Rastogi A, et al. "Randomized, double-blind placebo-controlled trial of coenzyme Q10 in patients with acute myocardial infarction." *Cardiovasc Drugs Ther.* 1998 Sep;12(4):347–53.

439 Langsjoen PH, Langsjoen AM. "Overview of the use of CoQ10 in cardiovascular disease." *Biofactors.* 1999;9(2):273–84.

440 Pourmoghaddas M, Rabbani M, Shahabi J, et al. "Combination of atorvastatin/coenzyme Q10 as adjunctive treatment in congestive heart failure: a double-blind randomized placebo-controlled clinical trial." *ARYA Atheroscler.* 2014 Jan;10(1):1–5.

441 Kocharian A, Shabanian R, Rafei-Khorgami M, et al. "Coenzyme Q10 improves diastolic function in children with idiopathic dilated cardiomyopathy." *Cardiol Young.* 2009 Sep;19(5):501–06.

442 Langsjoen H, Langsjoen P, Langsjoen P, et al. "Usefulness of coenzyme Q10 in clinical cardiology: a long-term study." *Mol Aspects Med.* 1994;15 Suppl;S165–75.

443 Prakash S, Sunitha J, Hans M. "Role of coenzyme Q(10) as an antioxidant and bioenergizer in periodontal diseases." *Indian J Pharmacol.* 2010 Dec;42(6):334–37.

444 Ravaglia G, Forti P, Maioli F, et al. "Effect of micronutrient status on natural killer cell immune function in healthy free-living subjects aged >/=90y." *Am J Clin Nutr.* 2000 Feb;71(2):590–98.

445 Yao LH, Jing YM, Shi J, et al. "Flavonoids in food and their health benefits." *Plant Foods Hum Nutr.* 2004 Summer;59(3):113–22.

446 Fuhman B, Aviram M. "Flavonoids protect LDL from oxidation and attenuate atherosclerosis." *Curr Opin Lipidol.* 2001 Feb;12(10):41–48.

447 McCullough M, Peterson J, Patel R, et al. "Flavanoid intake and cardiovascular disease mortality in a prospective cohort of US adults." *Am J Clin Nutr.* 2012 Feb;95(2):454–64.

448 Arai Y, Watanabe S, Kimira M, et al. "Dietary intakes of flavonoids, flavones and isoflavones by Japanese women and the inverse correlation between quercetin intake and plasma LDL cholesterol concentration." *J Nutr.* 2000;130:2243–50.

449 Gonzalez R, Ballester I, Lopez-Posadas R, et al. "Effects of flavonoids and other polyphenols on inflammation." *Crit Rev FoodSci Nutr.* 2011 Apr;51(4):331–62.

450 Romagnolo DF, Selmin OI. Flavonoids and cancer prevention: a review of the evidence." *J Nutr Gerontol Geriatr.* 2012;31(3):206–38.

451 Mead MN. "Diet and nutrition: temperance in green tea." *Diet Nutr.* 2007 Sep;115(9):A445.

452 Mashayehk A, Pham DL, Yousem DM, et al. "Effects of ginkgo biloba on cerebral blood flow assessed by quantitative MR perfusion imaging: a pilot study." *Neuroradiology.* 2011 Mar;53(3):185–91.

453 Yang M, Xu DD, Zhang Y, et al. "A systematic review on natural medicines for the prevention and treatment of Alzheimer's disease with meta-analyses of intervention effect of ginkgo." *Am J Clin Nutr.* 2014;42(3):505–21.

454 Vellas B, Coley N, Ousset PJ, et al. "Long-term use of standardized ginkgo biloba extract for the prevention of Alzheimer's disease (GuidAge): a randomized placebo-controlled trial." *Lancet Neurology.* 2012 Oct;11(10):851–59.

455 Hemmeter U, Annen B, Bischof R, et al. "Polysomnographic effects of adjuvant ginkgo biloba therapy in patients with major depression medicated with trimipramine." *Pharmacopsychiatry.* 2001 Mar;34(2):50–59.

456 Cybulska-Neinricj AK, Mozaffarieh M, Flammer J. "Ginkgo biloba: an adjuvant therapy for progressive normal and high tension glaucoma." *Mol Vis.* 2012;18:390–402.

457 McKay. "Nutrients and botanicals for erectile dysfunction: examining the evidence." *Altern Med Rev.* 2004 Mar;9(1):4–16.

458 Pebdani MA, Taavoni S, Seyedfatemi N, et al. "Triple-blind, placebo-controlled trial of ginkgo biolba extract on sexual desire in postmenopausal women in Tehran." *Iran J Nurs Midwifery Res.* 2014 May;19(3);262–5.

459 Kruis W, Pokrotnieks J, Lukas M, et al. "Maintaining remission of ulcerative colitis with the probiotic Escherichia coli Nissle 1917 is as effective as with standard mesalazine." *Gut.* 2004;53:1617–23.

460 Isolauri E, Sutas Y, Kankaanpaa P, et al. "Probiotics: effects on immunity." *Am J Clin Nutr.* 2001 Feb;73(2):444s–50s.

461 Logan AC, Katzman M. "Major depressive disorder: probiotics may be an adjuvant therapy." *Med Hypotheses.* 2005;64(3):533–38.

462 Lomax AR, Calder PC. "Probiotics, immune function, infection and inflammation: a review of the evidence from studies conducted in humans." *Curr Pharm Des.* 2009;15(13):1428–1518.

463 Alipour B, Homayouni-Rad A, Vaghef-Mehrabany E, et al. "Effects of Lactobacillus casei supplementation on disease activity and inflammatory cytokines in rheumatoid arthritis patients: a randomized double-blind clinical trial." *Int J Rhem Dis.* 2014 Jun;17(5):519–527.

464 Vaghef-Mehrabany E, Aipour B, Homayouni A, et al. "Probiotic supplementation improves inflammatory status in patients with rheumatoid arthritis." *Nutrition.* 2014 Apr;30(4):430–35.

465 Hataki K, Savilahti E, Ponka A, et al. "Effect of long term consumption of probiotic milk infections in children attending day care centres: double blind, randomized trial." *BMJ,* 2001 Jun 2;322(7298):1327.

466 Lever GJ, Li S, Mubasher ME, et al. "Probiotic effects on cold and influenza-like symptom incidence and duration in children." *Pediatrics.* 2009 Aug;124(2):e172–79.

467 Kumpu M, Kekkonen RA, Kautianen H, et al. "Milk containing probiotic Lactobacillus rhamnosus GG and respiratory illness in children: a randomized, double-blind, placebo-controlled trial." *Eur J Clin Nutr.* 2012 Sep;66(9):1020–23.

468 Indrio F, Mauro A, Riezzo G, et al. "Prophylactic use of probiotic in the prevention of colic, regurgitation, and functional constipation." A randomized clinical trial. *JAMA Pediatr.* 2014;168(3):228–33.

469 Falagas ME, Betsi GI, "Athanasiou S. Probiotics for prevention of recurrent vulvovaginal candidiasis: a review." *J Antimicrob Chemother.* 2006 Aug;58(2):266–72.

470 Vicariotto F, Del Piano M, Mogna L, et al. "Effectiveness of the association of 2 probiotic strains formulated in a slow release vaginal product, in women affected by vulvovaginal candidiasis: a pilot study." *J Clin Gastroenterol.* 2012 Oct;46 Suppl:S73–80.

471 Gallup. "America's desire to shed pounds outweighs effort." Accessed August 19, 2014, from http://www.gallup.com/poll/166082/americans-desire-shed-pounds-outweighs-effort.aspx.

472 Perry C, Heigenhauser G, Bonen A, Sprite L. "High-intensity aerobic interval training increases fat and carbohydrate metabolic capcities in human skeletal muscle." *Appl Physiol Nutr Metab.* 2008 Dec;33(6):1112–23.

473 Tesch P, Colliander E, Kaiser P. "Muscle metabolism during intense, heavy-resistance exercise." *Eur J Appl Physiol Occup Physiol.* 1986;55(4):362–6.

474 Heden T, Lox C, Rose P, Reid S, Kirk E. "One-set resistance training elevates energy expenditure for 72 h similar to three sets." *Eur J Appl Physiol.* 2011 Mar;111(3):477–84.

475 Hackney K, Engels H, Gretebeck R. "Resting energy expenditure and delayed-onset muscle soreness after full-body resistance training with an eccentric concentration." *J Strength Cond Res.* 2008 Sep;22(5):1602–9.

476 Gomez-Cabrera MC, Borras C, Pallardo FV, et al. "Decreasing xanthine oxidase-mediated oxidative stress prevents useful cellular adaptations to exercise in rats." *J Physiol.* 2005 Aug 15;567(Pt. 1):113–20.

477 Ristow M, Zarse K, Oberbach A, et al. "Antioxidants prevent health-prmoting effects of physical exercise in humans." *PNAS.* 2009 May;106(21):8665–70.

478 Tsai CL, Wang CH, Pan CY, et al. "Executive function and endocrinological responses to acute resistance exercise." *Front Behav Neurosci.* 2014 Aug 1;8:262.

479 Strohle A. "Physical activity, exercise, depression and anxiety disorders." *J Neural Transmission.* 2009 June;116(6):777–784.

480 Melancon MO, Lorrain D, Dionne IJ. "Exercise increases tryptophan availability to the brain in older men age 57–70 years." *Med Sci Sports Exerc.* 2012 May;44(5):881–87.

481 Melancon MO, Lorrain D, Dionne IJ. "Changes in markers of brain serotonin activity in response to chronic exercise in senior men." *Appl Physiol Nutr Metab.* 2014 Jun 23:1–7. [Epub ahead of print]

482 Burns, J. *Neurology.* July 15, 2008;71:210–216. American Academy of Neurology news release.

483 Nascimento CM, Pereira JR, Pires de Andrade L, et al. "Physical exercise improves peripheral BDNF levels ad cognitive functions in elderly mild cognitive impairment individuals with different BDNF Val66Met genotypes." *J Alzheimers Dis.* 2014 Jul 25. [Epub ahead of print]

484 Smith JC, Nielson KA, Woodward JL, et al. "Physical activity reduces hippocampal atrophy in elders at genetic risk for Alzheimer's disease." *Front Aging Neurosci.* 2014 Apr 23:6:61.

485 Radak Z, Hart N, Sarga L, et al. "Exercise plays a preventive role against Alzheimer's disease." *J Alzheimer's Disease.* 2010;20(3):777–83.

486 Yau SY, Gil-Mohapel J, Christie BR, et al. "Physical exercise-induced adult neurogenesis: a good strategy to prevent cognitive decline in neurodegenerative diseases?" *Biomed Res Int.* 2014;2014:403120.

487 Wong-Goodrich SJ, Pfau ML, Flores CT, et al. "Voluntary running prevents progressive memory decline and increases adult hippocampal neurogenesis and growth factor expression after whole-brain irradiation." *Cancer Res.* 2010 Nov 15;70(22):9329–38.

488 Moore S, Patel A, Matthews C, et al. "Leisure time physical activity of moderate to vigorous intensity and mortality: a large pooled cohort analysis." *PLoS One.* 2012 Nov 6;10:1371.

489 Byberg L, Melhus H, Gedeborg R, et al. "Total mortality after changes in leisure time and physical activity in fifty year old men: 35 year follow-up of population based cohort." *Br J Sports Med.* 2009 Jul;43(7):482.

490 Matthews C, Jurj AL, Shu XO, et al. "Influence of exercise, walking, cycling, and overall nonexercise physical activity on mortality in Chinese women." *Am J Epidemiol.* 2007 Jun 15;165(12):1343–1350.

491 Loprinzi PD, Cardinal BJ. "Association between biologic outcomes and objectively measured physical activity accumulated in ≥ 10-minute bouts and < 10-minute bouts." *Am J Health Promot.* 2013 Jan–Feb;27(3):143–51.

492 Macfarlane DJ, Taylor LH, Cuddihy TF. "Very short intermittent vs. continuous bouts in sedentary adults." *Prev Med.* 2006 Oct;43(4):332–36.

493 Holman RM, Carson V, Janssen I. "Does the fractionalization of daily physical activity (sporadic vs. bouts) impact cardiometabolic risk factors in children and youth?" *PLoS One.* 2011;6(10):e25733.

494 Glazer NL, Lyass A, Esliger DW, et al. "Sustained and shorter bouts of physical acticity are related to cardiovascular health." *Med Sci Sports Exerc.* 2013 Jan;45(1):109–15.

495 Murphy MH, Blair SN, Murtagh EM. "Accumulated versus continuous exercise for health benefit: a review of empirical studies." *Sports Med.* 2009;39(1):29–43.

496 Clarke J, Janssen. "Sporadic and bouted physical activity and the metabolic syndrome in adults." *Med Sci Sports Exerc.* 214 Jan;46(1):76–83.

497 Mark AE, Jenssen I. "Influence of bouts of physical activity on overweight in youth." *Am J Prev Med.* 2009 May;36(5):416–21.

498 Schmidt WD, Biwer CJ, Kalscheuer LK. "Effects of long versus short bout exercise on fitness and weight loss in overweight females." *J Am Coll Nutr.* 2001 Oct;20(5):494–501.

499 DeBusk R, Stenestrand U, Sheehan M, et al. "Training effects of long versus short bouts of exercise in healthy subjects." *Am J Cardiology.* 1990 Apr;65(15):1010–13.

500 Miyashita M. "Effects of continuous versus accumulated activity patterns on postprandial tricylglycerol concentrations in obese men." *Int J Obesity.* 2008;32:1271–78.

501 Haskell W, Lee I-Min, Pate R, et al. "Physical activity and public health: updated recommendation for adults from the American College of Sports Medicine and the American Heart Association." *Med Sci Sports Exerc.* 2007 Aug;39(8):1423–34.

502 Mckinnon LT. "Chronic exercise training effect on immune function." *Med Sci Sports Exercise.* 2000;32(7 Suppl):S369–76.

503 Nieman D. "Marathon training and immune function." *Sports Med.* 2007 Apr;37(4–5):412–15.

504 Nieman, D, Weidner, T, Dick, E, American College of Sports Medicine. "Exercise and the common cold." Accessed August 6, 2014, from http://www.acsm.org/docs/current-comments/exerciseandcommoncold.pdf.

505 Spence L, Brown WJ, Pyne DB, et al. "Incidence, etiology, and symptomatology of upper respiratory illness in elite athletes." *Med Sci Sports Exerc.* 2007 Apr;39(4):577–86.

506 Neilan T, Yoerger D, Douglas P, et al. "Persistent and reversible cardiac dysfunction among amateur marathon runners." *Clin Res.* 2006;27:1079–84.

507 Knebel F, Schimke I, Schroeckh S, et al. "Myocardial function in older male amateur marathon runners: assessment by tissue Doppler echocardiography, speckle tracking, and cardiac biomarkers." *J AM Soc Echocardiogr.* 2009 Jul;22(7):803–09.

508 Higashi Y, Sasaki S, Kurisu S, et al. "Regular aerobic exercise augments endothelial-dependent vascular relaxation in normotensive as well as hypertensive subjects." *Circulation.* 1999;100:1194–1202.

509 Laaksonen DE, Atalay M, NJiskanen LK, et al. "Aerobic exercise and the lipid profile in type 1 diabetic men:a randomized controlled trial." *Med Sci Sports Exerc.* 2000 Sep;32(9):1541–8.

510 Fred Hutchinson Cancer Research Center. "Regular, moderate-vigorous aerobic exercise significantly reduces markers of increased colon-cancer risk in men." Accessed April 8, 2009, from http://www.fhcrc.org/about/ne/news/2006/09/12/aerobic_exercise.html.

511 Campbell K, McTiernan A. "Exercise and biomarkers for cancer prevention studies." *J Nutr.* 2007 Jan;137(1):1615–95.

512 Thune I, Brenn T, Lund E, et al. "Physical activity and the risk of breast cancer." *N Engl J Med.* 1997;336:1269–75.

513 National Diabetes Information Clearinghouse (NDIC). "Am I at risk for type 2 diabetes? Taking steps to lower your risk of getting diabetes." Accessed August 5, 2014, from http://diabetes.niddk.nih.gov/dm/pubs/riskfortype2/.

514 Colberg S, Sigal R, Fernhall B, et al. "Exercise and type 2 diabetes. The American College of Sports Medicine and the American Diabetes Association: joint position statement." *Diabetes Care.* 2010 Dec;33(12):e147–e167.

515 Evans W. "Skeletal muscle loss: cachexia, sarcopenia, and inactivity." *Am J Clin Nutr.* 2010 Apr;91(4):1123S–75.

516 Tlacuilo-Parra A, Morales-Zambrano R, Tostado-Rabago N, et al. "Inactivity is a risk factor for low bone mineral density among haemophilic children." *Br J Haematol.* 2008 Mar;140(5):562–67.

517 Menkes A, Mazel S, Redmon RA, et al. "Strength training increases regional bone mineral density and bone remodeling in middle-aged and older men." *J App Phys.* 1993 May;74:2478–84.

518 Paddon-Jones D, Rasmussen B. "Dietary protein recommendations and the prevention of sarcopenia." *Curr Opin Clin Nutr Metab Care.* 2009 Jan;12(1):86–90.

519 Ivey FM, Tracy BL, Lemmer JT, et al. "Effects of strength training and detraining on muscle quality." *J Gerontol A Biol Med Sci.* 2000;55(3):B152-B157.

520 Kubo K, Kanehisa H, Kawakami Y, et al. "Influence of static stretching on viscoelastic properties of human tendon structures in vivo." *J Appl Physiol.* 2001;90:520–27.

521 Michalsen A, Traitteur H, Ludtke R, et al. "Yoga for chronic neck pain: a pilot randomized controlled clinical trial." *J Pain.* 2012 Nov;13(11):1122–30.

522 Hartfiel N, Burton C, Rycroft-Malone J, et al. "Yoga for reducing perceived stress and back pain at work." *Occup Med (Lond).* 2012 Dec;62(8):606–12.

523 Tilbrook HE, Cox H, Hewitt CE, et al. "Yoga for chronic low back pain: a randomized trial." *Ann Int Med.* 2011 Nov 1;155(9):569–78.

524 Streeter C, Whitfield T, Owen L, et al. "Effects of yoga versus walking on mood, anxiety, and brain GABA levels: a randomized controlled MRS study." *J Alt Comp Med.* 2010;16(11):1145.

525 Balasurbamaniam M, Telles S, Doraiswamy PM. "Yoga on our minds: a systematic review of yoga for neuropsychiatric disorders." *Front Psychiatry.* 2013 Jan 25;3:117.

526 Vedanthan PK, Kesavalu LN, Murthy KC, et al. "Clinical study of yoga techniques in university students with asthma: a controlled study." *Allergy Asthma Proc.* 1998 Jan–Feb;19(1):3–9.

527 Agnihotri S, Kant S, Kumar S, et al. "Impact of yoga on biochemical profile of asthmatics: a randomized controlled study." *Int J Yoga.* 2014 Jan;7(1):17–21.

528 Thirthalli J, Naveen GH, Rao MG, et al. "Cortisol and antidepressant effects of yoga." *Indian J Psychiatry.* 2013 Jul;55(Suppl 3):S403–08.

529 Blackwell T, Yaffe K, Laffan A, et al. "Associations of objectively and subjectively measured sleep quality with subsequent cognitive decline in older community-dwelling men: the MrOS Sleep Study." *SLEEP.* 2014 Apr 1;37(4):655–63.

530 Halpern J, Cohen M, Kennedy G, et al. "Yoga for improving sleep quality and quality of life for older adults." *Altern Ther Health Med.* 2014 May–Jun;20(3):37–46.

531 Newby J, Howard V. "Environmental influences in cancer aetiology." *J Nutritional & Environ Med.* 2006;15(2–3):56–114.

532 Calle E, Rodriquez C, Walker-Thurmond K, et al. "Overweight, obesity, and mortality from cancer in prospectively studied cohort of U. S. adults." *N Engl J Med.* 2003;348:1625–38.

533 Genius SJ, Beesoon S, Lob RA, et al. "Human elimination of phthalate compounds: blood urine and sweat (BUS) study." *Scientific World Journal.* 2012;2012:615068.

534 Genius SJ, Birkholz D, Rodushkin I, et al. "Blood, urine, and sweat (BUS) study: monitoring and elimination of bioaccumulated toxic elements." *Arch Enviorn Contam Toxicol.* 2011 Aug;61(2):344–57.

535 Singer S, Grismaijer S. *Dressed to kill.* Connecticut: ISCD Press, 2005.

536 Tanridag T, Aktan S, Gunal D. "Toxic effects of aluminum on neuromuscular system." *J Neurol Sci.* 1997;150.

537 Perl DP. "Relationship of aluminum to Alzheimer's disease." *Environ Health Perspect.* 1985 Nov;63:149–53.

538 Bhattacharjee S, Zhao Y, Lukiw W, et al. "Aluminum and its potential contribution to Alzheimer's disease (AD)." *Front Aging Neurosci.* 2014;6:62.

539 Environmental Protection Agency. "Arsenic compounds. Hazard summary—created in April 1992, Revised in December 2012." Accessed April 9, 2009, from http://www.epa.gov/ttn/atw/hlthef/arsenic.html.

540 Occupational Safety Hazard Association. "Cadmium." Accessed August 14, 2014, from https://www.osha.gov/pls/oshaweb/owadisp.show_document?p_table=standards&p_id=10035.

541 Diamanti-Kandarakis E, Bourguignon JP, Giudice LC, et al. "Endocrine-disrupting chemicals: an Endocrine Society scientific statement." *Endocr Rev.* 2009 Jun;30(4):293–342.

542 Holman A, Silver R, Poulin M, et al. "Terrorism, acute stress, and cardiovascular health. A 3-year national study following the September 11th attacks." *Arch Gen Psychiatry.* 2008;65(1):73–80.

543 American Psychological Association. "Stress in the workplace. Meeting the challenge." Accessed August 7, 2014, from http://www.healthadvocate.com/downloads/webinars/stress-workplace.pdf.

544 Pew Research Center. "5 facts about prayer." Accessed August 22, 2014, from http://www.pewresearch.org/fact-tank/2014/05/01/5-facts-about-prayer/.

545 Carvalho CC, Chaves Ede C, Iunes DH, et al. "Effectiveness of prayer for reducing anxiety in cancer patients." *Rev Esc Enferm USP.* 2014 Aug;48(4):684–90.

546 Boelens PA, Reeves RR, Reploge WH, et al. "A randomized trial of the effect of prayer on depression and anxiety." *Int J Psychiatry Med.* 2009;39(4):377–92.

547 Boelens PA, Reeves RR, Relogle WH, et al. "The effect of prayer on depression and anxiety: maintenance of positive influence one year after prayer intervention." *Int J Phsychiatry Med.* 212;43(1):85–98.

548 Turakitwanakan W, Mekseepralad C, Busarakumtragul P. "Effects of mindfulness meditation on serum cortisol of medical students." *J Med Assoc Thai.* 2013 Jan;96 Suppl 1:S90–95.

549 Fan Y, Tang YY, Posner MI. "Cortsiol level modulated by integrative meditation in a dose-dependent fashion." *Stress Health.* 2014 Feb;30(1):65–70.

550 Fan Y, Tang YY, Tang R, et al. "Short term integrative meditation improves resting alpha activity and stroop performance." *Appl Phsychophysiol Biofeedback.* 2014 Sep 25. [Epub ahead of print]

551 Ding X, Tangh YY, Tang R, et al. "Improving creativity performance by short-term meditation." *Behav Brain Funct.* 2014 Mar 19;10:9.

552 Lengacher C, Bennett MP, Gonzalez L, et al. "Immune responses to guided imagery during breast cancer treatment." *Biol Res Nurs.* 2008 Jan;9(3):205–14.

553 Pawlow LA, Jones GE. "The impact of abbreviated progressive muscle relaxation on salivary cortisol." *Biol Psychol.* 2002;60(1):1–16.

554 Schroder A, Heider J, Zaby A, et al. "Cognitive behavioral therapy verus progressive muscle relaxation training for multiple somatoform symptoms:

results of a randomized controlled tiral." *Cog Ther Res.* 2013 Apr;37(2):296–306.

555 Kubzansky P, Sparrow D, Vokonas P, et al. "Is the glass half empty or half full? A prospective study of optimism and coronary heart disease in the normative aging study." *Psychosom Med.* 2001 Nov–Dec;63(6):910–16.

556 Boehm JK, Peterson C, Kubzansky L, et al. "A prospective study of positive psychological well-being and coronary heart disease." *Health Psychol.* 2011 May;30(3):259–67.

557 Seligman M. *Learned optimism.* Essex: Vintage Publishing, 2006.

558 Cousins LA, Cohen LL, Venable C. "Risk and resilience in pediatric chronic pain: exploring the protective role of optimism." *J Pediatr Psychol.* 2014 Oct 28. [Epub ahead of print]

559 Jobin J, Wrosch C, Scheier MF. "Associations between dispositional optimism and diurnal cortisol in a community sample: when stress is perceived as higher than normal." *Health Psychol.* 2014 Apr;33(4):382–91.

560 Lai JC, Evans PD, Ng SH, et al. "Optimism, positive affectivity, and salivary cortisol." 2005 Nov;10(Pt 4):467–84.

561 Nichols AR, Polman R, Levy AR, et al. "Mental toughness, optimism, pessimism, and coping among athletes." *Personality Ind Diff.* 2008 Apr;44(5):1182–92.

562 Dunbar RI, Baron R, Frangou A, et al. "Social laughter is correlated with an elevated pain threshold." *Proc Biol Sci.* 2012 Mar 22;279(1731):1161–67.

563 Berk L, Tan S. "[beta]-endorphin and HGH increase are associated with both the anticipation and experience of mirthful laughter." *FASEB J.* 2006 Mar;20:A382.

564 Miller M, Fry WF. "The effect of mirthful laughter on the human cardiovascular system." *Med Hypothesis.* 209 Nov;73(5):636–39.

565 Bennett MP, Lengacher C. "Humor and laughter may influence health IV. Humor and immune function." *Evid Based Complement Altern Med.* 29 Jun;6(2):159–64.

566 Bennett MP, Zeller JM, Rosenberg L, et al. "The effect of mirthful laughter on stress and natural killer cell activity." *Altern Ther Health Med.* 2003 Mar–Apr;9(2):38–45.

567 Hayashi K, Hayashi T, Iwanaga S, et al. "Laughter lowered the increase in postprandial blood glucose." *Diabetes Care.* 2003 May;20(5):1651–52.

568 Berk L, Tan S. "Mirthful laughter, as adjunct therapy in diabetic care, increases HDL cholesterol and attenuates inflammatory cytokines and C-RP and possible CVD risk." *FASEB J.* 2009 Apr 23; Meeting abstract supplemental (990):1.

569 Holt-Lunstad J, Smith T, Layton JB. "Social relationships and mortality risk: a meta-analytic review." *PLoS Med.* 2010 Jul 27;7(7):e1000316.

570 Froh J, fives C, Fuller JR, et al. "Interpersonal relationships and irrationality as predictors of life satisfaction." *J Pos Psych.* 2007;2(1):29–39.

571 Morhenn V, Beavin LE, Zak PJ. "Massage increases oxytocin and reduces adrenocorticotropin in humans." *Altern Ther Health Med.* 2010 Nov–Dec;18(6):11–18.

572 Kripke DF, Garfinkel L, Wingard DL, et al. "Mortality associated with sleep duration and insomnia." *Arch Gen Psychiatry.* 2002 Feb;59(2):131–36.

573 Warmsley EJ, Tucker M, Payne JD, et al. "Dreaming of a learning task is associated with enhanced sleep-dependent memory consolidation." *Curr Biol.* 2010 May;20(9):850–55.

574 National Institute of Mental Health. "Major depression among adults." Accessed August 22, 2014, from http://www.nimh.nih.gov/statistics/1mdd_adult.shtml.

575 National Institute of Mental Health. "Any anxiety disorder among adults." Accessed August 22, 2014, from http://www.nimh.nih.gov/statistics/1anyanx_adult.shtml.

576 National Institute of Mental Health. "Antidepressants: a complicated picture." Accessed August 22, 2014, from http://www.nimh.nih.gov/about/director/2011/antidepressants-a-complicated-picture.shtml.

577 Butterweck V. "Mechanism of action of St John's Wort in depression: what is known?" *CNS Drugs.* 2003;17(8):539–62.

578 Gaster B, Holoroyd J. "St John's wort for depression: a systematic review." *Arch Int Med.* 2000 Jan;160(2):152–56.

579 Woelk H. "Comparison of St John's wort and imipramine for treating depression: randomised controlled trial." *BMJ.* 2000;321:536.

580 Birdsall TC. "5-Hydroxytryptophan:a clinically-effective serotonin precursor." *Alt Med Rev.* 1998;2(4):271–80.

581 Jangid P, Malik P, Singh P, et al. "Comparative study of efficacy of l-5-hydroxytryptophan and fluoxetine in patients presenting with first depressive episode." *Asian J Psychaitr.* 2013 Feb;6(1):29–34.

582 Byerley WF, Judd LL, Reimherr FW, et al. "5-Hydroxytryptophan: a review of its antidepressant efficacy and adverse effects." *J Clin Psychopharmacol.* 1987 Jun;7(3):127–37.

583 Carney MW, Edeh J, Bottiglieri T, et al. "Affective illness and S-adenosyl methionine: a preliminary report." *Clin Neuropharmacol.* 1986;9(4):379–85.

584 Papakostas G, Mischoulon D, Shyu I, et al. "S-adenosyl methionine (SAMe) augmentation of serotonin reuptake inhibitors for antidepressant

nonresponders with major depressive disorder: a double-blind, randomized clinical trial." *Am J Psychiatry.* 2010;167:942–48.

585 Mischoulon D, Fava M. "Role of S-adenosyl-L-methionine in the treatment of depression: a review of the evidence." *Am J Clin Nutr.* 2002 Nov;76(5):1158S–61S.

586 Endocrine Society. "Treating vitamin d deficiency may improve depression." Accessed August 22, 2014, from http://www.newswise.com/articles/treating-vitamin-d-deficiency-may-improve-depression.

587 Penckofer S, Kouba J, Byrn M, et al. "Vitamin D and depression: where is all the sunshine?" *Issues Mental Health Nurs.* 2010 Jun;31(6):385–93.

588 Anglin RE, Samaan Z, Walter SD, et al. "Vitamin D deficiency and depression in adults: systematic review and meta-analysis." *Bt J Psychiatry.* 2013 Feb;202:100–07.

589 Ju SY, Lee YJ, Jeong SN. "Serum 25-hydroxyvitamin D levels and the risk of depression: a systematic review and meta-analysis." *J Nutr Health Aging.* 2013;17(5):447–55.

590 Li G, Mbuagbaw L, Samaan Z, et al. "Efficacy of vitamin D supplementation in depression in adults: a systematic review protocol." *Syst Rev.* 2013 Aug 8;2:64.

591 Li G, Mbuagbaw L, Samaan Z, et al. "Efficacy of vitamin D supplementation in depression in adults: a systematic review." *J Clin Endocrinol Metab.* 2014 Mar;99(3):757–67.

592 Jorde R, Snerve M, figenschau Y, et al. "Effects of vitamin D supplementation on symptoms of depression in overweight and obese subjects: randomizd double blind trial." *J Int Med.* 2008 Dec;264(6):599–609.

593 Sargolzaee MR, Faayyazi Bordbar MR, Shakiba M, et al. "The comparison of the efficacy of citrus fragrance and fluoxetine in the treatment of major depressive disorder." *J of Gonabad University of Med Sci and Health Sci.* 2004;10(3):43–48.

594 Sarris J, Stough C, Bousman CA, et al. "Kava in the treatment of generalized anxiety disorder: a double-blind, randomized, placebo-controlled study." *J Clin Psychopharmacol.* 2013 Oct;33(5):643–48.

595 Teschke R, Sarris J, Glass X, et al. "Kava, the anxiolytic herb: back to basics to prevent liver injury?" *Br J Clin Pharmacol.* 2011 Mar;71(3):445–48.

596 Sarris J, Stough C, Teschke R, et al. "Kava for the treatment of generalized anxiety disorder RCT: analysis of adverse reactions, liver function, addiction, and sexual effects." *Phytother Res.* 2013 Nov;27(11):1723–28.

597 Pittler MH, Ernst E. "Efficacy of kava extract for treating anxiety: a systematic review and meta-analysis." *J Clin Psychopharmacol.* 2000;20:84–89.

598 Akhondzadeh S, Naghavi HR, Vazirian M, et al. "Passionflower in the treatment of generalized anxiety: a pilot double-blind randomized controlled trial with oxazepam." *J Clin Pharm Ther.* 2001 Oct;26(5):363–67.

599 Kaviani N, Tavakoli M, et al. "The efficacy of Passiflora incarnata in reducing anxiety in patients undergoing periodontal treatment." *J Dent (Shiraz).* 2013 Jun;14(2):68–72.

600 Aslanargum P, Cuvas O, Dikmen B, et al. "Passiflora incarnata Linneaus as an anxiolytic before spinal anesthesia." *J Anesth.* 2012 Feb;26(1):39–44.

601 Ngan A, Conduit R. "A double-blind, placebo-controlled investigation of the effects of passiflora incarnate (passionflower) herbal tea on subjective sleep quality." *Phytother Res.* 2011 Aug;25(8):1153–59.

602 Muller SF, Klement S. "A combination of valerian and lemon balm is effective in the treatment of restlessness and dyssomnia in children." *Phytomedicine.* 2006 Jun;13(6):383–87.

603 Kennedy DD, Little W, Scholey AB. "Attenuation of laboratory-induced stress in humans after acute administration of Melissa officinalis (lemon balm)." *Psychosom Med.* 2004 Jul–Aug;66(4):607–13.

604 Cases J, Ibarra A, Feuillere N, et al. "Pilot trial of Melissa officinalis L. leaf extract in the treatment of volunteers suffering from mild-to-moderate anxiety disorders and sleep disturbances." *Med J Nutrition Metab.* 2011 Dec;4(3):211–18.

605 Chung MJ, Cho SY, Bhuiyan MJ, et al. "Anti-diabetic effects of lemon balm (Melissa officinalis) essential oil on glucose- and lipid-regulating enzymes in type 2 diabetic mice." *Br J Nutr.* 2010 Jul;104(2):180–88.

606 Kobayashi K, Nagato Y, Aoi N, et al. "Effects of L-theanine on the release of ALPHA-brain waves in human volunteers." *J Agric Chem Soc (Japan).* 1998;72(2):153–57.

607 Unno K, Tanida N, Ishii N, et al. "Anti-stress effect of theanine on students during pharmacy practice: positive correlation among salivary α-amylase activity, trait anxiety and subjective stress." *Pharmacol Biochem Behav.* 2013 Oct;111:128–35.

608 van Veen JF, van Vilet LM, DeRijk RH, et al. "Elevated alpha-amylase but not cortisol in generalized social anxiety disorder." *Psychoneuroendocrinology.* 2008 Nov;33(10):1313–21.

609 Ritsner MS, Miodownik C, Ratner Y, et al. "L-theanine relieves positive, activation, and anxiety symptoms with schizophrenia and schizoaffective disorder: an 8-week, randomized, double-blind, placebo-controlled, 2-center study." *J Clin Psychiatry.* 2011 Jan;72(1):34–42.

610 Kasper S, Gastpar M, Muller WE, et al. "Lavender oil preparation Silexan is effective in generalized anxiety disorder—a randomized, double-blind

comparison to placebo and paroxetine." *Int J Neuropsychopharmacol.* 2014 Jun 17(6):859–69.

611 Kasper S, Gastpar M, Muller WE, et al. "Silexan, an orally administered Lavandula oil preparation, is effective in the treatment of 'subsyndromal' anxiety disorder: a randomized, double-blind, placebo controlled trial." *Int Clin Psychopharmacol.* 2010 Sep;25(5):277–87.

612 Woelk H, Schlafke S. "A multi-center, double-blind, randomised study of the lavender oil preparation silexan in comparison to lorazepam for generalized anxiety disorder." *Phytomedicine.* 2010 Feb;17(2):94–99.

613 Field T, field T, Cullen C, et al. "Lavender bath oil reduces stress and crying and enhances sleep in very young infants." *Early Hum Dev.* 2008 Jun;84(6):399–4401.

614 Cho MY, Min ES, Hur MH, et al. "Effects of aromatherapy on the anxiety, vital signs, and sleep quality of percutaneous coronary intervention patients in intensive care units." *Evid Based Compliment Alternat Med.* 2013;2013:381381.

615 Amsterdam JD, Li Y, Soeller I, et al. "A randomized, double-blind, placebo-controlled trial of oral Matricaria recutita (chamomile) extract therapy for generalized anxiety disorder. *J Clin Psychopharmacol.* 2009 Aug;29(4):378–82.

616 Amsterdam JD, Shults J, Soeller I, et al. "Chamomile (Matricaria recutita) may provide antidepressant activity in anxious, depressed humans: an exploratory study." *Altern Ther Health Med.* 2012 Sep–Oct;18(5):44–49.

617 Sarris J, Panossian A, Schweitzer I, et al. "Herbal medicine for depression, anxiety and insomnia: a review of psychopharmacology and clinical evidence." *Eur Neuropsychopharmacol.* 2011 Dec;21(12):841–60.

618 Centers for Disease Control. "Heart disease facts and statistics." Accessed August 9, 2014, at http://www.cdc.gov/heartdisease/facts.htm.

619 Grundy S, Benjamin I, Burke G, et al. "Diabetes and cardiovascular disease. A statement for healthcare professionals from the American Heart Association." *Circulation.* 1999;100:1134–46.

620 Lazzarino AI, Hamer M, Gaze D, et al. "The association between cortisol response to mental stress and high-sensitivity cardiac troponin T plasma concentration in healthy adults." *J Am Coll Cardiol.* 2013 Oct 29;62(18):1694–1701.

621 Djousse L, Gaziano JM. "Alcohol consumption and heart failure: a systematic review." *Curr Atheroscler Rep.* 2008 Apr;10(2):117–20.

622 Harris WA, Kris-Etherton PM, Harris KA. "Intakes of long-chain omega-3 fatty acid associated with reduced risk for death from coronary heart disease in healthy adults." *Curr Atheroscler Rep.* 2008 Dec;10(6):503–09.

623 Kuimov AD, Murzina TA. Coenzyme "q10 in complex therapy of patients with ischemic heart disease." *Kardiologia.* 2013;53(8):40–3.

624 Fotino AD, Thompson-Paul AM, Bazzano LA. "Effect of coenzyme Q10 supplementation on heart failure: a meta-analysis." *Am J Clin Nutr.* 2013 Feb;97(2):268–75.

625 Lee BJ, Yen CH, Hsu HC, Lin JY, Hsia S, Lin PT. "A significant correlation between plasma levels of coenzyme Q10 and vitamin B-6 and a reduced risk of coronary artery disease." *Nutr Res.* 2012 Oct;32(10):751–6.

626 Mikhin VP, Kharchenko AV, Rosliakova EA, Cherniatina MA. "Application of coenzyme Q10 in combination therapy of arterial hypertension." *Kardiologia.* 2011;51(6):26–31.

627 McCarty CA, Berg RL, Rottscheit CM, Dart RA. "The use of dietary supplements and their association with blood pressure in a large Midwestern cohort." *BMC Complement Altern Med.* 2013 Nov 28;13:339.

628 Ivanov AV, Gorodetskaya EA, Kalenikova EI, et al. "Single intravenous injection of coenzyme Q10 protects the myocardium after irreversible ischemia." *Bull Exp Biol Med.* 2013 Oct;155(6):771–74.

629 Singh RB, Niaz MA, Rastogi V, et al. "Coenzyme Q in cardiovascular disease." *J Assoc Physicians India.* 1998 Mar;46(3):299–306.

630 Kuchemenko QB. "Physiological aspects of ubiquinone supplementation in cardiovascular disease." *fiziol Zh.* 2006;52(5):80–91.

631 Soongswang J, Sangtawesin C, Durongpisitkul K, et al. "The effect of coenzyme Q10 on idiopathic chronic dilated cardiomyopathy in children." *Pediatr Cardiol.* 2005;26:361–66.

632 Lee BJ, Lin YC, Huang YC, et al. "The relationship between coenzyme Q10, oxidative stress, and antioxidant activities and coronary artery disease." *Scientific World Journal.* 2012;212:792756.

633 Corted EP, Gupta M, Chou C, et al. "Adriamycin cardiotoxicity: early detection by systolic timer interval and possible prevention by coenzyme Q10." *Cancer Reports.* 1978;623(6):887–891.

634 Failla ML, Chitchumroonchokchai C, Aoki F. "Increased bioavailability of ubiquinol compared to ubiquinone is due to more efficient micellarization during digestion and greater GSH-dependent uptake and basolateral secretion by Caco-2 cells." *J Agric Food Chem.* 2014 Jul 23;62(29):7174–82.

635 Langsjoen P, Langsjoen A. "Supplemental ubiquinol in patients with advanced congestive heart failure." *BioFactors.* 2008;32(1–4):119–28.

636 Singh RB. "Effect of dietary magnesium supplementation in the prevention of coronary heart disease and sudden cardiac death." *Magnes Trace Elem.* 1990;9(3):143–51.

637 Mathers TW, Beckstrand RL. "Oral magnesium supplementation in adults with coronary heart disease risk." *J Am Acad Nurse Pract.* 2009 Dec;21(12):651–57.

638 Jing Ma, Folsom A, Melnick S, et al. "Associations of serum and dietary magnesium with cardiovascular disease, hypertension, diabetes, insulin, and carotid arterial wall thickness. The ARIC study." *J Clin Epid.* 1995 July;48(7):927–40.

639 Sueta CA, Clarke SW, Dunlap SH, et al. "Effect of acute magnesium administration on the frequency of ventricular arrhythmia in patients with heart failure." *Circulation.* 1994;89:660–66.

640 Martynov AI, Akatova EV. "Fifteen years experience of the use of magnesium preparations in patients with mitral valve prolapse." *Kardiologiia.* 2011;51(6):60–65.

641 Bobkowski W, Nowak A, Durlach J. "The importance of magnesium status in the pathophysiological of mitral valve prolapse." *Magnes Res.* 2005 Mar;18(1):35–52.

642 McKevoy GK. *AHFS drug information.* Bethesda, MD: American Society of Health-System Pharmacists. 1998.

643 Akhtar MS, Ramzan A, Ali A, Ahmad M. "Effect of Amla fruit (Embilica officianalis Gaertn.) on glucose and lipid profile of normal and type 2 diabetic patients." *Int J Food Sci Nutr.* 2011 Sep;62(6):609–16.

644 Antony B, Benny M, Kaimal TN. "A pilot clinical study to evaluate the effect of Emilica officinalis extract (Amlamax) on markers of systemic inflammation and dyslipidemia." *Indian J Clin Biochem.* 2008 Oct;23(4):378–81.

645 Antony B, Merina B, Sheeba V. "Amlamax in the management of dyslipidemia in humans." *Indian J Pharm Sci.* 2008 Jul–Aug;70(4):504–7.

646 Jacob A, Pandey M, Kapoor S, Saroja R. "Effect of the Indian gooseberry (amla) on serum cholesterol levels in men aged 35–55 years." *Eur J Clin Nutr.* 1988 Nov;42(11):939–44.

647 Gopa B, Bhatt J, Hemavathis KG, "A comparative clinical study of hypolipidemic efficacy of Amla (Embilica officinalis) and 3-hydroxy-3-methylglutaryl-coenzyme-A reductase inhibitor simvastatin." *Indian J Pharmcaol.* 2012 Mar;44(2):238–42.

648 Mathur R, Sharma A, Dixit VP, Varma M. "Hypolipidaemic effect of fruit juice of Embilica officinalis in cholesterol-fed rabbits." *J Ethnopharmacol.* 1996 Feb;50(2):61–8.

649 Usharani P, Fatima N, Muralidhar N. "Effects of Phyllanthus embilica extract on endothelial dysfunction and biomarkers of oxidative stress in

patients with type 2 diabetes mellitus: a randomized, double-blind, controlled study." *Diabetes Metab Syndr Obes.* 2013 Jul 26;6:275–84.

650 Wongpradabchai S, Chularojmontri L, Phornchirasilp S, Wattanapitayakul SK. "Protective effect of Phyllanthus embilica fruit extract against hydrogen peroxide-induced endothelial cell death." *J Med Assoc Thai.* 2013 Jan;96 Suppl 1:S40–8.

651 Chularojmontri L, Suwatronnakorn M, Wattanapitayakul SK. "Phyllanthus embilica L. enhances human umbilical vein endothelial would healing and sprouting." *Evid Based Compliment Altern Med.* 2013;2013:720728.

652 Fatima N, Pingali U, Muralidhar N. "Study of pharmacodynamics interaction of Phyllanthus embilica extract with clopidogrel and ecosprin in patients with type II diabetes mellitus." *Phytomedicine.* 2013 Nov 28; Pii:S0944-7113(13)00433-9.

653 Ihantola-Vormisto A, Summanen J, Kankaanranta H, Vuorela H, Asmawi ZM, Moilanen E. "Anti-inflammatory activity of extracts from leaves of Phyllanthus embilica." *Planta Med.* 1997 Dec;63(6):518–24.

654 Movahed A, Yu L, Thandapilly SJ, Louis XL, Netticadan T. "Resveratrol protects adult cardiomyocytes against oxidative stress mediated cell injury." *Arch Biochem Biophys.* 2012 Nov 15;527(2):74–80.

655 Thuc LC, Teshima Y, Takahashi N, et al. "Inhibition of Na+ -H+ exchange as mechanism of rapid cardioprotection by resveratrol." *Br J Pharmacol.* 2012 Jul;166(6):1745–55.

656 Tsai YF, Liu FC, Lau YT, Yu HP. "Role of Akt-dependent pathway in resveratrol-mediated cardioprotection after trauma-hemorrhage." *J Surg Res.* 2012 Jul;176(1):171–7.

657 Wu JM, Hsieh TC. "Resveratrol: a cardioprotective substance." *Ann N Y Acad Sci.* 2011 Jan;1215:16–21.

658 Magyar K, Halmosi R, Ralfi A, et al. "Cardioprotection by resveratrol: A human clinical trial in patients with stable coronary artery disease." *Clin Hemorheol Micorcirc.* 2012;50(3):179–87.

659 Wu JM, Hsieh TC, Yang CJ, Olson SC. "Resveratrol and its metabolites modulate cytokine-mediated induction of eotaxin-1 in human pulmonary artery endothelial cells." *Ann N Y Acad Sci.* 2013 Jul;1290:30–6.

660 Da Luz PL, Tanaka L, Brum PC, et al. "Red wine and equivalent oral pharmacological doses of resveratrol delay vascular aging but do not extend life span of rats." *Atherosclerosis.* 2012 Sep;224(1):136–42.

661 Das DK, Mukherjee S, Ray D. "Resveratrol and red wine, healthy heart and longevity." *Heart Fail Rev.* 2012 Sep;15(5):467–77.

662 Voloshyna I, Hussaini SM, Reiss AB. "Resveratrol in cholesterol metabolism and atherosclerosis." *J Med Food.* 2012 Sep;15(9):763–73.

663 Tome-Carneiro J, Gonzalez M, Larrosa M, et al. "Consumption of grape extract supplement containing resveratrol decreases oxidized LDL and ApoB in patients undergoing primary prevention of cardiovascular disease: a triple-blind, 6 month follow-up, placebo-controlled, randomized study." *Mol Nutr Food Res.* 2012 May;56(5):810–21.

664 Fan E, Zhang L, Jiang S, Bai Y. "Beneficial effects of resveratrol on atherosclerosis." *J Med Food.*2008 Dec;11(4):610–4.

665 Toliopoulos IK, Simos YV, Oikonomidis S, Karkabounas SC. "Resveratrol diminishes platelet aggregation and increases susceptibility of K562 tumor cells to natural killer cells." *Indian J Biochem Biophys.* 2013 Feb;50(1):14–8.

666 Lango R, Smolenski RT, Narkiewicz M, et al. "Influence of L-carnitine and its derivatives on myocardial metabolism and function in ischemic heart disease and during cardiopulmonary bypass." *Cardiovasc Res.* 2001 Jul;51(1):21–29.

667 Ferrari R, Merli E, Cicchitelli G, et al. "Therapeutic effects of L-carnitine and propionyl-L-carnitine on cardiovascular diseases: a review." *Ann N Y Acad Sci.* 2004 Nov;1033:79–91.

668 Dinicolantonio JJ, Niazi AK, McCarty MF, et al. "L-carnitine for the treatment of acute myocardial infarction." *Rev Cardiovasc Med.* 2014;15(1): 52–62.

669 Vescovo G, Ravara B, Gobbo V, et al. "L-carnitine: a potential treatment for blocking apoptosis and preventing skeletal muscle myopathy in heart failure." *Am J Physiol.* 2002 Sep;283(3):C802–10.

670 DiNicolantonio JJ, Lavie CJ, Fares H, et al. "L-carnitine in the secondary prevention of cardiovascular disease: systematic review and meta-analysis." *Mayo Clin Proc.* 2013 Jun;88(6):544–51.

671 Bloomer RJ, Smith WA, fisher-Wellman KH. "Glycine propionyl-L-carnitine increases plasma nitrate/nitrite in resistance trained men." *J Int Sports Nutr.* 2007 Dec 3;4:22.

672 Mahmoodi M, Islami MR, Asadi Karam GR, et al. "Study on the effects of raw garlic consumption on the level of lipids and other blood biochemical factors in hyperlipidemic individuals." *Pak J Pharm Sci.* 2006 Oct;19(4):295–98.

673 Kojuri J, Vosoughi AR, Akrami M. "Effects of anethum graveolens and garlic on lipid profile in hyperlipidemic patients." *Lipids Health Dis.* 2007 Mar 1;6:5.

674 Ried K, Frank O, Stocks N, et al. "Effect of garlic on blood pressure: a systematic review and meta-analysis. *BMC Cardiovasc Disord.* 2008 Jun 16;8:13.

675 Popping S, Rose H, Ionescu I, fishcer Y, Kammermeier H. "Effect of hawthorn extract on contraction and energy turnover of isolated rat cardiomyocytes." *Arzneimittelforschung.* 1995 Nov;45(11):1157–61.

676 Von Holubarsch CJ, Niestroj M, Wassmer A, Gaus W, Meinertz T. "Hawthorn extract WS 1442 in the treatment of patients with heart failure and LVEF of 25-35%." *MMW Fortschr Med.* 2012 Jul 1;152 Suppl 2:56–61.

677 Koch E, Malek FA. "Standardized extracts from hawthorn leaves and flowers in the treatment of cardiovascular disorders—preclinical and clinical studies." *Planta Med.* 2011 Jul;77(11):1123–8.

678 Schmidt U, et al. "Wirksamkeit des Extrak-tes LI 132 (600 mg/Tag) bei achitowchiger Therapie." *Munch Med Wschr.* 1994;136:S13–19.

679 Weng WL, Zhang WQ, Liu FZ, et al. "Therapeutic effect of Crataegus pinnatifida on 46 cases of angina pectoris—a double blind study." *J Trad Chin Med.* 1984 Dec;4(4):293–4.

680 Dalli E, Colomer E, Tormos MC, et al. "Crataegus laevigata decreases neutrophil elastase and has hypolipidemic effect: a randomized, double-blind, placebo-controlled trial." *Phytomedicine.* 2011 Jun 15;18(8-9):769–75.

681 Chularojmontri L, Suwatronnakorn M, Wattanapitayakul SK. "Phyllanthus embilica L. enhances human umbilical vein endothelial would healing and sprouting." *Evid Based Compliment Altern Med.* 2013;2013:720728.

682 Zhang Y, Zhang L, Geng Y, et al. "Hawthorn fruit attenuates atherosclerosis by improving the hyperlipidemic and antioxidant activities in apolipoprotective e-deficient mice." *J Atheroscler Thromb.* 2012;21(2):119–28.

683 Hong Xu, Hou-En Xu, Ryan D. "A study of the comparative effects of hawthorn fruit compound and silvastatin on lowering blood lipid levels." *Am J Clin Med.* 2009;37(5):903–08.

684 Zick S, Gillespie B, Aaronson K. "The effect of Crataegus oxycantha special extract WSS 1442 on clinical progression in patients with mild to moderate symptoms of heart failure." *Eur J Heart Fail.* 28 Jun;10(6):587–93.

685 Hobbs C. "Hawthorn: for the heart." Accessed November 2, 2014, from http://www.christopherhobbs.com/library/articles-on-herbs-and-health/hawthorn-for-the-heart/.

686 American Cancer Society. "Lifetime risk of developing or dying from cancer." Accessed August 11, 2014, from http://www.cancer.org/cancer/cancerbasics/lifetime-probability-of-developing-or-dying-from-cancer.

687 American Cancer Society. "Cancer facts & figures 2014." Accessed August 11, 2014, from http://www.cancer.org/acs/groups/content/@research/documents/webcontent/acspc-042151.Pdf.

688 US Centers for Disease Control. "Cancer prevention and control." Accessed August 11, 2014, from http://www.cdc.gov/cancer/dcpc/resources/features/WorldCancerDay/.

689 US Centers for Disease Control and Prevention. "Cancer among men." Accessed August 11, 2014, from http://www.cdc.gov/cancer/dcpc/data/men.htm.

690 US Centers for Disease Control. "Cancer among women." Accessed August 11, 2014, http://www.cdc.gov/cancer/dcpc/data/women.htm.

691 US Centers for Disease Control and Prevention. "Cancer among children." Accessed August 11, 2014, at http://www.cdc.gov/cancer/dcpc/data/children.htm.

692 Stanford Cancer Genetics Program. "Care and treatment of hereditary cancers." Accessed August 11, 2014, from http://stanfordhealthcare.org/medical-clinics/cancer-genetics-program/understanding-genetics.html.

693 Doll R, Peto R. "The causes of cancer: quantitative estimates of avoidable risks of cancer in the United States today." *J Natl Cancer Inst.* 1981 Jun;66(6):1191–1308.

694 Baade P, Xingqiong M, Sincalir C, et al. "Estimating the future burden of cancers preventable by better diet and physical activity in Australia." *Med J Aust.* 2012;196(5):337–40.

695 Giovannucci E. "Modifiable risk factors for colon cancer." *Gastroenterol Clin North Am.* 2002 Dec;31(4):925–43.

696 National Cancer Institute, US National Institutes of Health. "Cancer prevention overview." Accessed August 11, 2014, from http://www.cancer.gov/cancertopics/pdq/prevention/overview/patient/page3.

697 American Cancer Society. "Tobacco-related cancers fact sheet." Accessed August 11, 2014, from http://www.cancer.org/cancer/cancercauses/tobaccocancer/tobacco-related-cancer-fact-sheet.

698 Fazel R, Krumholz HM, Wang Y, et al. "Exposure to low-dose ionizing radiation from medical imaging procedures." *N Engl J Med.* 2009;361(9): 849–57.

699 Berrington de González A, Mahesh M, Kim KP, et al. "Projected cancer risks from computed tomographic scans performed in the United States in 2007." *Arch Intern Med.* 2009 Dec 14;169(22):2071–77.

700 Smith-Bindman R, Lipson J, Marcus R, et al. "Radiation dose associated with common computed tomography examinations and the

associated lifetime attributable risk of cancer." *Arch Intern Med.* 2009 Dec 14;169(22):2078–86.

701 Miller A, Wall C, Baines C, et al. "Twenty five year follow-up for breast cancer incidence and mortality of the Canadian National Breast Screening Study: randomised screening trial." *BMJ.* 2014 Feb 11;384:g366.

702 Weedon-Fekaer H, Romundstat PR, Vatten LJ. "Modern mammography screening and breast cancer mortality: population study." *BMJ.* 2014 Jun 17;348:g3701.

703 Brkljacic B, Miletric D, Sardanelli. "Thermography is not a feasible method for breast cancer screening." *Coll Antropol.* 2013 Jun;37(2):589–93.

704 Suganthi SS, Ramakrishnan S. "Analysis of breast thermograms using Gabor wavelet anistopy index." *J Med Syst.* 2014 Sep;38(9):101.

705 Lin W, Xu Y, Huan CC, et al. "Toxicity of nano- and micro-sized ZnO particles in human lung epithelial cells." *J Nano Res.* 2009 Jan;11(1):25–39.

706 Environmental Working Group. "What not to take on vacation." Accessed August 11, 2014, from http://www.ewg.org/2014sunscreen/what-not-to-bring-on-vacation/.

707 Heinrich U, Gartner C, Weibusch M, et al. "Supplementation with beta-carotene or similar amount of mixed carotenoids protects humans from UV-induced erythema." *J Nutr.* 2003 Jan;133(1):98–101.

708 Lyons NM, O'Brien NM. "Modulatory effects of an algal extract containing astaxanthin on UVA-irradiated cells in culture." *J Dermatol Sci.* 2002 Oct;30(1):73–84.

709 Beral V, Banks E, Reeves G, et al. "Breast cancer and hormone-replacement therapy: the Million Women Study." *The Lancet.* 2003 Oct 18;362(9392):1330–31.

710 Grady D, Gebretsadik T, Kerlikowske K, et al. "Hormone replacement therapy and endometrial cancer risk: a meta-analysis. *Obstet Gynecol.* 1995 Feb;85(2):304–13.

711 Nelson HD, Humphrey LL, Nygren P, et al. "Postmenopausal hormone replacement therapy: scientific review." *JAMA.* 2002 Aug 21;288(7):872–81.

712 Li C, Malone K, Porter P, et al. "Relationship between long durations and different regimens of hormone replacement therapy and risk of breast cancer." *JAMA.* 2003;289(24):3254–63.

713 Daley AJ, Stokes-Lampard HJ, MacArthur C. "Exercise to reduce vasomotor and other menopausal symptoms: a review." *Maturitas.* 2009 Jul 20;63(3):176–80.

714 Slaven L, Lee C. "Mood and symptom reporting among middle-aged women: the relationship between menopausal status, hormone

replacement therapy, and exercise participation." *Health Psychology.* 1997 May;16(3):203–08.

715 Stojanovska L, Apostolopoulos V, Polman R, et al. "To exercise, or, not to exercise, during menopause and beyond." *Maturitas.* 2014 Apr;77(4): 318–23.

716 Van Die MD, Burger HG, Teede HJ, et al. "Vitex agnus-castus (Chaste-Tree/Berry) in the treatment of menopause-related complaints." *J Altern Complement Med.* 2009 Aug;15(8):853–62.

717 Mohammad-Alizadeh-Charandabi S, Shahnazi M, Nahaee J, et al. "Efficacy of black cohosh (Cimicifuga racemosa L.) in treating early symptoms of menopause: a randomized clinical trial." *Chin Med.* 2013 Nov 1;8(1):20.

718 Ruiz AD, Daniels KR. "The effectiveness of sublingual and topical compounded bioidentical hormone replacement therapy in postmenopausal women: an observational cohort study." *Int J Pharm Compd.* 2014 Jan–Feb;18(7):70–77.

719 Medline Plus. "Wild yam." Accessed August 12, 2014, from http://www.nlm.nih.gov/medlineplus/druginfo/natural/970.html.

720 Vucenik I, Stains J. "Obesity and cancer risk: evidence, mechanisms, and recommendations." *Ann NY Acad Sci.* 2012 Oct;1271:27–43.

721 American Cancer Society. "Cancer facts & figures 2013." Accessed August 12, 2014, from http://www.cancer.org/acs/groups/content/@epidemiologysurveilance/documents/document/acspc-036845.pdf.

722 American Cancer Society. "Non-small cell lung cancer survival rates by stage." Accessed August 12, 2014, from http://www.cancer.org/cancer/lungcancer-non-smallcell/detailedguide/non-small-cell-lung-cancer-survival-rates.

723 American Lung Association. "Lung cancer fact sheet." Accessed August 12, 2014, from http://www.lung.org/lung-disease/lung-cancer/resources/facts-figures/lung-cancer-fact-sheet.html.

724 American Cancer Society. "Cancer facts & figures 2014." Accessed August 12, 2014, from http://www.cancer.org/cancer/cancercauses/tobaccocancer/tobacco-related-cancer-fact-sheet.

725 Konickova R, Vankova K, Vanikova K, et al. "Anti-cancer effects of blue-green alga Spirulina platensis, a natural source of bilirubin-like tetrapyrrolic compounds." *Ann Hepatol.* 2014 Mar–Apr;13(2):273–83.

726 Matthew B, Sankaranarayanan R, Nair PP, et al. "Evaluation of chemoprevention of oral cancer with Spirulina fusiformis." *Nutr Cancer.* 1995;24(2):197–202.

727 Renju GL, Muraleedhara Kurup G, Bandugula VR. "Effect of lycopene isolated from Chlorella marina on proliferation and apoptosis in human prostate cancer cell line PC-3." *Tumour Biol.* 2014 Jul 30. [Epub ahead of print]

728 Yusof YA, Saad SM, Makpol S, et al. "Hot water extract of Chlorella vulgaris induced DNA damage and apoptosis." *Clinics (SAO Paulo).* 2010;65(12):1371–77.

729 Pope III C., et al. "Lung cancer, cardiopulmonary mortality, and long-term exposure to fine particulate pollution." *JAMA.* 2002;287:1132–1141.

730 Vargas AJ, Burd R. "Hormesis and synergy: pathways and mechanisms of quercetin in cancer prevention and management." *Nutr Rev.* 2010 Jul;68(7):418–28.

731 Yang JH, Hsia TC, Kuo HM, et al. "Inhibition of lung cancer cell growth by quercetin glucuronides via G2/M arrest and induction of apoptosis." *Drug Metab Dispos.* 2006 Feb;34(2):296–304.

732 Mendoza EE, Burd R. "Querceitn as a systemic chemopreventative agent: structural and functional mechanisms." *Mini Rev Med Chem.* 2011 Dec;11(14):1216–21.

733 Murakami A, Ashida H, Terao J. "Multitargeted cancer prevention by quercetin." *Cancer Lett.* 2008 Oct 8;269(2):315–25.

734 Cufi S, Bonavia R, Vazquez-Martin A, Corominas-Faja B, et al. "Silibinin meglumine, a water soluble form of milk thistle silymarin, is an orally active anti-cancer agent that impedes the epithelial-to-mesenchymal transition (EMT) in EGFR-mutant non-small-cell lung carcinoma cells." *Food Chem Toxicol.* 2013 Oct;60:360–68.

735 Liang Z, Yang Y, Wang H. "Inhibition of SIRT1 signaling sensitizes the antitumor activity of silybin against lung adenocarcinoma cells in vitro and in vivo." *Mol Cancer Ther.* 2014 Jul;13(7):1860–72.

736 Sadava D, Kane SE. "Silibinin reverses drug resistance in human small-cell lung carcinoma cells." *Cancer Lett.* 2013 Oct;339(1):102–06.

737 American Cancer Society. "How many men get prostate cancer?" Accessed August 12, 2014, http://www.cancer.org/cancer/prostatecancer/overview-guide/prostate-cancer-overview-key-statistics.

738 American Cancer Society. "Survival rates for prostate cancer." Accessed August 12, 2014, from http://www.cancer.org/cancer/prostatecancer/detailedguide/prostate-cancer-survival-rates.

739 Joshi AD, Corral R, Catsburg C, et al. "Red meat and poultry, cooking practices, genetic susceptibility and risk of prostate cancer: results from a multiethnic case-controlled study." *Carcinogenesis.* 2012 Nov;33(11):2108–18.

740 John EM, Stern MC, Sinha R, et al. "Meat consumption, cooking practices, meat mutagens, and risk of prostate cancer." *Nutr Cancer.* 2011;63(4):525–37.

741 Koutros S, Cross AJ, Sandler DP, et al. "Meat and meat mutagens and risk of prostate cancer in the Agricultural Health Study." *Cancer Epidemiol Biomarkers Prev.* 2008 Jan;17(1):80–87.

742 Abid Z, Cross AJ, Sinha R. "Meat, dairy, and cancer." *Am J Clin Nutr.* 2014 May 21;100(Supplement 1):386S–93S.

743 Nagata Y, Sonoda T, Mori M, et al. "Dietary isoflavones may protect against prostate cancer in Japanese men." *J Nutr.* 2007 Aug;137(8):1974–79.

744 Brooks J. Metter E, Chan D, et al. "Plasma selenium level before diagnosis and the risk of prostate cancer development." *J Urol.* 2001 Dec;166(6):2034–38.

745 Mandair D, Rossi RE, Pericleous M, et al. "Prostate cancer and the influence of dietary factors and supplements: a systematic review." *Nutr Metab (Lond).* 2014 Jun 16;11:30.

746 Li H, Stampfer MJ, Giovannucci EI, et al. "A prospective study of plasma selenium levels and prostate cancer risk." *J Natl Cancer Inst.* 2004 May 5;96(9):645–7.

747 Clark LC, Combs GF Jr., Turnbull BW, et al. "Effects of selenium supplementation for cancer prevention in patients with carcinoma of the skin. A randomized controlled trial." *JAMA.* 1996;276:1957–63.

748 Lippmann SM, Klein EA, Goodman PJ, et al. "Effect of selenium and vitamin E on risk of prostate cancer and other cancers: the selenium and vitamin E cancer prevention trial (SELECT)." *JAMA.* 2009;301:39–51.

749 Aliaev IuG, Vinarov AZ, Demidko, et al. "The results of the 10-year study of efficacy and safety of Serenoa repens extract in patients at risk of progression of benign prostatic hyperplasia." *Urologia.* 2013 Jul–Aug;(4):32–36.

750 Goepel M, Hecker U, Krege S, et al. "Saw palmetto extracts potently and noncompetitively inhibit human a1-adrenoceptors in vitro." *The Prostate.* 1999 Feb 15;38(3):208–15.

751 Gerber G, Kuznetsov D, Johnson B, et al. "Randomized, double-blind, placebo-controlled trial of saw palmetto in men with lower urinary tract symptoms." *Urology.* 2001 Dec;58(6):960–63.

752 Bent S, Kane C, Shinohara K, et al. "Saw palmetto for benign prostatic hyperplasia." *N Eng J Med.* 2006 Feb 9;35(6):557–66.

753 Gossel-Williams M, Davis A, O'Connor N, et al. "Inhibition of testosterone-induced hyperplasia if the prostate of Sprague-Dawley rats by pumpkin seed oil." *J Med Food.* 2006 Summer;9(2):284–86.

754 Hong H, Kim CS, Maeng S. "Effects of pumpkin seed oil and saw palmetto oil in Korean men with symptomatic benign prostatic enlargement." *Nutr Res Pract.* 209 Winter;3(4):323–27.

755 American Cancer Society. "What are the key statistics about breast cancer?" Accessed August 12, 2014, from http://www.cancer.org/cancer/breastcancer/detailedguide/breast-cancer-key-statistics.

756 American Cancer Society. "What are the risks for breast cancer?" Accessed August 12, 2014, from http://www.cancer.org/cancer/breastcancer/detailedguide/breast-cancer-risk-factors.

757 Formby B, Wiley TS. "Progesterone inhibits growth and induces apoptosis in breast cancer cells: inverse effects on Bcl-2 and p53." *Ann Clin Lab Sci.* 1998 Nov 1;28(6):360–69.

758 Zheng JS, Hu XJ, Zhao YM, et al. "Intake of fish and marine n-3 polyunsaturated fatty acids and risk of breast cancer: meta-analysis of data from 21 independent prospective cohort studies." *BMJ.* 2013 Jun 27;346:f3706.

759 Collaborative Group on Hormonal Factors in Breast Cancer, ICRF Cancer Epidemiology Unit, Radcliffe Infirmary, Oxford UK. "Breast cancer and hormonal contraceptives: collaborative reanalysis of individual data on 53,297 women with breast cancer and 100,239 women without breast cancer from 54 epidemiological studies." *Lancet.* 1996 Jun 22;347(9017):1713–27.

760 Mamun AA, Hayatbakhsh MR, O'Callaghan M, et al. "Early overweight and pubertal maturation—pathways of association with young adults' overweight: a longitudinal study." *Int J Obes (Lond).* 2009 Jan;33(1):14–20.

761 Pasquali R, Pelusi C, Genhini S, et al. "Obesity and reproductive disorders in women." *Hum Reprod Update.* 2003 Jul–Aug;9(4):359–72.

762 Lorincz AM, Sukumar S. "Molecular links between obesity and breast cancer." *Endocr Relat Cancer.* 2006 June 1;13:279–92.

763 Akahoshi M, Soda M, Nakashima E, et al. "The effect of body mass index on age at menopause." *Int J Obes Relat Metab Disord.* 2002 Jul;26(7):961–68.

764 Lee SH, Akuete K, Fulton J, et al. "An increased risk of breast cancer after delayed first parity." *Am J Surg.* 2003 Oct;186(4):409–12.

765 Woodman I. "Breast feeding reduces risk of breast cancer, says study." *BMJ.* 2002 July 27;325(7357):184.

766 Awad AB, Downie A, fink CS, et al. "Dietary phytosterol inhibits the growth and metastasis of MDA-MB-231 human breast cancer cells grown in SCID mice." *Anticancer Res.* 2000 Mar–Apr;20(2A):821–24.

767 Woyengo TA, Ramprasath VR, Jones PJ. "Anticancer effect of phytosterols." *Eur J Clin Nutr.* 2009 Jul;63(7):813–20.

768 Lugasi A. "Foods fortified with phytosterins: their role in decreasing serum cholesterol level, their European Community authorization and requirements for placing them on the market." *Orv Hetil.* 2009 Mar 15;150(11):483–96.

769 Liu RH. "Potential synergy of phytochemicals in cancer prevention: mechanism of action." *J Nutr.* 2004 Dec;134(12):3479S–85S.

770 Collett ED, Davidson LA, Fan YY, et al. "n-6 and n-3 polyunsaturated fatty acids differentially modulate oncogenic RAS activation in colonocytes." *Am J Physiol Cell Physiol.* 2001 May;280(5):C1066–75.

771 Hsieh C, Trichopoulos D. "Breast size, handedness and breast cancer risk." *Eur J Cancer.* 1991;27(2):131–35.

772 Steck SE, Chalecki AM, Miller P, et al. "Conjugated linoleic acid supplementation for twelve weeks increases lean body mass in obese humans." *J Nutr.* 2007 May;137(5):1188–93.

773 Park HS, Ryu JH, Ha YL, et al. "Dietary conjugated linolenic acid (CLA) induces apoptosis of colonic mucosa in 1,2-dimethylhydrazine-treated rats: a possible mechanism of the anticarcinogenic effect by CLA." *Br J Nutr.* 2001 Nov;86(5):549–55.

774 Kelley N, Hubbard N, Erickson K. "Conjugated linoleic acid isomers and cancer." *J Nutr.* 2007 Dec;137(12):2599–2607.

775 Tanmahasamut P, Liu J, Hendry LB, et al. "Conjugated linoleic acid blocks estrogen signaling in human breast cancer cells" *J Nutr.* 2004 Mar;134(3):674–80.

776 Rakib MA, Lee WS, Kim GS, et al. "Antiproliferative action of conjugated linoleic acid on human MCF-7 breast cancer cells mediated by enhancement of gap junctional intercellular communication through inactivation of NF-kB." *Evid Based Complement Alterat Med.* 2013;2013:429393.

777 Kawamori T, Lubet R, Steele VE, et al. "Chemopreventive effect of curcumin, a naturally occurring anti-inflammatory agent, during the promotion/progression stages of colon cancer." *Cancer Res.* 1999 Feb 1;59(3):597–61.

778 Chen L, Tian G, Shao C, et al. "Curcumin modulates eukaryotic initiation factors in human lung adenocarcinoma epithelial cells." *Mol Biol Rep.* 2010 Oct;37(7):3105–10.

779 Liu D, Chen Z. "The effect of curcumin on breast cancer cells." *J Breast Cancer.* 2013 Jun;16(2):133–37.

780 MD Anderson Cancer Center. "Curcumin halts spread of breast cancer in mice." Accessed August 12, 2014, from http://www.mdanderson.org/newsroom/news-releases/2005/10-14-05-curcumin-halts-spread-of-breast-cancer-in-mice-news-release.html.

781 Sharma RA, McLelland HR, Hill KA, et al. "Pharmacodynamic and pharmacokinetic study of oral Curcuma extract in patients with colorectal cancer." *Clin Cancer Res.* 2001;7:1894–1900.

782 Haggar FA, Boushey RP. "Colorectal cancer epidemiology: incidence, mortality, survival, and risk factors." *Clin Colon Rectal Surg.* 2009 Nov;22(4):191–97.

783 Dong-Hyun K. "Risk factors of colorectal cancer." *J Korean Soc Coloprotocol.* 2009 Oct;25(5):356–62.

784 US Centers for Disease Control and Prevention. "Colorectal cancer, what are the risk factors?" Accessed August 12, 2014, from http://www.cdc.gov/cancer/colorectal/basic_info/risk_factors.htm.

785 Giovannucci E, Willet WC. "Dietary factors and risk of colon cancer." *Ann Med.* 1994 Dec;26(6):443–52.

786 Slattery M, Benson J, Berry TD, et al. "Dietary sugar and colon cancer." *Cancer Epidemiol Biomarkers Prev.1997* Sep;6:677.

787 Bingham S, Day NE, Luben R, et al. "Dietary fibre in food and protection against colorectal cancer in the European Prospective Investigation into Cancer and Nutrition (EPIC): an observational study." *Lancet.* 2003 May;361(9368):1496–1501.

788 de Vogel J, Jonker-Termont DS, van Liershout EM, et al. "Green vegetables, red meat, and colon cancer: chlorophyll prevents the cytotoxic and hyperproliferative effects of haem in rat colon." *Carcinogenesis.* 2005 Feb;26(2):387–93.

789 Kojima M, Wakai K, Tokudome S, et al. "Bowel movement frequency and risk of colorectal cancer in a large cohort study of Japanese men and women." *Br J Cancer.* 2004;90:1397–1401.

790 Shanahan F. "Probiotics and inflammatory bowel disease: is there a scientific rationale?" *Inflam Bowel Dis.* 2000 May;6(2):107–15.

791 Hedin C, Whelan K, Lindsay J. "Evidence for the use of probiotics and prebiotics in inflammatory bowel disease: a review of clinical trials." *Proc Nutr Soc.* 2007 Aug;66(3):307–15.

792 Meijer BJ, Dieleman LA. "Probiotics in the treatment of human inflammatory bowel disease: update 2011." *J Clin Gatroenterol.* 2011 Nov;45 Suppl:S139–44.

793 Perdigon G, Alvarez S, Rachid M, et al. "Immune system stimulation by probiotics." *J Dairy Sci.* 1995 Jul;78(7):1597–1606.

794 Perez Martinez G, Bauerl C, Collado MC. "Understanding gut microbiota in elderly's health will enable intervention through probiotics." *Benef Microbes.* 2014 Sep;6(3):235–46.

795 Vieira AT, Teixeira MM, Martins FS. "The role of probiotics and prebiotics in inducing gut immunity." *Front Immunol.* 2013 Dec;12:4:445.

796 Kalliomaki M, Salminen S, Arvilommi H, et al. "Probiotics in primary prevention of atopic disease: a randomized placebo-controlled trial." *Lancet.* 2001 Apr 7;357(9262):1076–79.

797 Kalliomaki M, Salminen S, Poussa T, et al. "Probiotics and prevention of atopic disease: 4-year follow-up of a randomized placebo-controlled trial. *Lancet.* 2003 May;361(9372):1869–71.

798 Rayes N, Seehofer D, Muller AR, et al. "Influence of probiotics and fibre on the incidence of bacterial infections following major abdominal surgery—results of a prospective trial." *Zeitschrif fur Gastroenterolgie.* 2002;40(10):869–76.

799 Weizman Z, Asli G, Alsheikh A. "Effect of a probiotic infant formula on infections in child care centers: comparison of two probiotic agents." *Pediatrics.* 2005 Jan 1;115:5–9.

800 Khosravi A, Yanez A, Price JG, et al. "Gut microbiota promote hematopoiesis to control bacterial infection." *Cell Host Microbe.* 2014 Mar 12;15(3):374–81.

801 Lever GJ, Li S, Mubasher ME, et al. "Probiotic effects on cold and influenza-like symptom incidence and duration in children." *Pediatrics.* 2009 Aug;124(2):e172–79.

802 Kumpu M, Kekkonen RA, Kautiainen H, et al. "Milk containing probiotic Lactobacillus rhamnosus GG and respiratory illness in children: a randomized, double-blind, placebo-controlled trial." *Eur J Clin Nutr.* 2012 Sep;66(8):1020–23.

803 Rafter J. "The effects of probiotics on colon cancer development." *Nutr Res Rev.* 2004 Dec;17(2):277–84.

804 Zhong L, Zhang X, Covasa M. "Emerging roles of lactic acid bacteria in protection against colorectal cancer." *World J Gastroenterol.* 2014 Jun 28;20(24):7878–85.

805 Uccello M, Malaguarnera G, Basile F, et al. "Potential role of probiotics on colorectal cancer prevention." *BMC Surgery.* 2012;12(Suppl 1):S35.

806 Moos P, Edes K, Mullally J, et al. "Curcumin impairs tumor suppressor p53 function in colon cancer cells." *Carcinogenesis.* 2004 Sep;25(9):1611–17.

807 Tsvetkov P, Asher G, Reiss V, et al. "Inhibition of NAD(P)H: quinone oxidoreductase 1 activity and induction of p53 degradation by the natural phenolic compound curcumin." *Proc Natl Acad Sci U S A.* 2005 Apr;102(15):5535–40.

808 Banerji A, Chakrabarti J, Mitra A, et al. "Effect of curcumin on gelatinase A (MMP-2) activity in B16F10 melanoma cells." *Cancer Lett.* 2004 Aug 10;211(2):235–42.

809 Alappat L, Awad A. "Curcumin and obesity: evidence and mechanisms." *Nutr Rev.* 2010 Dec;68(12):729–38.

810 Shehzad A, Lee J, Huh TL, et al. "Curcumin induces apoptosis in human colorectal carcinoma (HCT-15) cells by regulating expression of Prp4 and p53." *Mol Cells.* 2013 Jun;35(6):526–32.

811 Ejaz A, Wu D, Kwan P, et al. "Curcumin inhibits angiogenesis in 3T3-L1 adipocytes and angiogenesis and obesity in C57/BL mice." *J Nutr.* 2009 May;139(5):919–25.

812 Gururaj A, Belakavadi M, Venkastesh D, et al. "Molecular mechanisms of anti-angiogenic effect of curcumin." *Biochem Biophys res Comm.* 2002 Oct 4;297(4):934–42.

813 Pettan-Brewer C, Morton J, Angalindan R, et al. "Curcumin suppresses intestinal polyps in APC Min mice fed fat diet." *Pathobiol Aging Age Relate Dis.* 2011;1.

814 Chinary R, Brockman JA, Peeler MO, et al. "Antioxidants enhance the cytotoxicity of chemotherapeutic agents in colorectal cancer." *Nat Med.* 1997 Nov;3(11):1233–41.

815 National Heart, Lung, and Blood Institute. "Who is at risk of stroke?" Accessed August 12, 2014, from http://www.nhlbi.nih.gov/health/health-topics/topics/stroke/atrisk.html.

816 Canadian Stroke Congress. "'Cafeteria diet' hastens stroke risk." 2012. Accessed August 25, 2014, from http://www.eurekalert.org/pub_releases/2012-10/hasf-dh092712.php.

817 Azevedo J, Fernandes I, Faria A, et al. "Antioxidant properties of antho-cyanidins, anthocyanidins-3-glucosides and respective portisins." *Food Chemistry.* 2010 Mar;119(2):518–23.

818 Walalce T. "Amthocyanins in cardiovascular disease." *Adv Nutr.* 2011 Jan;2:1–7.

819 Mursu J, Voutilainen S, Nurmi T, et al. "Flavanoid intake and the risk of ischaemic stroke and CVD mortality in middle-aged finnish men: the Kuopip Ischaemic Heart Disease Risk Factor Study." *Br J Nutr.* 2008 Oct;100(4):890–95.

820 Ascherio A, Rimm EB, Hernan MA, et al. "Intake of potassium, magne-sium, calcium, and fiber and risk of stroke among US men." *Circulation.* 1998 Sep 22;98(12):1198–1204.

821 Larsson SC, Virtamo J, Wolk A. "Potassium, calcium, and magnesium intakes and risk of stroke in women." *Am J Epidemiol.* 2011 Jul 1;174(1):35–43.

822 Yeung A, Vershtein V, Krantz D, et al. "The effect of atherosclerosis on the vasomotor response of coronary arteries to mental stress." *N Engl J Med.* 1991 Nov 28;325(22):1551–56.

823 Inoue N. "Stress and atherosclerotic cardiovascular disease." *J Atheroscler Thromb.* 2014;21(5):391–401.

824 Matthews K, Katholi C, McCreath H, et al. "Blood pressure reactivity to psychological stress predicts hypertension in the CARDIA study." *Circulation.* 2004;110:74–78.

825 McDonnel MN, Esterman AJ, Williams RS, et al. "Physical activity habits and preferences in the month prior to first ever stroke." *Peer J.* 214 Jul 10;2:e489.

826 Inman WH, Vessey MP. "Investigation of deaths from pulmonary, coronary, and cerebral thrombosis and embolism in women of child-bearing age." *Br Med J.* 1968;2(5599):193–99.

827 Gillium L, Mamidipudi S, Johnston S. "Ischemic stroke risk with oral contraceptives: a meta-analysis." *JAMA.* 2000 July 5;284(1):72–78.

828 Kemmeren J, Tanis B, van den Bosch M, et al. "Risk of Arterial Thrombosis in Relation to Oral Contraceptives (RATIO) study." *Stroke.* 2002;33:122–08.

829 Grodstein F, Manson J, Stampfer M, et al. "Postmenopausal hormone therapy and stroke:role of time since menopause and age at initiation of hormone therapy." *Arch Intern Med.* 2008 Apr 28;168(8):861–68.

830 Gu H, Zhao X, Zhao X, et al. "Risk of stroke in healthy postmenopausal women during and after hormone therapy: a meta-analysis." *Menopause.* 2014 Mar 31. [Epub ahead of print]

831 Wassertheil-Smoller S, Hendrix S, Limacher M, et al. "Effect of estrogen plus progestin on stroke in postmenopausal women." *JAMA.* 2003;289(2):2673–84.

832 Reynolds K, Lewis B, David J, et al. "Alcohol consumption and risk of stroke: a meta-analysis." *JAMA.* 2003;289(5):579–88.

833 Puddey I, Beilin L, Rakic V. "Alcohol, hypertension and the cardiovascular system: a critical appraisal." *Addiction Biol.* 1997 Apr;2(2):159–70.

834 Grogan JR, Kochar MS. "Alcohol and hypertension." *Arch Fam Med.* 1994 Feb;3(2):150–4.

835 Holmes MV, Dale CE, Zuccolo L, et al. "Association between alcohol and cardiovascular disease: Mendelian randomisation analysis based on individual participant data." *BMJ.* 2014 Jul 10;349:g4164.

836 Berthold HK, Sudhop T. "Garlic preparations for prevention of atherosclerosis." *Curr Opin Lipidol.* 1998 Dec;9(6):565–69.

837 Lau BH. "Suppression of LDL oxidation by garlic." *J Nutr.* 2001 Mar;131(3s):985S–88S.

838 Ide N, Lau BH. "Garlic compounds protect vascular endothelial cells from oxidized low density lipoprotein-induced injury." *J Pharm Pharmacol.* 1997 Sep;49(9):908–11.

839 Lau KK, Chan YH, Wong YK, et al. "Garlic intake is an independent predictor of endothelial function in patients with ischemic stroke." *J Nutr Health Aging.* 2013 Jul;17(7):600–04.

840 Williams MJ, Sutherland WH, McCormick MP, et al. "Aged garlic extract improves endothelial function in men with coronary artery disease." *Phytother Res.* 2005 Apr;19(4):314–9.

841 Chan JY, Yuen AC, Chan RY, et al. "A review of the cardiovascular benefits and antioxidant properties of allicin." *Phytother Res.* 2013 May;27(5):637–46.

842 American Lung Association. "Disease data 2008. Chronic obstructive pulmonary disease (COPD)." Accessed August 13, 2014, from http://www.lung.org/assets/documents/publications/lung-disease-data/ldd08-chapters/LDD-08-COPD.pdf.

843 World Health Organization. "Risk factors for chronic respiratory diseases." Accessed August 13, 2014, from http://www.who.int/gard/publications/Risk%20factors.pdf.

844 US Centers for Disease Control and Prevention. Accessed August 17, 2014, from http://www.cdc.gov/media/pressrel/2010/r101022.html.

845 American Diabetes Association. "Statistics about diabetes. Overall numbers, diabetes and prediabetes." Accessed August 13, 2014, from http://www.diabetes.org/diabetes-basics/statistics/.

846 Mayo Clinic. "Type 1 diabetes. Risk factors." Accessed August 13, 2014, from http://www.mayoclinic.org/diseases-conditions/type-1-diabetes/basics/risk-factors/con-20019573.

847 Farshchi H, Taylor M, MacDonald I. "Beneficial metabolic effects of regular meal frequency on dietary thermogenesis, insulin sensitivity, and fasting lipid profiles in healthy obese women." *Am J Clin Nutr.* 2005 Jan;81(1):16–24.

848 Jenkins DJ, Ocana A, Jenkins AL, et al. "Metabolic advantages of spreading the nutrient load: effects of increased meal frequency in non-insulin-dependent diabetes." *Am J Clin Nutr.* 1992 Feb;55(2):461–67.

849 Bertelsen J, Christiansen C, Thomsen C, et al. "Effect of meal frequency on blood glucose, insulin, and free fatty acids in NIDDM subjects." *Diabetes Care.* 1993 Jan;16(1):4–7.

850 Calorie King. "M&M's Peanut chocolate candies." Accessed August 13, 2014, from http://www.calorieking.com/foods/calories-in-chocolate-peanut_f-ZmlkPTE5MTQw.html.

851 Calorie King. "Snickers Fun Size Snickers chocolate bar." Accessed August 13, 2014, from http://www.calorieking.com/foods/calories-in-chocolate-bar-fun-size_f-ZmlkPTIwMDM1NQ.html.

852 Self Nutrition Data. "Bread, whole wheat, commercially prepared." Accessed August 13, 2014, from http://nutritiondata.self.com/facts/baked-products/4876/2.

853 Franz M. "Protein controversies in diabetes." *Diabetes Spectrum.* 2000;13(3):132.

854 Moore M, Coate K, Winnick J, et al. "Regulation of hepatic glucose uptake and storage in vivo." *Adv Nutr.* 2012 May;3:286–94.

855 DeFronzo R, Ferannini E, Sato Y, et al. "Synergistic interaction between exercise and insulin on peripheral glucose uptake. *J Clin Invest.* 1981 Dec;68(6):1468–74.

856 Goodyear L, Kahn B. "Exercise, glucose transport, and insulin sensitivity." *Ann Rev Med.* 1998;49:235–61.

857 Winncik JJ, Sherman WM, Habash DL, et al. "Short-term aerobic exercise training in obese humans with type 2 diabetes mellitus improves whole-body insulin sensitivity through gains in peripheral, not hepatic insulin sensitivity." *J Clin Endocrinol Metab.*2008 Mar;93(3):771–78.

858 Heijden G, Toffolo G, Manesso E, Sauer P, Sunehag A. "Aerobic exercise increases peripheral and hepatic insulin sensitivity in sedentary adolescents." *J Clin Endocrinol Metab.*2009 Nov;94(11):4292–99.

859 Klimcakova E, Polak J, Moro C, et al. "Dynamic strength training improves insulin sensitivity without altering plasma levels and gene expression of adipokines in subcutaneous adipose tissue in obese men." *J Clin Endocrinol Metab.* 2006;91(12):5107–12.

860 Brooks N, Layne JE, Gordon PL, et al. "Strength training improves muscle quality and insulin sensitivity in Hispanic older adults with type 2 diabetes." *Int J Med Sci.* 2006 Dec 18;4(1):19–27.

861 Miller JP, Pratley RE, Goldberg AP, et al. "Strength training increases insulin action in healthy 50- to 65-yr-old men." *J Appl Physiol.* 1994 Sep;77:1122–27.

862 Gang H, Jousilahti P, Barengo NC, et al. "Physical activity, cardiovascular risk factors, and mortality among finnish adults with diabetes." *Diabetes Care.* 2005 Apr;28(4):799–805.

863 Murphy JC, McDaniel JL, Mora K, et al. "Preferential reductions in intramuscular and visceral adipose tissue with exercise-induced weight loss compared with calorie restriction." *J Appl Physiol (1985).* 2012 Jan;112(1):79–85.

864 Hamman R, Wing R, Edelstein S, et al. "Effect of weight loss with lifestyle intervention on risk of diabetes." *Diabetes Care.* 2006 Sep;29(9):212–07.

865 Weiss EP, Racette SB, Villareal DT, et al. "Improvements in glucose tolerance and insulin action induced by increasing energy expenditure or decrease energy intake: a randomized controlled trial." *Am J Clin Nutr.* 2006 Nov;84(5):133–42.

866 Anderson RA. "Chromium in the prevention and treatment of diabetes." *Diabetes Metab.* 2000 Feb;26(1):22–27.

867 Suksomboon N, Poolsup N, Yuwanakorn A. "Systematic review and meta-analysis of the efficacy and safety of chromium supplementation in diabetes." *J Clin Pharm Ther.* 2014 Jun;39(3)292–306.

868 Linday LA. "Trivalent chromium and the diabetes prevention program." *Med Hypotheses.* 1997 Jul;49(1):47–49.

869 John-Kalarickal J, Pearlman G, Carlson HE. "New medications which decrease levothyroxine absorption." *Thyroid.* 2007;17:763–65.

870 Ansar H, Mazloom Z, Kazemi F, et al. "Effect of alpha-lipoic acid on blood glucose, insulin resistance and glutathione peroxidase of type 2 diabetic patients." *Saudi Med J.* 2011 Jun;32(6):584–86.

871 Vallianou N, Evangelopoulos A, Koutalas P. "Alpha-lipoic acid and diabetic neuropathy." *Rev Diabet Stud.* 2009 Winter;6(4):230–36.

872 Anton S, Martin C, Han H, et al. "Effects of stevia, aspartame, and sucrose on food intake, satiety, and postprandial glucose and insulin levels." *Appetite.* 2010 Aug;55(1):37–43.

873 Mellis MS. "A crude extract of Stevia rebaudiana increases the renal plasma flow of normal and hypertensive rats." *Braz J Med Biol Res.* 1996;29: 669–75.

874 Davis PA, Yokoyama W. "Cinnamon intake lowers fasting blood glucose: meta-analysis." *J Med Food.* 2011 Sep;14(9):884–89.

875 Ping H, Zhang G, Ren G. "Antidiabetic effects of cinnamon oil in diabetic KK-Ay mice." *Food Chem Toxicol.* 2010 Aug–Sep;48(8–9):2344–49.

876 Mishra A, Bhatti R, Singh A, et al. "Ameliorative effect of the cinnamon oil from Cinnamon zeylanicum upon early stage diabetic nephropathy." *Planta Med.* 2010 Mar;76(5):412–17.

877 Alzheimer's Association. "Alzheimer's facts and figures." Accessed August 13, 2014, from http://www.alz.org/alzheimers_disease_facts_and_figures.asp#quickFacts.

878 Alzheimer's Association. "Risk factors." Accessed August 13, 2014, from http://www.alz.org/alzheimers_disease_causes_risk_factors.asp.

879 Tomljenovic L. "Aluminum and Alzheimer's disease: after a century of controversy, is there a plausible link?" *J Alzheimers Dis.* 2011;23(4):567–98.

880 Miu AC, Benga O. "Aluminum and Alzheimer's disease: a new look." *J Alzheimer's Dis.* 2006 Nov;10(2–3)179–201.

881 Campbell A. "The potential role of aluminum in Alzheimer's disease." *Nephrol Dial Transplant.* 2002;17(Suppl 2):17–20.

882 Lemire J, Appanna V. "Aluminum toxicity and astrocyte dysfunction: a metabolic link to neurological disorders." *J Inorganic Biochem.* 2011 Nov;105(11):1513–17.

883 Poulose S, Bielinski D, Shukitt-Hale. "Neuronal housekeeping via activation of autophagy by blueberry, strawberry, acai berry and walnut extracts." *FASEB J.* 2011 Apr;(Meeting abstract supplement):213.8.

884 "Berry fruit enhances beneficial signaling in the brain." *J Agric Food Chem.* 2012;60(23):5709–15.

885 Shukitt-Hale B, Lau FC, Joseph JA. "Berry fruit supplementation and the aging brain." *J Agric Food Chem.* 2009 Feb 13;56(3):636–41.

886 Willis LM, Shukitt-Hale B, Joseph JA. "Recent advances in berry supplementation and age-related cognitive decline." *Curr Opin Clin Nutr Metab Care.* 2009 Jan;12(1):91–94.

887 Joseph JA, Shukitt-Hale B, Willis LM. "Grape juice, berries, and walnuts affect brain aging and behavior." *J Nutr.* 209 Sep;139(9):1813S–17S.

888 Johnson M, de Mejia E, Fan J, et al. "Anthocyanins and proanthocyanidins from blueberry-blackberry fermented beverages inhibit markers of inflammation in macrophages and carbohydrate-utilizing enzymes in vitro." *Mol Nutr Food Res.* 2013 July;57(7):1182–97.

889 Kidd PM. "Omega-3 DHA and EPA for cognition, behavior, and mood:- clinical findings and structural-functional synergies with cell membrane phospholipids." *Altern Med Rev.* 2007 Sep;12(3):207–27.

890 Birch EE, Garfield S, Casteneda Y, et al. "Visual acuity and cognitive outcomes at 4 years of age in a double-blind, randomized trial of long-chain polyunsaturated fatty acid-supplemented infant formula." *Early Hum Dev.* 2007 May;83(5):279–84.

891 Innis SM, Friesen RW. "Essential n-3 fatty acids in pregnant women and early visual acuity maturation in term infants." *Am J Clin Nutr.* 2008;87:548–57.

892 Yurko-Mauro K, McCarthy D, Rom D, et al. "Beneficial effects of docosahexaenoic acid on cognition in age-related cognitive decline" *Alzheimer's and Dementia.* 2010;6(6):456.

893 Mizwicki MT, Liu G, fiala, et al. "1α-25-dihydroxyvitamin D3 and resolving D1 retune the balance between amyloid-β phagocytosis and inflammation in Alzheimer's disease patients." *J Alzheimer's Dis.* 2013 Jan 1;34(1):155–70.

894 Sando SB, Melquist S, Cannon A, et al. "Risk-reducing effect of education in Alzheimer's disease." *Int J Geriatr Psychiatry.* 2008 Nov;23(11):1156–62.

895 Roe CM, Xiong C, Miller P, et al. "Education and Alzheimer's disease without dementia: support for the cognitive reserve hypothesis." *Neurology.* 2007 Jan 16;68(3):223–28.

896 Kennedy D, Pace S, Haskell C, et al. "Effects of cholinesterase inhibiting sage 9 Salvia officinalis) on mood, anxiety and performance on a psychological stressor battery." *Neuropsychopharmacology.* 2006 Apr;31(4):845–52.

897 Moss L, Rouse M, Wesnes KA, et al. "Differential effects of the aromas of Salvia species on memory and mood." *Hum Psychopharmacol.* 2010 Jul;25(5):388–96.

898 Kennedy DO, Dodd Fl, Robertson BC, et al. "Monoterpenoid extract of sage (Salvia lavendulaefolia) with cholinesterase inhibiting properties improves cognitive performance and mood in healthy adults. *J Psychopharmacol.* 2011 Aug;25(8):1088–1100.

899 Akhondzadeh S, Noroozian M, Mohammadi M, Ohadinia S, Akhondzadeh S, Noroozian M, Mohammadi M, et al. "Salvia officinalis extract in the treatment of patients with mild to moderate Alzheimer's disease: a double blind, randomized and placebo-controlled trial." *J Clin Pharm Ther.* 2003 Feb;28(1):53–59.

900 Tildesley NT, Kennedy DO, Perry EK, et al. "Salvia lavandulaefolia (Spanish sage) enhances memory in healthy young volunteers." *Pharmacol Biochem Behav.* 2003 Jun;75(3):669–74.

901 Burkhard PR, Burkhard K, Haenggeli CA, et al. "Plant-induced seizures: reappearance of an old problem." *J Neurol.* 1999 Aug;246(8):667–70.

902 Perry NB, Anderson RE, Brennan NJ, et al. "Essential oils from Dalmatian (Salvia officinalis l.) variations among individuals, plant parts, seasons, and sites." *J Agric Food Chem.*1999;47:2048–54.

903 Yoshida H, Meng P, Matsumiya T, et al. "Carnosic acid suppressed the production of amyloid-β 1-42 and 1-43 by inducing an α-secretase TACE/ADAM17 in U373MG human astrocytoma cells." *Neurosci Res.* 2014 Feb;79:83–93.

904 Moss M, Cook J, Wesnes K, et al. "Aromas of rosemary and lavender essential oils differentially affect cognition and mood in healthy adults." *Int J Neurosci.* 2003 Jan;113(1):15–38.

905 Jimbo D, Kimura Y, Taniguchi M, et al. "Effect of aromatherapy with Alzheimer's disease." *Psychogeriatrics.* 2009 Dec;9(4):173–79.

906 Hope J. "Why a whiff of rosemary does help you remember: Sniffing the herb can increase memory by 75%." Accessed August 14, 2014, from http://

www.dailymail.co.uk/health/article-2306078/Why-whiff-rosemary-does-help-remember.html.

907 Perry G, Nunomura A, Hirai K, et al. "Oxidative damage in Alzheimer's disease: the metabolic dimension." *Int J Dev Neurosci.* 2000 Jul–Aug; 18(4–5):417–21.

908 Butterfield A, Drake J, Pocernich C, et al. "Evidence of oxidative damage in Alzheimer's disease brain: central role for amyloid B-peptide." *Trends Mol Med.* 2001 Dec;7(12):548–54.

909 Zhao Y, Zhao B. "Oxidative stress and pathogenesis of Alzheimer's disease." *Oxidative Medicine and Cellular Longevity.* 2013;2013:Article ID 316523.

910 Frank B, Gupta S. "A review of antioxidants and Alzheimer's disease." *Ann Clin Psychiatry.* 2005 Oct–Dec;17(4):269–86.

911 Jama J, Launer LJ, Witteman JC, et al. "Dietary antioxidants and cognitive function in a population-based sample of older persons." *Am J Epidemiology.* 1996 Aug 1;144(3):275–80.

912 Prasad KN, Bondy SC. "Inhibition of early upstream events in prodromal Alzheimer's disease by use of targeted antioxidants." *Curr Aging Sci.* 2014 Aug 4. [Epub ahead of print]

913 Rinaldi P, Polidori MC, Metastasio A, et al. "Plasma antioxidants are similarly depleted in mild cognitive impairment and in Alzheimer's disease." *Neurobiol Aging.* 2003 Nov;24(7):915–19.

914 Frank B, Supta S. "A review of antioxidants and Alzheimer's disease." 2005;17(4):269–86.

915 Morris M, Beckett L, Scherr P, et al. "Vitamin E and vitamin C supplement use and risk of incident Alzheimer's disease." *Alzheimer Dis Assoc Disord.* 1998 Sep;12(3):121–26.

916 Engelhart M, Geerlings M, Ruitenberg A, et al. "Dietary intake of antioxidants and risk of Alzheimer's disease." *JAMA.* 2002 June 26;287(24):3223–3229.

917 Zandi PP, Anthony JC, Khachaturian AS, et al. "Reduced risk of Alzheimer's disease in users of antioxidant vitamin supplements: the Cache County Study." *Arch Neurol.* 2004 Jan;61(1):82–88.

918 Dysken M, Sano M, Asthana S, et al. "Effect of vitamin E and memantine on functional decline in Alzheimer Disease. The TEAM-AD VA Cooperative Randomized trial." *JAMA.* 2014 Jan 1;311(1):33–44.

919 Fukui K, Masuda A, Hosono A, et al. "Changes in microtubule-related proteins and autophagy in long-term vitamin E-deficient mice." *Free Radic Res.* 2014 Jun;48(6):649–58.

920 Kontush K, Schekatolina S. "Vitamin E in neurodegenerative disorders: Alzheimer's disease." *Ann N Y Acad Sci.* 2004 Dec;1031:249–61.

921 Schippling S, Kontush A, Arlt S, et al. "Increased lipoprotein oxidation in Alzheimer's disease." *Free Radic Biol Med.* 2000 Feb 1;28(3):351–60.

922 Kook SY, Lee KM, Kim Y, et al. "High-dose of vitamin C supplementation reduces amyloid plaque burden and ameliorates pathologic changes in the brain of 5XFAD mice." *Cell Death Dis.* 2014 Feb 27;5:e1083.

923 Heo JH, Hyon-Lee, Lee Km. "The possible role of antioxidant vitamin C in Alzheimer's disease treatment and prevention." *Am J Alzheimers Dis Other Demen.* 2013 Mar;28(2):120–25.

924 Kontush A, Mann U, Arlt S, et al. "Influence of vitamin E and C supplementation on lipoprotein oxidation in patients with Alzheimer's disease." *Free Radic Biol Med.* 2001 Aug 1;31(3):345–54.

925 Li FJ, Shen L, Ji HF. "Dietary intakes of vitamin E, vitamin C, and β-carotene and risk of Alzheimer's disease: a meta-analysis." *J Alzheimers Dis.* 2012;31(2):253–58.

926 US Centers for Disease Control and Prevention. "Pneumonia." Accessed August 14, 2014, from http://www.cdc.gov/nchs/fastats/pneumonia.htm.

927 US Centers for Disease Control and Prevention. "Seasonal influenza Q&A." Accessed August 14, 2014, from http://www.cdc.gov/flu/about/qa/disease.htm.

928 US Centers for Disease Control and Prevention. "Influenza." Accessed August 14, 2014, from http://www.cdc.gov/nchs/fastats/flu.htm.

929 Mayo Clinic. "Influenza. Risk factors." Accessed August 14, 2014, from http://www.mayoclinic.org/diseases-conditions/flu/basics/risk-factors/con-20035101.

930 National Heart, Lung, and Blood Institute. "Who is at risk for pneumonia?" Accessed August 14, 2014, from http://www.nhlbi.nih.gov/health/health-topics/topics/pnu/atrisk.html.

931 Puri A, Saxena R, Saxena RP, et al. "Immunostimulant agents from Andrographis paniculata." *J Nat Prod.* 1993;56:995–99.

932 Caceres DD, Hancke JL, Burgos RA et al. "Prevention of common colds with Andrographis Paniculata dried extract: a pilot, double-blind trial." *Phytomedicine.* 1997;4:101–104.

933 Roxas M, Jurenka J. "Colds and influenza: a review of diagnosis and conventional, botanical, and nutritional considerations." *Alternat Med Rev.* 2007;12(10):25–48.

934 Lindenmuth G, Lindenmuth E. "The efficacy of Echinacea compound herbal tea preparation on the severity and duration of upper respiratory and flu symptoms: a randomized, double-blind placebo-controlled study." *J Alernat Comp Med.* 2004 Jun 30;6(4):327–34.

935 Sharma SM, Anderson M, Schoop SR, et al. "Bactericidal and anti-inflammatory properties of standardized Echinacea extract (Echinaforce®): dual actions against respiratory bacteria." *Phytomedicine.* 2010 Jul;17(8–9):563–68.

936 Gorski JC, Huang S, Zaheer NA, et al. "The effect of Echinacea (Echinacea purpurea root) on cytochrome P450 activity in vivo." *Clin Pharmacol Ther.* 2003;73:P94.

937 Zakay–Rones Z, Varsona N, Zlotnik M, et al. "Inhibition of several strains of influenza virus in vitro and reduction of symptoms by an elderberry extract (Sambucus nigra L.) during an outbreak of Influenza B Panama." *J Alternat Comp Med.* 2007 Aug;1(4):361–69.

938 Roschek B, fink RC, McMichael MD, et al. "Elderberry flavonoids bind to and prevent H1N1 infection in vitro." *Phytochemistry.* 2009;70:1255–61.

939 Rehman J, Dillow JM, carter SM, et al. "Increased production of antigen-specific immunoglobulins G and M following in vitro treatment with the medicinal plants Echinacea angustifolia and Hydrastis Canadensis." *Immunon Lett.* 1999;68:391–95.

940 Kaneda Y, Torii M, Tanaka T, et al. "In vitro effects of berberine sulphate on the growth and structure of Entanoeba histolytica, Giardia lambilia and Trichomonas vaginalis." *Ann Trop Med Parasitol.* 1991;85:417–25.

941 Gupte S. "Use of berberine in treatment of giardiasis." *Am J Dis Child.* 1975;129:966.

942 Cech NB, Junio HA, Ackermann LW, et al. "Quorum quenching and antimicrobial activity of goldenseal (Hydrastis canadensis) against methicillin-resistant Staphylococcus aureus (MRSA)." *Planta Med.* 2012 Sep;78(14):1556–61.

943 Cecil Ce, Davis JM, Cech NB, et al. "Inhibition of H1N1 Influenza A virus growth and induction of inflammatory mediators by the isoquinoline alkaloid berberine and extracts of goldenseal (Hydrastis canadensis)." *Int Imunopharmacol.* 2011 Nov;11(11):1706–14.

944 Frost C. "A double-blind study on the comparative efficacy of influenza vaccination and influenzinum 7 CH." *Am Homeopath.* 2006 Jan;12:9.

945 Mathie RT, Frye J, fisher P. "Homeopathic oscillococcinum for preventing and treating influenza and influenza-like illness." *Cochrane Database Syst Rev.* 2012 Dec 12;12:CD001957.

946 Mroninski C, Adriano E, Mattos G. "Meningococcinum: its protective effect against meningococcal disease." *Homoeopathic Links.* Winter, 2001;14(4);230–4.

947 Golden I. *Homoeoprophylaxis—a fifteen year clinical study.* Daylesford: Isaac Golden Publications. 2004.

948 Cannell JJ, Vieth R, Umhau JC, et al. "Epidemic influenza and vitamin D." *Epidemiol Infect.* 2006 Dec;134(6):1129–40.

949 Aloia JF, Ling M. "Re: epidemic influenza and vitamin D." *Epidemiol Infect.* 2007 Oct;135(7):1095–96.

950 Bergman P, Lindh AU, Bjorkhem-Bergman L, et al. "Vitamin D and respiratory tract infections: a systematic review and meta-analysis of randomized controlled trials." *PLoS One.* 2013 Jun 19;8(6):e65835.

Index

Fat, 39–46, 55, 57, 62, 67, 69, 72, 73,
74, 75, 78, 81, 86, 90, 91, 99, 104,
111, 112, 118–120, 161, 162, 164,
165, 166, 167, 172, 173
Fiber, 20, 32–39, 46, 57, 119, 125, 164,
167, 172, 175
Fiber, soluble, 20, 36
Fish oil, 43, 96–97, 162, 167, 175
Flexibility, 108, 113–115, 136
Folate, 33, 38, 78–80, 81
Folic acid, 32, 35, 73, 78–80, 166
Food additives, 47, 52, 118, 123, 124, 176
Food quality, 65
Fruits, 18–24, 37, 46, 52, 55, 63–65, 69,
84, 92, 125, 148, 157, 162, 164, 167,
172, 185

Garlic, 21, 37, 74, 125, 151–152, 168–169
Gastrointestinal system, 20, 28, 57, 99,
126
Ginkgo biloba, 99
Glucose, 33, 39, 45, 46, 47, 56, 74, 78, 80,
86, 139, 145, 171, 173, 174
Gluten, 35–38, 171
Goldenseal, 170, 181, 182
Grains, 18–20, 32–39, 57, 72, 91, 172

Hawthorn, 125, 152
Healing, 3–5, 8–11, 72, 77, 82, 117,
120, 132, 134, 136
Heart disease, 17, 18, 28, 30, 31, 33–38,
40, 43, 46, 54, 76, 88, 93, 94, 97,
136, 137, 139, 147–152, 167, 168,
173, 176, 180, 186
Heartburn, 47, 51, 58
Heavy metals, 46, 85, 93, 96, 97,
118–124, 175, 186
Herbalism, 9–10
Herbs, standardization of, 10
High blood pressure, 70, 74, 82, 89, 92,
94, 130, 136, 148, 149, 158, 167–
168, 173, 176
High-fructose corn syrup, 37, 46–47, 53,
148, 185
Hippocrates, 9

Holistic, 5, 187
Homeopathy, 7–9, 14
Homeostasis, 1, 2, 5, 9, 101, 186
Homeoprophylaxis, 183
Hormone replacement therapy, 155, 161
Hormones, 26, 29, 63, 65, 75, 76, 82,
87, 93–95, 108, 114, 119, 120, 129,
139, 151, 155, 161, 163
Hypertension, 47, 149, 150, 152

Immune system, 21, 30, 33, 35, 38, 39,
42, 45, 46, 56, 72, 77, 82, 93–95, 98,
99, 106, 108, 109, 119–121, 123,
125, 128, 134, 139, 141, 165, 171,
175, 180–182, 184
Indian gooseberry (Amla, Amalaki), 150
Influenza, 147, 180–184
Inflammation, 20, 32, 35, 42, 43, 52,
56, 57, 62, 78, 84, 90, 95, 98, 122,
139, 150, 158, 167, 175, 181
Insomnia, 47, 49, 135
Intestines, 9, 11, 12, 20, 30, 35–36, 39,
51, 56, 69, 73, 100, 105, 117–119,
126, 163, 165, 171
Iodine, 23, 84, 87–88, 93
Iron, 32, 35, 36, 38, 50, 59, 65, 75, 78,
83, 84, 87, 88–89, 91, 93

Joints, 24, 63, 64, 73, 82, 87, 91, 95, 96,
104, 113–115, 136, 186

Kava-kava, 144–145
Kidneys, 24, 26, 39, 45, 64, 117,
119–120, 174, 186

Lactose, 8, 30–31, 57
Laughter, 138–139, 186
Lavender, 131, 141, 144, 146, 177
Lead, 26, 27, 85, 121, 123
Lemon balm, 131, 144, 145
Lifestyle, 18, 29, 34, 60, 79, 103, 111,
131, 147–149, 153, 172, 187
Liver, 11, 12, 24, 26, 28, 46, 47, 49, 51,
52, 54, 55, 69, 72, 75, 76, 79, 81, 97,